Diseases of the Rectum and Anus - A Concise Guide

Edited by Alberto Vannelli

Published in London, United Kingdom

Diseases of the Rectum and Anus - A Concise Guide
http://dx.doi.org/10.5772/intechopen.1005995
Edited by Alberto Vannelli

Contributors
ad, Adriana Jovanov, Andrea Sagnotta, Ante Jerković, Arum Linangkung, Ashley Parks, Atheer Alotaibi, Augusto Belardi, Ayyob Alqarni, Benedetto Battaglia, Dagmara Adamska-Tomaszewska, Damir Karlović, Despoina Papageorgiou, Di Qiu, Dorian Kršul, Eleni Polyzou, Farah Slaczka, Filippo Maria Michele Frederick Dentice Di Accadia Capozzi, Francesk Mulita, Glora Folliero, Hadeel Helmi, Haibo Yu, Jinhuan Zhang, Jin K. Kim, Jorge Marcet, Joyce El-H, Karolina Akinosoglou, Kaylee Smith, Lucia Klarica, Luigi Solinas, Luisa Berto, Marcos Marton, Margherita Loponte, Maria Francesca Russo, Maria Gavatha, Mario Milotić, Marko Zelić, Mateusz Slaczka, Nikola Simičić, Omar Alhafidh, Parshottambhai Patel, Sabina Więcek, Sara Lazzaro, Stefano Mancini, Tingyu Wang, Xingxian Huang, Yongfeng Liu, Yusif Aliyarov

First published in London, United Kingdom, 2025 by IntechOpen
IntechOpen is the global imprint of INTECHOPEN LIMITED, registered in England and Wales, registration number: 11086078, 167-169 Great Portland Street, London, W1W 5PF, United Kingdom

For EU product safety concerns: IN TECH d.o.o., Prolaz Marije Krucifikse Kozulić 3, 51000 Rijeka, Croatia, info@intechopen.com or visit our website at intechopen.com.

British Library Cataloguing-in-Publication Data
A catalogue record for this book is available from the British Library

Diseases of the Rectum and Anus - A Concise Guide
Edited by Alberto Vannelli
p. cm.
Print ISBN 978-1-83634-590-9
Online ISBN 978-1-83634-589-3
eBook (PDF) ISBN 978-1-83634-591-6

If disposing of this product, please recycle the paper responsibly.

Meet the editor

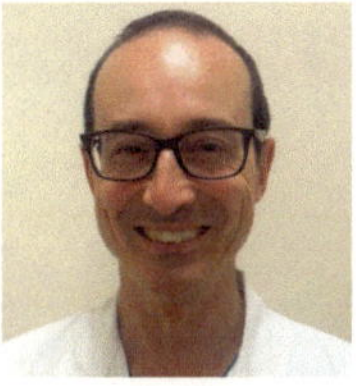

Dr. Alberto Vannelli completed medical school, postgraduate research, and general surgical training in Milan, Italy, before pursuing specialized training in colorectal surgery at the National Cancer Institute. He later worked at Valduce Hospital in Como, where he established a leading division of gastrointestinal oncologic surgery and subsequently served as Director of General Surgery. His clinical practice focuses on advanced minimally invasive techniques and the multidisciplinary management of colorectal cancer. His division became a referral center for colorectal disease, particularly sphincter-preserving procedures in rectal cancer and inflammatory bowel disease (IBD). In 2012, Dr. Vannelli founded Erone Onlus, a non-profit organization supporting cancer patients and their families. He also collaborates with the University of Milan in postgraduate surgical training.

Contents

Preface

Diseases of the Rectum and Anus – A Concise Guide was conceived to provide a clear, accessible, and authoritative reference on the wide spectrum of anorectal diseases. This volume brings together international experts who share both clinical experience and academic insight, offering readers state-of-the-art knowledge as well as practical guidance.

The opening section, **Fistulas and Rare Rectal Disorders**, explores conditions that remain particularly challenging in daily practice. The authors review established surgical strategies and present updated perspectives on perianal fistulas, while also drawing attention to solitary rectal ulcer syndrome in children, a rare but clinically significant entity. Collectively, these chapters provide valuable insights into pathologies that demand nuanced and individualized management.

The second section, **Hemorrhoids: Evidence-Based and Special Settings**, addresses one of the most prevalent anorectal conditions worldwide. Contributions range from evidence-based guidelines, including a perspective on traditional Chinese medicine, to innovative surgical approaches and the management of hemorrhoids in pregnancy and breastfeeding. These chapters underscore the importance of tailoring treatment to diverse patient populations and cultural contexts.

The third section, **Rectal and Anal Tumors**, moves into the oncological domain. The authors examine the interplay between biology and social determinants in HPV-related disease, evaluate predictive factors of response to neoadjuvant chemoradiotherapy, and discuss the complex management of presacral tumors. This section reflects the collaborative efforts of surgeons, oncologists, and researchers to improve both survival and quality of life.

In the fourth section, **Anatomy, Emergencies, and Diagnostics**, readers are guided back to the essentials. A review of anorectal anatomy and physiology lays the foundation for understanding disease, while chapters on anorectal emergencies and modern diagnostic modalities emphasize timely recognition and appropriate intervention. These contributions are highly practical, bridging fundamental knowledge with decision-making in both acute and routine settings.

The final section, **Functional Disorders and Anorectal Infections**, focuses on conditions that often have a profound impact on quality of life. The authors provide guidance on the evaluation and management of fecal incontinence, describe the rare entity of internal anal sphincter achalasia, and review the treatment of perianal abscesses. Together, these chapters highlight the balance between technical expertise and compassionate care required in the management of functional and infectious anorectal disease.

Across all sections, the book emphasizes the importance of multidisciplinary collaboration, engaging surgeons, gastroenterologists, oncologists, radiologists, pathologists, and specialized nurses. By combining established evidence with emerging perspectives, the contributors have created a concise yet comprehensive guide that will serve as a valuable resource for both specialists and trainees.

I am deeply grateful to all the authors for their dedication and expertise, and to the publishing team for their support in bringing this project to completion. I also want to acknowledge IntechOpen, whose commitment to open-access publishing recalls the vision of Denis Diderot and the Enlightenment encyclopedists. Diderot believed that "an encyclopedia ought to change the common way of thinking". In the same spirit, IntechOpen provides a model of free and collaborative publishing, ensuring that knowledge can circulate without barriers and serve the progress of medicine and science worldwide.

Alberto Vannelli
Valduce Hospital,
Department of Surgery,
Como, Italy

Section 1

Fistulas and Rare Rectal Disorders

Chapter 1

Anal Fistulas: Surgical Treatment

Luigi Solinas, Maria Francesca Russo,
Filippo Maria Michele Frederick Dentice Di Accadia Capozzi,
Augusto Belardi, Benedetto Battaglia, Andrea Sagnotta,
Glora Folliero, Margherita Loponte, Sara Lazzaro
and Stefano Mancini

Abstract

Perianal disease with abscesses and fistulas is a commonly encountered condition, but one that is complex to manage, requiring careful diagnosis and appropriate surgical management. A thorough preoperative diagnostic evaluation is crucial to understand the specific characteristics of the condition and the patient, as well as to identify any underlying chronic inflammatory bowel diseases, such as Crohn's disease, which may complicate the clinical picture. Surgery, primarily involving the incision and removal of the fistulous tracts, is often the only option to treat perianal fistulas. However, managing this condition may require more than one procedure, particularly to address any recurrences, which are quite common. Modern surgical techniques and the use of advanced technologies, such as ultrasound or fistulography, have improved outcomes and reduced the risks of postoperative complications. Treatment must be tailored to each patient's specific characteristics, taking into account the complexity of the disease and the potential for recurrences. The main challenge remains achieving complete healing while reducing the risk of long-term complications and improving the patient's quality of life. Additionally, postoperative management and long-term monitoring are essential to prevent new infections and ensure the success of the surgery.

Keywords: anal abscess, anal, rectal fistula, perineal abscess, anal fistula

1. Introduction

Anal fistula is a frequent and challenging scenario for a general surgeon, with an estimated prevalence of 8.6–10/100,000 in the general population per year [1, 2]. Usually, the patient is examined in an outpatient scenario, with the first clinical diagnosis made after anorectal examination. Diagnostic evaluation can involve a transperineal ultrasonography and perineal magnetic resonance. A preoperative classification is mandatory to plan a tailored surgical procedure, but the final diagnosis is usually performed in the operating room. However, perineal and anorectal evaluation under anesthesia allows the surgeon to conduct a real exploration and identification of fistula tracks. Many surgical techniques have now been developed to obtain a complete or partial fistula excision [3, 4].

In most cases, recurrences that require complex surgical solutions occur. In case of associated inflammatory bowel disease (IBD), the management of perineal fistula and abscess is more complex and limited to allow bio-pharmacological treatment.

2. Surgical anatomy and classification

Anatomical landmarks for surgical treatment of anal fistulas include anal and rectal anatomy, sphincteric muscle complex, levator ani muscle, and ischiorectal space.

2.1 Anorectal anatomy

The anal canal represents the final segment of the lower gastrointestinal (GI) tract, specifically the large intestine. It is situated between the anal verge, also known as the anal orifice or anus, located in the perineum below, and the rectum above. This canal extends from the pelvic diaphragm to the anal orifice [5].

The boundary separating the rectum from the anal canal is referred to as the anorectal ring or anorectal flexure. This structure is characterized by the puborectalis muscle, which creates a sling around the posterior side of the anorectal junction, resulting in an anterior kink. The anal canal is entirely located outside the peritoneal cavity. Its length measures approximately 4 cm. Almost two-thirds of this length is situated above the pectinate line, while the remaining one-third is located below it [6, 7].

The anal valves, which are transverse mucosal folds located at the lowest extremities of the anal columns, give the pectinate line its scalloped appearance. Above the anal valves, the anal glands release their contents into the anal sinuses. Despite not being apparent during standard clinical examinations, the pectinate line can be identified under anesthesia by slightly retracting the anal canal. The anal pecten or transitional zone is the section of the anal canal that is situated right above the pectinate line and measures roughly 1–2 cm. The columnar epithelium that lines the anal canal in this region is not sensitive to cutting. The top portion of the anal canal has six to ten longitudinal mucosal folds that make up the anal columns, also referred to as Morgagni's columns [8, 9].

At the base of these columns are anal sinuses or crypts, which function as openings for the anal glands and anal papillae. The infection of the anal glands is likely the initial event that leads to the formation of perianal abscess and fistula-in-ano. Three of these columns—namely, the left lateral, right posterior, and right anterior, positioned at the 3-, 7-, and 11-o'clock locations when the individual is lying supine—are particularly notable. These structures are known as anal cushions and encompass branches and tributaries of the superior rectal (hemorrhoidal) artery and vein. When these veins become engorged, they can result in internal hemorrhoids. The anorectal junction, also referred to as the anorectal ring, is situated approximately 5 cm from the anus. At the anorectal flexure or angle, this junction is elevated anterosuperiorly by the puborectal sling, which continues downward as the anal canal. The pelvic diaphragm is composed of the levator ani and coccygeus muscles. Flanking the anal canal are the pyramidal ischioanal (ischiorectal) fossae, located beneath the pelvic diaphragm and above the perianal skin. These paired ischioanal fossae are interconnected posteriorly to the anal canal. The anterior structures associated with the anal canal include the seminal vesicles, prostate, and urethra in males, as well as the cervix and vagina with the perineal body situated in between in females. Anterior to the anal canal is the rectovesical fascia (of Denonvilliers), while posteriorly lies the presacral endopelvic fascia (of Waldeyer), beneath which is a dense network of presacral veins. The tip of the coccyx, which is linked to the anal canal by the anococcygeal ligament, is positioned posterior to the anal canal, along with the lower sacrum (**Figure 1**).

2.2 Vascularization and innervation

2.2.1 Arterial supply and lymphatic drainage

The anal canal above the pectinate line receives its blood supply from the terminal branches of the superior rectal artery, which is a branch of the inferior mesenteric artery. Lymphatic fluid from this area is transported to the inferior mesenteric lymph nodes (**Figure 2**).

The anal canal below the pectinate line receives its blood supply from the middle and inferior rectal arteries. The middle rectal artery originates from the internal iliac artery, whereas the inferior rectal artery is a branch of the internal pudendal artery, which itself branches from the internal iliac artery. Lymphatic drainage in this region predominantly flows to the superficial inguinal lymph nodes [5, 9].

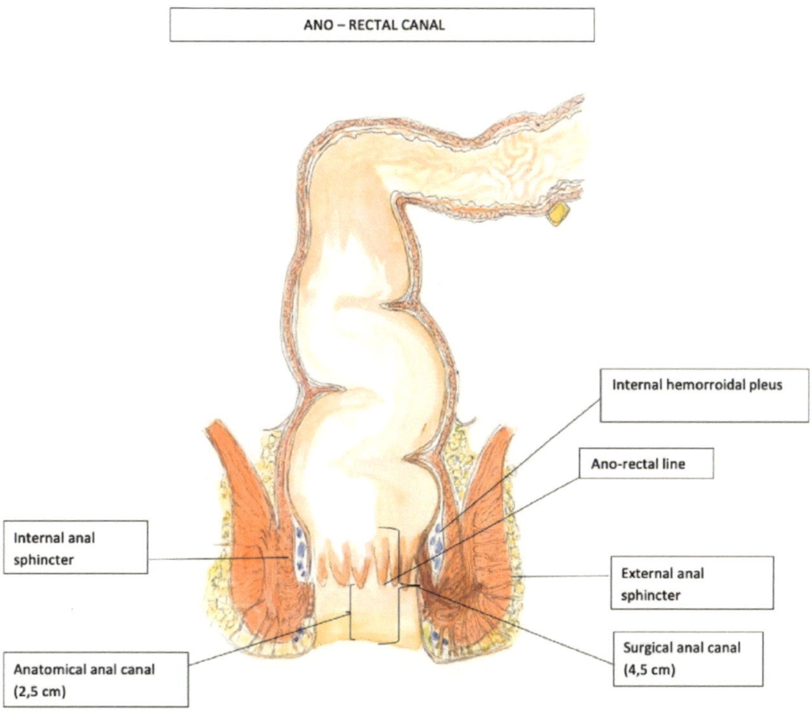

Figure 1.
Anatomy of the anal canal.

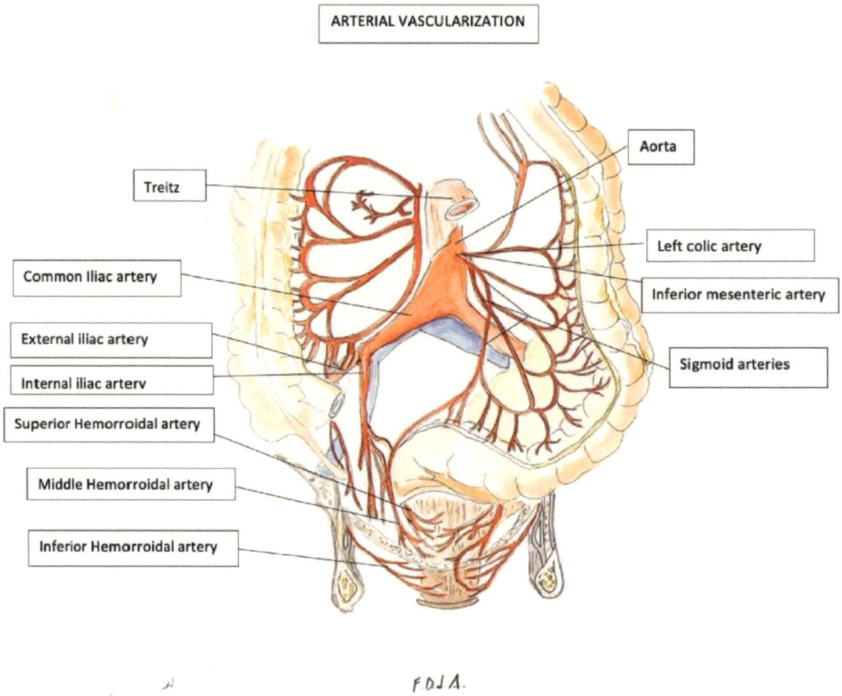

Figure 2.
Arterial supply of the anal canal.

2.2.2 Venous drainage

The venous drainage of the anal canal above the pectinate line occurs through the superior rectal veins, which ultimately drain into the inferior mesenteric vein (refer to **Figure 3**). These veins are components of the hepatic portal venous system, responsible for transporting oxygen-depleted, nutrient-rich blood to the liver for metabolic processing. In contrast, the venous drainage of the anal canal below the pectinate line is facilitated by the internal pudendal veins, which direct their flow to the internal iliac vein. These veins belong to the systemic venous system, which carries oxygen-depleted, nutrient-poor blood back to the heart. The presence of anastomoses between the portal and systemic venous systems within the anorectal canal provides potential alternative circulatory pathways. In individuals with portal hypertension, the presence of anorectal varices may be observed. It is important to note that these portosystemic anastomoses are not limited to the anal canal but can also be identified in other regions of the body [5, 9].

3. Nerves

It is pertinent to examine the nervous system of the anal canal both above and below the pectinate line, in conjunction with the blood supply and lymphatics. These two areas exhibit distinct innervation patterns and respond differently to various stimuli. In the region above the pectinate line, the anal canal is autonomically innervated by the inferior hypogastric plexus (**Figure 4**). The parasympathetic fibers

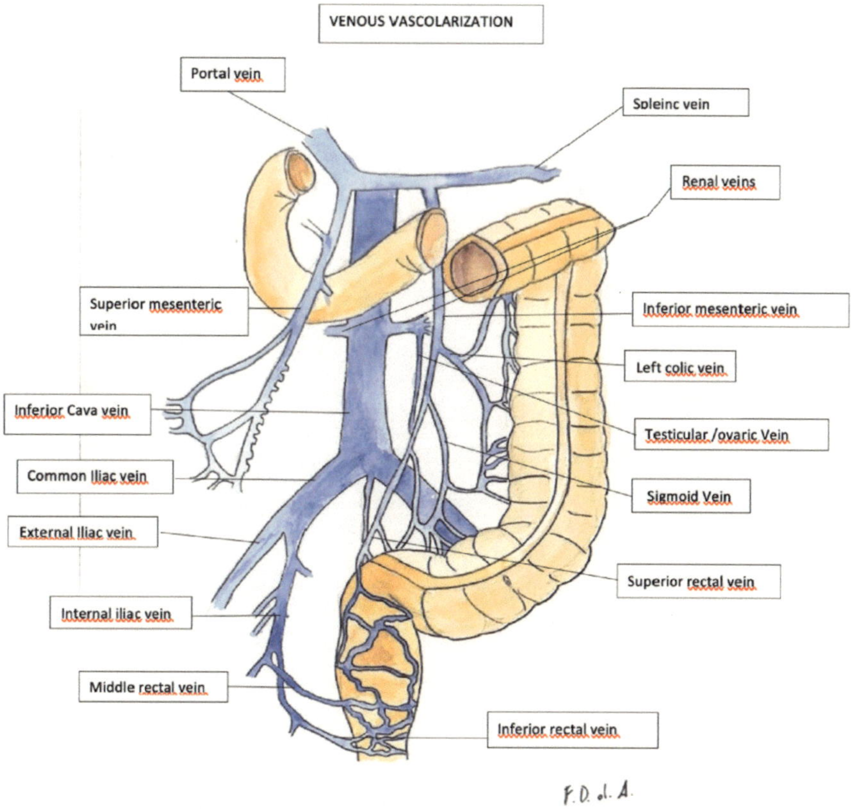

Figure 3.
Venous supply of the anal canal.

reduce the tone of the internal anal sphincter and trigger peristaltic contractions to facilitate defecation. Conversely, sympathetic innervation serves to maintain the tone of the internal anal sphincter, thereby aiding in the preservation of continence. The superior portion of the anal canal is particularly responsive to viscerosensory signals, making it highly sensitive to stretch and distention. In contrast, the area below the pectinate line is innervated somatically by branches of the pudendal nerve (**Figure 4**). Consequently, the inferior section of the anal canal exhibits heightened sensitivity to pain, temperature, and tactile stimuli [5, 9].

4. Anorectal fistula

An anorectal fistula refers to an abnormal passage that links the anorectal canal to the perianal region. This condition is often associated with significant morbidity and frequently arises after the drainage of a perianal abscess. Comprehensive follow-up is essential for accurate diagnosis and effective treatment. Proper classification of fistulas plays a crucial role in determining the appropriate therapeutic approach. Surgical intervention remains the primary method of treatment.

The most widely used classification is the Park's Classification System that categorizes anal fistulas based on their anatomical location in relation to the sphincter

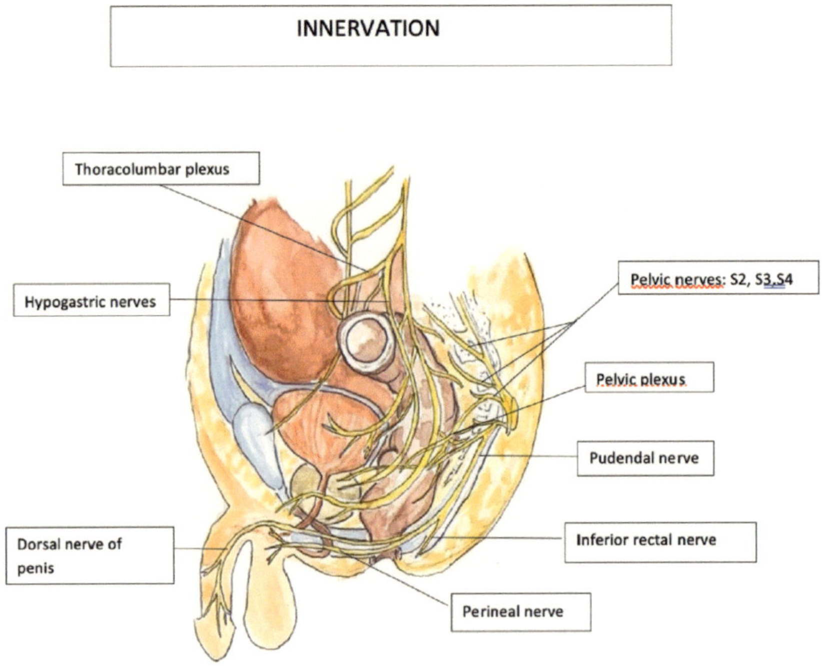

Figure 4.
Innervation of the anal canal.

complex (**Figure 5**) [10]. It was first described by Parks, Gordon, and Hardcastle, in 1976. Fistulas are classified as intersphinteric (45%), trans-sphinteric (30%), supra-sphincteric (20%), and extrasphincteric (5%).

4.1 Park's classification of anorectal fistulas

4.1.1 Intersphincteric fistulas

The intersphinteric fistula is the most frequent type since the majority of abscesses develop in the space between the two sphincters. It passes through the internal sphincter and then has a tract to the outside of the anus without crossing the external sphincter. A fistulotomy or the opening of the fistulous tract is effective in this kind of fistula and rarely causes incontinence, as the disease does not affect the external sphincter.

4.1.2 Trans-sphincteric fistulas

Trans-sphincteric fistula refers to a condition that traverses from the intersphincteric plane within the mid-anal canal, passing through the external sphincter to the ischiorectal fossa and ultimately reaching the skin [10]. The management of such fistulas typically necessitates more intricate or staged treatment approaches. This often involves the application of a seton to gradually "lower" the fistulous tract, thereby reducing its involvement with the external sphincter, which facilitates the possibility of performing a fistulotomy while maintaining anal continence. Depending on the extent of the external sphincter's involvement, a partial sphincterotomy may be

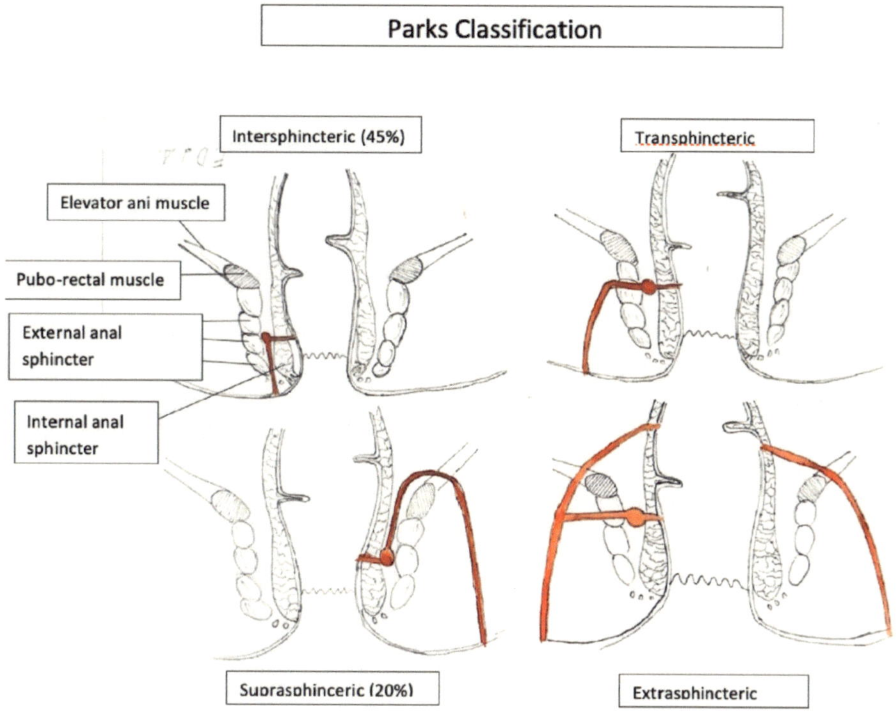

Figure 5.
Park's classification system.

indicated. Conversely, a complete division of the external sphincter could lead to fecal incontinence.

4.1.3 Suprasphincteric fistulas

This fistula originates in the intersphincteric plane of the mid-anal canal and ascends within the same plane to a location above the puborectalis muscle level, subsequently descending into the ischiorectal fossa [10]. Due to the elevated nature of these tracts, the application of a seton may be deemed appropriate prior to performing a fistulotomy.

4.1.4 Extrasphincteric fistulas

These fistulas are uncommon: a channel extends from the skin of the perineal region, traversing the adipose tissue of the ischiorectal fossa, subsequently passing through the levator ani muscle, and ultimately penetrating the rectal wall. This tract is located outside the complete circumference of the sphincter muscle, which is the reason for the designation "Extrasphincteric."

5. Etiology

A well-known, commonly used, acronym for remembering the factors responsible for the formation of the fistula is "FRIENDs of the fistula": foreign body, radiation, infection or inflammatory bowel disease, epithelialization, neoplasm, and distal obstruction.

Foreign bodies in the rectum often are those placed intentionally.

Radiation proctitis is a very well-known cause of fistulae formation and lesions to the vagina, urethra, and bladder can be a common complication.

Infection is the primary factor contributing to the development of anorectal fistulas, typically arising from a blockage of the anal glands and crypts. Frequently, an abscess forms within the avascular fatty plane situated between the two anal sphincters, which may subsequently drain spontaneously through a fistula. The obstruction of the anal glands facilitates bacterial growth, leading to the formation of perirectal, anorectal, or perianal abscesses. In such instances, the likelihood of fistula formation is significantly heightened.

A precise knowledge of the anorectal anatomy and accurate localization of the fistulous tract is crucial for a correct management and treatment of this disease.

The essential structures in the anorectal region include the rectum itself, anal glands, anal sphincters, and the levator ani muscles (puborectalis, pubococcygeus, and iliococcygeus).

Anal fistulae are rarely a presentation of anal tuberculosis and should be suspected in endemic regions or in recurrent fistulas [11, 12].

In young patients, complex or multiple fistulas should be investigated for Crohn's disease (CD).

Sexually transmitted infections (STIs) of the anus and rectum, such as gonorrhea, chlamydia, syphilis (*Treponema pallidum*), and herpes simplex [13], usually secondary to anal intercourse, may predispose individuals to perianal abscess and fistula.

Complicated vaginal deliveries that result in third- or fourth-degree perineal tears or necessitate an episiotomy may increase the likelihood of developing anal fistulas; however, these fistulas frequently resolve on their own. In cases of obstetric-related anal fistulas that do not heal, the surgical approach is determined by the fistula's location and any involvement of the vagina. When the fistula is located distal to the dentate line, a rectovaginal fistula may evolve into an ano-rectovaginal fistula. The primary causes are typically obstetric trauma linked to difficult vaginal deliveries. Patients who have undergone an episiotomy face a heightened risk of sphincter damage and subsequent fecal incontinence [14].

Also, another possible scenario is congenital fistula. Over 96% of cases are observed in infants under the age of 1 year. The typical manifestation includes a recurrent perianal abscess, which may or may not have undergone surgical intervention [15].

6. Pathophysiology

The pathophysiology of an anal fistula is characterized by a chronic turnover of the inflammatory and epithelial cells, with a constant residue in the fistula tract that causes obstruction and prevents the fistula from healing.

7. Diagnosis, imaging, and laboratory findings

Typical symptoms include itching, drainage, discomfort, and pain with defecation.

A perianal examination and anoscopy are essential for the diagnosis of an anorectal fistula. On inspection, one or more external secondary orifices may be identified, sometimes with the appearance of a granulation button secreting pus, blood, serum, or feces. On palpation, the perianal fistula can appear as a cord-like and fibrous subcutaneous lesion, moving from the fistulous orifice toward the anus.

In other cases, the digital rectal examination is necessary to assess the location of the internal orifice that can be suspected by the presence of an induration and the palpation of any tenderness may suggest the location of an occult abscess.

While the diagnosis of the anorectal fistula is clinical, the imaging is fundamental to define its course and origin.

7.1 Endorectal ultrasound

Endorectal ultrasound is an effective modality to evaluate for an abscess or a fistulous tract with similar sensitivity but less specificity than magnetic resonance imaging (MRI) [16]. The use of hydrogen peroxide into the external fistulous orifice aids in identifying both fistulous tracts and occult abscesses [17–20]. It is a less expensive modality than MRI, helpful for patients with chronic fistula, such as Crohn's disease patients who require long-term follow-up; on the other hand, it is totally operator dependent.

7.2 CT scan and CT-fistulography

Computed tomography (CT scan) is a helpful technique for identifying abscesses and fluid collections that could be drainable, as it is fast and easily accessible. CT scan may be the choice in case of an acute infection or when an abscess is suspected [21, 22].

CT-fistulography is a useful and efficient modality for identifying fistula tracts preoperatively [23]. It is less expensive than the MRI but it requires an expert radiologist and surgeons to perform. It should be considered in complex anal fistula preoperative planning or in patients who are unable to undergo an MRI [24].

7.3 Magnetic resonance imaging (MRI)

Magnetic resonance imaging (MRI) of the pelvis plays a crucial role in detecting fistulous tracts and hidden abscesses, as well as in assessing the relationship of these tracts to the internal and external sphincters during preoperative planning. Various studies have demonstrated that MRI is more sensitive than computed tomography (CT) scans in identifying fistulous tracts, enabling surgeons to prepare for more extensive surgical interventions when required [25].

MRI serves as a valuable preoperative imaging tool, particularly for complex fistulas and those with an external opening exceeding 2 cm from the anus [26]. In research conducted by Garg et al., involving 229 patients, the implementation of MRI altered the preoperative diagnosis in half of the cases of simple fistulas and in over one-third of complex cases [27].

Additionally, MRI is effective in detecting postoperative complications, such as abscesses or recurrent fistulas, at or beyond 12 weeks following surgery [28]. Buchanan et al. have found that utilizing MRI for surgical planning was linked to a reduction in fistula recurrence by ensuring a thorough initial operation. In a case-controlled study involving 41 patients, a comparison between CT-fistulography and MRI revealed that internal openings were identified more effectively by MRI (85.3% compared to 68.2% for CT-fistulography). The findings from both imaging modalities were most consistent with the actual operative results [21, 29].

7.4 Laboratory findings

Basic laboratory panels, such as a complete blood count and metabolic profile, are essential. A low hemoglobin level may indicate anemia, potentially linked to inflammatory bowel disease or gastrointestinal cancer. Additionally, leukocytosis may suggest an underlying infection or hidden abscess, along with an increase in C-reactive protein (CRP) levels.

8. Surgical management

The surgical management of these fistulas varies based on the underlying etiology, fistula complexity, and involvement of sphincter muscles. Crohn's disease-associated fistulas are typically more complex and often require more specialized treatment to manage the inflammation and preserve anal function. Conversely, fistula sine causa refers to idiopathic fistulas (IFs) that are less complicated and generally have a better prognosis with simpler surgical approaches.

8.1 Perianal fistulas in Crohn's disease

Perianal fistulas in CD occur as a result of transmural inflammation, leading to abscess formation and the subsequent development of abnormal fistulous tracts between the anal canal and the skin or other areas.

Fistulas associated with CD are often complex, involving multiple tracts, and may be high, trans-sphincteric, or involve the rectovaginal space [30]. The development of these fistulas is influenced by the active disease state, and their management is complicated by factors, such as the involvement of anal sphincters, recurrence, and the need for sphincter preservation to avoid incontinence [31].

8.2 Idiopathic fistula (IF)

These fistulas typically follow a more straightforward clinical course than those associated with Crohn's disease and are usually less prone to recurrence or complications. In most cases, simple fistulas involve only a single tract, and the internal opening is located in the anal canal. Imaging studies and clinical examination play a crucial role in diagnosing and planning treatment for IF, which typically responds well to surgical intervention.

8.3 Disease control in Crohn's disease

For Crohn's disease-associated fistulas, the priority is to achieve disease remission. Surgical interventions performed during periods of active disease are associated with poorer outcomes and higher recurrence rates due to ongoing inflammation. The use of biologic therapies, such as tumor necrosis factor (TNF) inhibitors (infliximab, adalimumab), immunosuppressants (azathioprine, mercaptopurine), and corticosteroids, is essential for achieving disease control before undergoing surgical treatment [32].

Combination therapy (biologics and corticosteroids) has been implemented in controlling perianal fistulas and resulted in a significant reduction in the need for surgical interventions, emphasizing the importance of medical management prior to surgery.

Preoperative imaging studies are pivotal in assessing the complexity of the fistula and determining its relationship to surrounding structures. MRI, endorectal ultrasound, and fistulography are commonly used to evaluate the fistula tract and abscesses [33]. In Crohn's disease, MRI is the preferred imaging modality due to its ability to provide detailed anatomical views, allowing for accurate assessment of sphincter involvement, trans-sphincteric fistulas, and multifocal disease.

9. Surgical approaches in Crohn's disease

9.1 Seton placement

Seton placement is considered the cornerstone of managing high, complex, or trans-sphincteric fistulas in Crohn's disease, particularly when the fistulas are active or associated with abscesses [34]. Setons help in drainage, reduce the risk of abscess formation, and facilitate healing in inflamed tissue (**Figure 6**).

In patients with chronic, draining fistulas, setons serve as a bridging strategy for further procedures, such as fistulotomy or advancement flap surgery, after disease control is achieved.

The seton is threaded through the fistula tract, with the initial placement often being loose to allow for drainage. Over time, the seton is tightened gradually to induce fibrosis of the fistula tract, promoting closure. Seton placement can be temporary or permanent, depending on the specific needs of the patient.

Seton placement is typically associated with partial fistula closure and symptom relief in approximately 60% of cases.

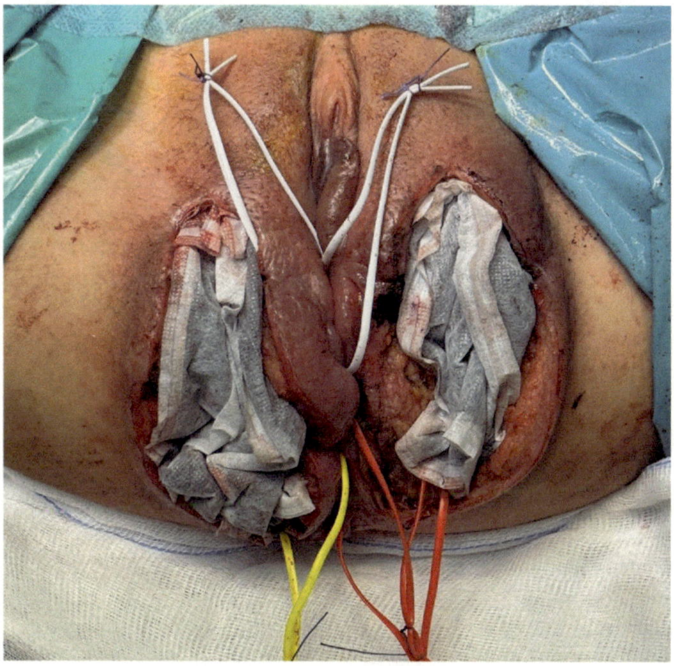

Figure 6.
Seton placement in Crohn's disease with concurrent fistulotomy.

Common complications include infection, seton dislodgement, and prolonged drainage. In Crohn's disease, there is a higher risk of incomplete healing, especially in cases of active inflammation [35].

9.2 Fistulotomy

While fistulotomy is highly effective for simple, low fistulas, its application in Crohn's disease is more controversial due to the risk of incontinence and poor healing [36].

The fistula tract is incised from the internal to external opening, and the wound is left open to heal by secondary intention. This technique is preferred in non-Crohn's disease patients and for patients with noncomplicated fistulas.

In simple fistulas, fistulotomy has an 80–90% success rate. However, in Crohn's disease, success rates drop significantly, with recurrence occurring in 50–70% of cases.

The main complications include infection, abscess formation, and incontinence, especially in patients with trans-sphincteric fistulas.

9.3 Advancement flap surgery

Advancement flap surgery is typically used for high, trans-sphincteric fistulas in Crohn's disease when fistulotomy is not appropriate due to the risk of sphincter damage. This is preferred when maintaining sphincter function is paramount [37].

The procedure involves mobilizing rectal mucosa or skin to create a flap, which is advanced and sutured over the internal opening of the fistula. The flap promotes healing by covering the fistula tract and preventing recurrent infection. The external opening is generally left open to facilitate drainage. Clinical studies indicate that this method yields satisfactory healing rates, with recurrence observed in less than 10% of cases, making it a viable option for patients with a history of previous fistula surgeries [38].

Success rates range from 60% to 80%, with higher failure rates in patients with active disease. Failure is often attributed to inadequate vascular supply to the flap in the context of active inflammation.

Flap necrosis, infection, and recurrence are common complications in Crohn's disease. Postoperative stricture formation and sphincter dysfunction can also occur. Evidence suggests that Crohn's disease patients who receive immunologic treatment may experience enhanced outcomes following this surgical intervention [39].

9.4 Bioprosthetic collagen plugs

Collagen plugs made from biologic materials, such as porcine collagen, are used in simple, low anorectal fistulas. However, their use in Crohn's disease is limited due to the chronic inflammatory nature of the disease.

The collagen plug is inserted into the internal opening of the fistula and secured to promote granulation tissue formation and closure. Success rates range from 50% to 60% in Crohn's disease, which is significantly lower than in idiopathic fistulas. The plug can dislodge or be expelled in cases of active inflammation. The primary complications include dislodgement, infection, and recurrence [40].

9.5 Stem cell therapy

Stem cell therapy represents a novel approach for refractory perianal fistulas in Crohn's disease, especially in cases where conventional surgeries have failed or in patients who do not wish to undergo further surgery [41].

Mesenchymal stem cells (MSCs) are injected into the fistula tract, where they promote tissue regeneration and healing. MSCs are usually harvested from the patient's bone marrow or adipose tissue.

Early studies show success rates of 50–60%, but further research is required to determine long-term efficacy and potential for wound healing.

The main risks include infection at the injection site and failure of tissue regeneration.

10. Surgical management of idiopathic fistula (IF)

10.1 Fistulotomy and fistulectomy

In idiopathic fistulas (IFs), fistulotomy remains the gold standard surgical treatment.

Simple, low anorectal fistulas are ideal candidates for fistulotomy, which can lead to complete resolution in 80–90% of cases.

The first step in the procedure is to identify the fistula tract using a probe. The patient is positioned in either a lithotomy or prone jackknife position. Deep sedation or general anesthesia is provided for the duration of the procedure. The anal and perianal areas are prepared with betadine. Initially, a local anesthetic is administered to reduce postoperative pain and assist in the separation of tissue planes. A digital rectal examination is performed. A Lonestar retractor or Park's retractor is then employed. The external opening of the fistula is probed with a lacrimal probe to locate the tract. Following this, methylene blue or hydrogen peroxide is injected into the external opening through a small angio-catheter to identify the internal opening and ascertain the presence of any additional internal openings. While keeping the probe in both the external and internal openings, the sphincters are carefully identified and assessed for involvement. If the external sphincter is unaffected, a fistulotomy is performed. It is generally preferable to avoid cutting the external sphincter to preserve continence; however, if division of the lower segment is required, it is typically associated with acceptable rates of postoperative continence [35].

Care must be taken to steer clear of the external sphincter while gently opening the fistulous tract, either with Bovie cautery or through sharp dissection. Subsequently, electrocautery is employed to eliminate the epithelialized tract to the greatest extent feasible, and the wound is allowed to heal in an open manner. Some studies have indicated that healing rates for fistulotomy can reach as high as 94% [33].

Success rates are higher in IF than in Crohn's disease, with low recurrence rates and minimal complications. The risk of infection and delayed healing remains, but the occurrence of incontinence is rare in IF.

In case of high transphincteric or supra-sphincteric fistulas, fistulectomy accompanied by sphincter reconstruction is the intervention of choice. This method involves the division of the sphincter at the site of the fistula tract, followed by the excision of the tract itself. Subsequently, the sphincter is re-approximated using absorbable sutures. Recent research indicates that this approach yields encouraging outcomes for high and complex fistulas, with healing rates nearing 90% and a reported incontinence rate of only 2% [36].

10.2 Ligation of the intersphincteric fistula tract (LIFT)

The LIFT technique is a newer approach for low anorectal fistulas, with the potential to preserve sphincter function. This procedure was initially introduced by Rojanasakul et al. in 2007, demonstrating successful treatment in 18 patients suffering from intersphincteric fistulas through this innovative approach [42].

The LIFT technique is ideal for intersphincteric fistulas, typically low-lying and simple, without significant involvement of the sphincter muscles.

The fistula tract is isolated between the internal and external anal sphincters, and the tract is ligated. This allows the fistula to heal from the inside out while preserving the surrounding sphincter muscles.

This method involves locating the intersphincteric groove (ISG) along with the internal and external openings of the fistula, followed by careful dissection of the fistula tract situated within the intersphincteric groove. The dissection can be carried out using either cautery or small scissors. Once the tract has been dissected and secured with a right angle clamp, it may be safely ligated with sutures within the ISG, in proximity to the internal sphincter, while ensuring the integrity of both the internal and external sphincter muscles is maintained. An absorbable suture is utilized for the ligation. The tract is then sharply cut distal to the ligation, which is confirmed by injecting saline or hydrogen peroxide through the external opening. Any residual portion of the intersphincteric tract is excised, and a small incision is created at the external opening to facilitate drainage. Finally, the wound over the ISG is meticulously approximated with several simple absorbable sutures.

The LIFT technique offers 70–80% success in uncomplicated cases with minimal recurrence [43].

Recurrence is the main complication, typically duc to incomplete ligation [44].

10.3 Anal fistula plug

An anal fistula plug is a technique designed to preserve the sphincter, suitable for patients at a heightened risk of incontinence or those with complex fistulas. These plugs can be composed of materials, such as fibrin, porcine tissue, or other biologically absorbable substances. Before the insertion of any plugs, it is crucial to ensure adequate drainage of the fistula to minimize the risk of anal sepsis. The procedure begins with the identification of the internal and external openings of the fistula, followed by the introduction of a probe through these openings. This may be accompanied by a minor debridement of the tract using a "fistula brush." A suture is then threaded through the tract, facilitating the insertion of the plug. The plug is anchored within the internal opening to the mucosa and the internal anal sphincter, ensuring that the mucosa envelops it. In contrast, the external opening of the fistula is deliberately left open to promote drainage. The application of anal fistula plugs has sparked significant discussion, as research has yielded inconsistent outcomes. These plugs are associated with higher recurrence rates compared to alternative surgical methods for anal fistulas. In a randomized controlled trial that compared the fistula plug to a mucosal advancement flap, the recurrence rate for the fistula plug was reported to be 66% [45].

10.4 Surgical novelties

A novel minimally invasive and sphincter-saving technique for treating complex anal fistulas is the video-assisted anal fistula treatment (VAAFT).

The procedure is conducted in two distinct phases: diagnostic and operative.

During the diagnostic phase, the fistuloscope is introduced into the fistula to pinpoint the internal opening within the anus and to detect any secondary tracts or abscess cavities. A speculum is employed to maintain the anal canal in an open position, while an irrigation solution is utilized to enhance visibility of the fistula tract. The illumination from the fistuloscope is observable from within the anal canal at the site of the internal opening of the fistula, facilitating the identification of this opening.

During the operative phase, the fistula tract undergoes cleansing, and the internal opening of the fistula is occluded. To achieve this, the surgeon employs a unipolar electrode, guided by video, to cauterize the tissue within the fistula tract. Concurrently, necrotic material is extracted utilizing a fistula brush and forceps, along with continuous irrigation. Subsequently, the surgeon sutures and staples the internal opening from within the anal canal [46].

Moreover, in the last decade laser treatment for fistula-in-ano, also known as FiLaCR (fistula laser closure) or LAFT (laser ablation of fistula tract), has gained increasing attention. The procedure involves the application of laser energy at a full 360° within the lumen of fistulas, utilizing a radial fiber that is gradually retracted from the external opening. The process of laser ablation is confined to the lumen of the fistulas, thereby preserving the sphincter [47].

11. Conclusion

The surgical treatment of anorectal fistulas requires a personalized approach based on the underlying etiology, the complexity of the fistula, and the involvement of sphincter muscles. In Crohn's disease, managing fistulas involves techniques that prioritize disease control, such as seton placement, advancement flap surgery, and stem cell therapies. For idiopathic fistulas, simpler procedures such as fistulotomy and LIFT are often effective, leading to excellent outcomes.

The future of anorectal fistula treatment will likely involve continued advancements in biologic therapies, regenerative medicine, and minimally invasive surgical techniques, offering hope for improved healing and quality of life for patients suffering from this challenging condition.

However, anal fistulas impose a significant economic burden through high treatment costs, lost productivity, and social impacts. Surgery, postoperative care, and specialist visits can be expensive, while individuals often miss work and face reduced efficiency during recovery. Stigma and caregiver burdens add further costs, straining the healthcare system. Timely treatment and prevention could help reduce these financial burdens.

Author details

Luigi Solinas[1*], Maria Francesca Russo[2],
Filippo Maria Michele Frederick Dentice Di Accadia Capozzi[1], Augusto Belardi[1],
Benedetto Battaglia[1], Andrea Sagnotta[1], Glora Folliero[1], Margherita Loponte[1],
Sara Lazzaro[1] and Stefano Mancini[1]

1 General and Oncologic Surgery Department, San Filippo Neri Hospital, Rome, Italy

2 Department of Surgery, Università La Sapienza, Rome, Italy

*Address all correspondence to: luigi73solinas@gmail.com

References

[1] García-Olmo D, Van Assche G, Tagarro I, et al. Prevalence of anal fistulas in Europe: Systematic literature reviews and population-based database analysis. Advances in Therapy. 2019;**36**:3503-3518

[2] Sarveazad A, Bahardoust M, Shamseddin J, et al. Prevalence of anal fistulas: A systematic review and meta-analysis. Gastroenterology and Hepatology from Bed to Bench. 2022;**15**:1-8

[3] Guntz M, Parnaud E, Bernard A, Chome J, Regnier J, Toulemonde JL. Vascularisation sanguine du canal anal [Vascularization of the anal canal]. Bulletin de L'association des Anatomistes (Nancy). 1976;**60**(170):527-538. French

[4] Ahmed A, Arbor TC, Qureshi WA. Anatomy, Abdomen and Pelvis: Anal Canal. Treasure Island, Florida: StatPearls Publishing; 2024

[5] Standring S. Gray's Anatomy: The Anatomical Basis of Clinical Practice. 42nd ed. Amsterdam, Holland: Elsevier Health Sciences; 2021

[6] Agur AMR, Lee MJ, Grant JCB. Grant's Atlas of Anatomy. 10th ed. London, UK: Lippincott Williams and Wilkins; 1999

[7] Sinnatamby CS. Last's Anatomy: Regional and Applied. 10th ed. Edinburgh: Churchill Livingstone; 1999

[8] Romanes GJ. Thorax and Abdomen. Cunningham's Manual of Practical Anatomy. 15th ed. Vol. II. New York, NY: Medical Publications, Oxford University Press; 1986

[9] Nikolouzakis TK, Mariolis-Sapsakos T, Triantopoulou C, et al. Detailed and applied anatomy for improved rectal cancer treatment. Annals of Gastroenterology. 2019;**32**(5):431-440

[10] Parks AG, Gordon PH, Hardcastle JD. A classification of fistula-in-ano. The British Journal of Surgery. 1976;**63**(1):1-12

[11] Garg P, Garg M, Das BR, Khadapkar R, Menon GR. Perianal tuberculosis: Lessons learned in 57 patients from 743 samples of histopathology and polymerase chain reaction and a systematic review of literature. Diseases of the Colon and Rectum. 2019;**62**(11):1390-1400

[12] Choi YS, Kim DS, Lee JB, Kim JK, Jung HJ, Lee SD, et al. Clinical features of tuberculous versus Crohn's anal fistulas, in Korea. Journal of Crohn's & Colitis. 2015;**9**(12):1132-1137

[13] Assi R, Hashim PW, Reddy VB, Einarsdottir H, Longo WE. Sexually transmitted infections of the anus and rectum. World Journal of Gastroenterology. 2014;**20**(41):15262-15268

[14] Do NL, Nagle D, Poylin VY. Radiation proctitis: Current strategies in management. Gastroenterology Research and Practice. 2011;**2011**:917941

[15] Afşarlar CE, Karaman A, Tanır G, Karaman I, Yılmaz E, Erdoğan D, et al. Perianal abscess and fistula-in-ano in children: Clinical characteristic, management and outcome. Pediatric Surgery International. 2011;**27**(10):1063-1068. DOI: 10.1007/s00383-011-2956-7

[16] Siddiqui MR, Ashrafian H, Tozer P, Daulatzai N, Burling D, Hart A,

et al. A diagnostic accuracy meta-analysis of endoanal ultrasound and MRI for perianal fistula assessment. Diseases of the Colon and Rectum. 2012;**55**(5):576-585

[17] Felt-Bersma RJ. Endoanal ultrasound in benign anorectal disorders: Clinical relevance and possibilities. Expert Review of Gastroenterology & Hepatology. 2008;**2**(4):587-606

[18] Karanikas I, Koutserimpas C, Siaperas P, Skarpas A, Karoubalis J, Velimezis G. Transrectal ultrasonography of perianal fistulas: A single center experience from a surgeon's point of view. Il Giornale di Chirurgia. 2018;**39**(4):258-260

[19] Felt-Bersma RJ. Endoanal ultrasound in perianal fistulas and abscesses. Digestive and Liver Disease. 2006;**38**(8):537-543

[20] Visscher AP, Felt-Bersma RJ. Endoanal ultrasound in perianal fistulae and abscesses. Ultrasound Quarterly. 2015;**31**(2):130-137

[21] Soker G, Gulek B, Yilmaz C, Kaya O, Arslan M, Dilek O, et al. The comparison of CT fistulography and MR imaging of perianal fistulae with surgical findings: A case-control study. Abdominal Radiology (New York). 2016;**41**(8):1474-1483

[22] Khati NJ, Sondel Lewis N, Frazier AA, Obias V, Zeman RK, Hill MC. CT of acute perianal abscesses and infected fistulae: A pictorial essay. Emergency Radiology. 2015;**22**(3):329-335

[23] Liang C, Jiang W, Zhao B, Zhang Y, Du Y, Lu Y. CT imaging with fistulography for perianal fistula: Does it really help the surgeon? Clinical Imaging. 2013;**37**(6):1069-1076

[24] Baskan O, Koplay M, Sivri M, Erol C. Our experience with MR imaging of perianal fistulas. Polish Journal of Radiology. 2014;**79**:490-497

[25] Liang C, Lu Y, Zhao B, Du Y, Wang C, Jiang W. Imaging of anal fistulas: Comparison of computed tomographic fistulography and magnetic resonance imaging. Korean Journal of Radiology. 2014;**15**(6):712-723

[26] Konan A, Onur MR, Özmen MN. The contribution of preoperative MRI to the surgical management of anal fistulas. Diagnostic and Interventional Radiology. 2018;**24**(6):321-327

[27] Garg P, Singh P, Kaur B. Magnetic resonance imaging (MRI): Operative findings correlation in 229 fistula-in-ano patients. World Journal of Surgery. 2017;**41**(6):1618-1624

[28] Garg P. Comparison of preoperative and postoperative MRI after fistula-in-ano surgery: Lessons learnt from an audit of 1323 MRI At a single centre. World Journal of Surgery. 2019;**43**(6):1612-1622

[29] Buchanan G, Halligan S, Williams A, Cohen CR, Tarroni D, Phillips RK, et al. Effect of MRI on clinical outcome of recurrent fistula-in-ano. Lancet. 2002;**360**(9346):1661-1662

[30] Sica GS, Di Carlo S, Tema G, Montagnese F, Del Vecchio BG, Fiaschetti V, et al. Treatment of peri-anal fistula in Crohn's disease. World Journal of Gastroenterology. 2014;**20**(37):13205-13210. DOI: 10.3748/wjg.v20.i37.13205

[31] Takesue Y, Ohge H, Yokoyama T, Murakami Y, Imamura Y, Sueda T. Long-term results of seton drainage on complex anal fistulae in patients with Crohn's disease. Journal of Gastroenterology. 2002;**37**(11):912-915

[32] Singh A, Midha V, Kochhar GS, Shen B, Sood A. Management of perianal fistulizing Crohn's disease. Inflammatory Bowel Diseases. 2024;**30**(9):1579-1603. DOI: 10.1093/ibd/izad195

[33] Hall JF, Bordeianou L, Hyman N, Read T, Bartus C, Schoetz D, et al. Outcomes after operations for anal fistula: Results of a prospective, multicenter, regional study. Diseases of the Colon and Rectum. 2014;**57**(11):1304-1308

[34] Whiteford MH, Kilkenny J 3rd, Hyman N, Buie WD, Cohen J, Orsay C, et al. Practice parameters for the treatment of perianal abscess and fistula-in-ano (revised). Diseases of the Colon and Rectum. 2005;**48**(7):1337-1342. DOI: 10.1007/s10350-005-0055-3

[35] Garcés-Albir M, García-Botello SA, Esclapez-Valero P, Sanahuja-Santafé A, Raga-Vázquez J, Espi-Macías A, et al. Quantifying the extent of fistulotomy. How much sphincter can we safely divide? A three-dimensional endosonographic study. International Journal of Colorectal Disease. 2012;**27**(8):1109-1116

[36] Farag AFA, Elbarmelgi MY, Mostafa M, Mashhour AN. One stage fistulectomy for high anal fistula with reconstruction of anal sphincter without fecal diversion. Asian Journal of Surgery. 2019;**42**(8):792-796

[37] Soltani A, Kaiser AM. Endorectal advancement flap for cryptoglandular or Crohn's fistula-in-ano. Diseases of the Colon and Rectum. 2010;**53**(4):486-495

[38] Bessi G, Siproudhis L, Merlini l'Héritier A, Wallenhorst T, Le Balc'h E, Bouguen G, et al. Advancement flap procedure in Crohn and non-Crohn perineal fistulas: A simple surgical approach. Colorectal Disease. 2019;**21**(1):66-72

[39] Yellinek S, Krizzuk D, Moreno Djadou T, Lavy D, Wexner SD. Endorectal advancement flap for complex anal fistula: Does flap configuration matter? Colorectal Disease. 2019;**21**(5):581-587

[40] Senéjoux A, Siproudhis L, Abramowitz L, Munoz-Bongrand N, Desseaux K, Bouguen G, et al. Groupe d'Etude thérapeutique des affections inflammatoires du tube digestif [GETAID] fistula plug in fistulising ano-perineal Crohn's disease: A randomised controlled trial. Journal of Crohn's & Colitis. 2016;**10**(2):141-148

[41] Cao Y, Su Q, Zhang B, Shen F, Li S. Efficacy of stem cells therapy for Crohn's fistula: A meta-analysis and systematic review. Stem Cell Research & Therapy. 2021;**12**(1):32. DOI: 10.1186/s13287-020-02095-7

[42] Rojanasakul A, Pattanaarun J, Sahakitrungruang C, Tantiphlachiva K. Total anal sphincter saving technique for fistula-in-ano; the ligation of intersphincteric fistula tract. Journal of the Medical Association of Thailand. 2007;**90**(3):581-586

[43] Kang WH, Yang HK, Chang HJ, Ko YT, Yoo BE, Lim CH, et al. High ligation of the anal fistula tract by lateral approach: A prospective cohort study on a modification of the ligation of the intersphincteric fistula tract (LIFT) technique. International Journal of Surgery. 2018;**60**:9-14

[44] Emile SH, Khan SM, Adejumo A, Koroye O. Ligation of intersphincteric fistula tract (LIFT) in treatment of anal fistula: An updated systematic review, meta-analysis, and meta-regression

of the predictors of failure. Surgery. 2020;**167**(2):484-492

[45] Bondi J, Avdagic J, Karlbom U, Hallböök O, Kalman D, Šaltytė Benth J, et al. Randomized clinical trial comparing collagen plug and advancement flap for trans-sphincteric anal fistula. The British Journal of Surgery. 2017;**104**(9):1160-1166

[46] VAAFT for Treating anal Fistulae. Available from: www.nice.org.uk/guidance/mib102

[47] Giamundo P. Laser treatment for anal fistulas: What are the pitfalls? Techniques in Coloproctology. 2020;**24**(7):663-665. DOI: 10.1007/s10151-020-02225-6. Epub 2020 May 2

Chapter 2

Perianal Fistula (Fistula-in-Ano): Latest Update and Knowledge

Omar Alhafidh

Abstract

Perianal fistulas are abnormal tracts connecting the anal canal to the perianal skin. Anatomy involves the anal glands, which, when blocked, lead to infection and abscess formation. Pathology progresses from abscess to fistula, with epithelialization of the tract. Clinically, patients experience pain, swelling, and purulent discharge. Examination reveals external openings. Investigations include physical examination, often under anesthesia, to map the fistula's course. MRI or endoanal ultrasound helps visualize complex tracts and assess sphincter involvement. Proctoscopy aids in identifying internal openings. These methods guide surgical planning and treatment. Tissue engineering presents a promising avenue for treating diseases using tissue-like structures from biomaterials, scaffolds, nanoparticles, biomolecules, and stem cells. This advanced approach aims to improve perianal fistula treatment, surpassing traditional seton therapy. Advances in stem cell biology, genetics, biomaterials, fabrication, and nanotechnology enable this multidisciplinary method to repair damaged tissue during seton procedures. Tissue engineering offers nanostructured biomaterials for setons, enhancing mechanical and biological properties like antibacterial and anti-inflammatory effects. This review explores tissue engineering's applications, advantages, and future in improving seton techniques, offering a novel fistula treatment. *In vivo* and *in vitro* studies on tissue engineering in fistula treatment are reported. Surgical procedures and different setons are summarized. Finally, challenges and future directions for tissue engineering in seton-based perianal fistula therapy are presented.

Keywords: perianal fistula, tissue engineering, stem cells, biomaterials, seton therapy, nanotechnology, fistula laser closure (FiLaC), video-assisted anal fistula treatment (VAAFT), ligation of the intersphincteric fistula tract (LIFT)

1. Introduction

A fistula-in-ano is an abnormal, granulation tissue-lined tract connecting a primary opening within the anal canal to a secondary opening on the perianal skin. Multiple secondary tracts may arise from a single primary opening [1, 2].

It is important to distinguish this condition from other processes that do not communicate with the anal canal, such as hidradenitis suppurativa, infected inclusion cysts, pilonidal disease, and Bartholin gland abscesses in females.

Most fistulas are believed to originate from cryptoglandular infections leading to perirectal abscess formation. The abscess represents the acute phase, while the fistula signifies the chronic stage. Symptoms significantly impact quality of life, ranging from minor discomfort and drainage to severe sepsis.

Pioneering surgeons like Goodsall, Miles, Milligan, Morgan, Thompson, and Lockhart-Mummery, in the late nineteenth and early twentieth centuries, significantly advanced anal fistula treatment by developing pathogenesis theories and classification systems.

Despite these early advances, the fundamental understanding of the disease has remained relatively stable. Parks further refined the classification system in 1976, which is still commonly used [3]. In recent decades, numerous surgical techniques have been proposed to reduce recurrence and incontinence, but fistula-in-ano remains a complex surgical challenge despite extensive experience spanning millennia [4].

Currently, there is no definitive medical treatment for fistula-in-ano. However, long-term antibiotic prophylaxis and infliximab may be considered for recurrent fistulas in Crohn's disease patients. Surgery remains the preferred treatment approach, aiming to drain infection, eradicate the fistulous tract, and prevent recurrence while preserving anal sphincter function [5, 6].

2. Anatomy

A solid understanding of pelvic floor and sphincter anatomy is essential for comprehending the classification system associated with fistulous disease (Refer to the image below, **Figure 1**).

The external anal sphincter consists of striated muscle under voluntary control and is divided into three components: submucosal, superficial, and deep. The deep segment merges with the puborectalis muscle, forming the anorectal ring that can be palpated during digital examination [7].

In contrast, the internal anal sphincter is composed of smooth muscle under autonomic control and extends from the circular muscle layer of the rectum.

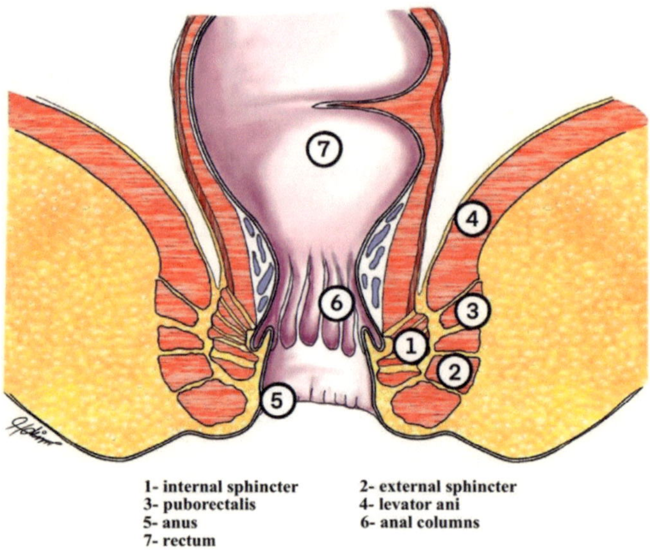

Figure 1.
Anatomy of the anal canal and pelvic floor.

For uncomplicated cases, the *Goodsall rule* (**Figure 2**) provides guidance in predicting fistula-in-ano anatomy. This rule indicates that if an external opening is located anterior to a transverse plane through the center of the anus, it will typically follow a straight radial path toward the dentate line. Conversely, openings situated posterior to this line generally take a curved route toward the posterior midline (see image below). Exceptions occur when external openings are more than 3 cm from the anal verge; these usually originate as primary or secondary tracts from the posterior midline due to prior horseshoe abscess formation [8].

2.1 Parks classification system

For fistula-in-ano classification, developed by Parks, Gordon, and Hardcastle. It is the most common system used and categorizes fistulas into four types based on their relationship to the sphincter muscles: [3]

- *Intersphincteric:* The fistula tract remains between the internal and external sphincter muscles.
- *Transsphincteric:* The tract crosses through the external sphincter muscle.
- *Supra-sphincteric:* The tract extends upward and above the puborectalis muscle (part of the levator ani muscle group), then down to the perianal skin.
- *Extra-sphincteric:* The tract originates outside the external sphincter, extends upward, and then tracks down to the perianal skin (**Figures 3** and **4**).

This is a description of the four types of fistula-in-ano based on the *Parks classification system:*

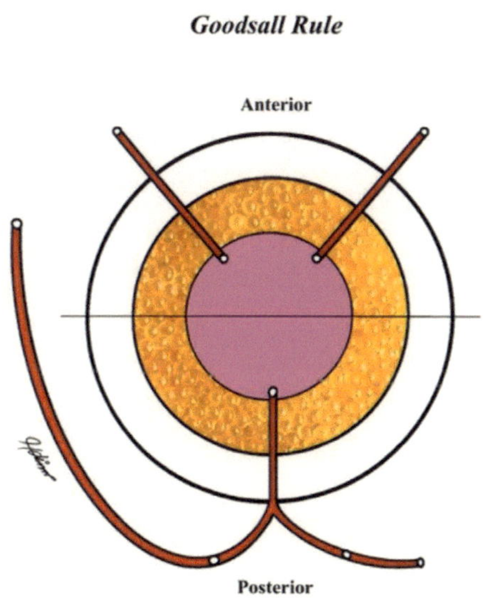

Figure 2.
Fistula-in-ano. Goodsall rule.

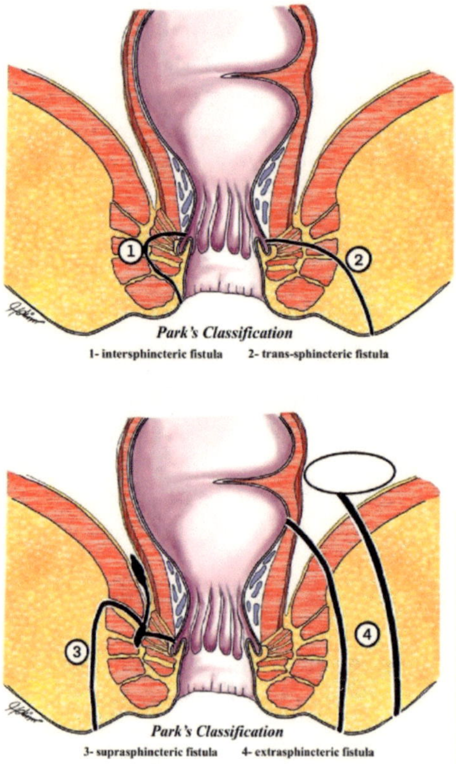

Figure 3.
Parks classification of fistula-in-ano.

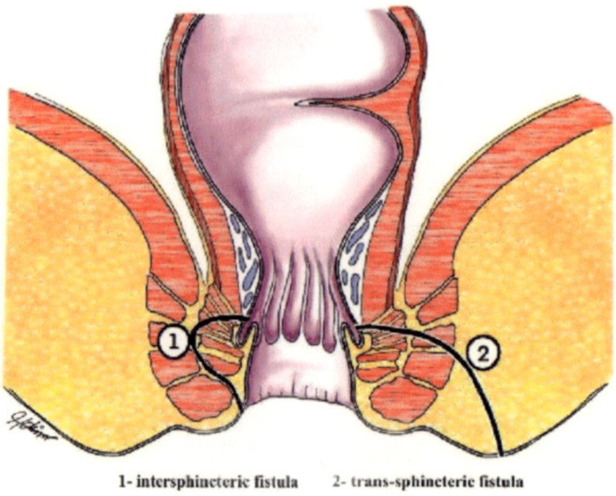

Figure 4.
Simplified classification.

1. Intersphincteric fistula:

    - Origin: Perianal abscess.
    - Course: Dentate line → internal sphincter → intersphincteric space → perianal skin.

- Prevalence: 70% (most common).
- Variations: No perineal opening, or high blind tract.

2. Transsphincteric fistula:
    - Origin: Ischiorectal fossa abscess.
    - Course: Dentate line → internal & external sphincters → ischiorectal fossa → perianal skin.
    - Prevalence: 25%.
    - Variations: High tract with perineal opening or high blind tract.
3. Supra-sphincteric fistula:
    - Origin: Supralevator abscess.
    - Course: Dentate line → intersphincteric space → above puborectalis → external sphincter → ischiorectal fossa → perianal skin.
    - Prevalence: 5%.
    - Variations: High blind tract (palpable through rectal wall).
4. Extra-sphincteric fistula:
    - Origin: Foreign body, injury, Crohn's, cancer, or pelvic inflammatory disease.
    - Course: Perianal skin → ischiorectal fossa → levator ani → rectal wall (outside sphincter complex). May or may not connect to dentate line.
    - Prevalence: 1% (least common).

This text discusses the differences between *the Current Procedural Terminology (CPT) coding* for anal fistulas and the Parks classification system.

Here is a breakdown:

CPT coding:

- Subcutaneous: This is a superficial fistula, not included in the Parks classification.
- Submuscular: (Includes intersphincteric and low transsphincteric fistulas in Parks classification).
- Complex/Recurrent: (Includes high transsphincteric, supra-sphincteric, extra-sphincteric, multiple tracts, and recurrent fistulas in Parks classification).
- Second stage: Refers to procedures done in stages.

Key difference:

- Subcutaneous fistulas: CPT coding includes subcutaneous fistulas, but the Parks classification does *not*. Subcutaneous fistulas are typically caused by non-cryptoglandular issues like unhealed anal fissures or anorectal procedures (hemorrhoidectomy, sphincterotomy), whereas the Parks system focuses on cryptoglandular origin.

In essence:

- CPT coding is more comprehensive for billing purposes, including superficial fistulas and staged procedures.
- The Parks classification is specifically for classifying fistulas based on their anatomical relationship to the sphincter muscles, focusing on those originating from the anal glands.

Pathophysiology of perianal fistula:

- Definition: An abnormal connection between the anorectal tract and the perineal skin [1].
- Incidence: 2 to 9 cases per 100,000 people annually, more common in men aged 20-40 [9, 10].
- Impact: While rarely life-threatening, it can be debilitating and socially embarrassing, affecting quality of life due to pain, discharge, abscesses, and tissue damage [11–13].
- Origin: Often arises without prior disease, but 30-50% follow an anorectal abscess [1].

Classification:

1. Parks classification, mentioned above.
2. Simplified classification:
    - Simple: Single intersphincteric or low transsphincteric tract without branching.
    - Complex: High transsphincteric, supra-sphincteric, extra-sphincteric, branched (multiple openings), horseshoe (extending to both ischiorectal fossae) [14]. Also, low fistulas in high-risk patients (recurrent, incontinent) and those with IBD, malignancy, incontinence, diarrhea, or prior radiation are considered complex [15, 16].

Epidemiology:

- True prevalence is unknown.
- Incidence after anal abscess: 26 to 38% of anal abscesses develop into fistulas.

- Prevalence: 8.6 cases per 100,000 population.
    - Men: 12.3 per 100,000
    - Women: 5.6 per 100,000
- Male-to-female ratio: 1.8:1
- Mean age: 38.3 years [17]

In summary: While the exact number of people with fistula-in-ano is not known, studies suggest it affects roughly 8.6 out of every 100,000 people, with men being nearly twice as likely to be affected as women. A significant portion of anal abscesses leads to fistula formation, and the average age of those affected is just under 40.

History:

Common symptoms (in order of prevalence):

- Perianal discharge: This is the most common symptom.
- Pain: Often described as throbbing or constant.
- Swelling: Inflammation and abscess formation can lead to noticeable swelling.
- Bleeding: May be associated with bowel movements or due to local trauma.
- Diarrhea: Altered bowel habits can occur.
- Skin excoriation: The constant moisture and discharge can irritate the surrounding skin.
- External opening: The visible opening of the fistula on the skin.

Factors suggesting a complex fistula:

- Inflammatory bowel disease (IBD): Conditions like Crohn's disease can increase the risk of complex fistulas.
- Diverticulitis: Inflammation of pouches in the colon wall can lead to fistula formation.
- Previous radiation therapy: Radiation to the pelvic area can damage tissues and increase fistula risk.
- Tuberculosis: This infection can cause complex fistulas.
- Steroid therapy: Long-term steroid use can weaken the immune system and increase the risk of infections.
- HIV infection: Compromised immune function makes individuals more susceptible to complex infections and fistulas [16, 17].

Key takeaway: A thorough patient history, including symptoms and any underlying conditions, is crucial for diagnosing and managing fistula-in-ano, especially in identifying potentially complex cases that may require specialized treatment.

Physical examination.

Visual inspection:

- Perineum: The examiner should carefully look for any external openings, which may appear as open sinuses or raised areas of granulation tissue.
- Discharge: Note any spontaneous drainage of pus or blood from the external opening.

Digital rectal examination (DRE):

- Tract palpation: A fibrous tract or cord may be felt beneath the skin.
- Inflammation: DRE helps identify any additional areas of acute inflammation that have not yet drained.
- Induration: Lateral or posterior firmness may suggest deeper extension into the postanal or ischiorectal space.

Other important aspects:

- Relationship to anorectal ring: The examiner should determine the tract's location to the anorectal ring *before* the patient's muscles are relaxed under anesthesia (as this helps determine the fistula's path).
- Sphincter assessment: Assess sphincter tone and voluntary squeeze pressure *before* surgery to determine if preoperative manometry (a test of anal muscle function) is needed.
- Anoscopy: Visual examination of the anal canal using an anoscope is usually necessary to locate the *internal* opening of the fistula.
- Proctoscopy: If there is suspicion of rectal disease (like Crohn's), a proctoscopy (examination of the rectum with a scope) is recommended.
- Probing: Gently probing the fistula tract in the office setting is generally *not* advised as it is usually too painful for the patient [15–17].

Key takeaway: The physical exam relies heavily on visual inspection and DRE to identify the external opening, assess the tract, and determine the fistula's relationship to surrounding structures. Anoscopy and possibly proctoscopy help visualize the internal opening and rule out other rectal issues. Assessing sphincter function is crucial for planning treatment and minimizing the risk of incontinence.

Investigations:

1. Imaging studies

   - Usually not a routine: Imaging is not typically used for initial fistula evaluation as the anatomy can usually be determined during surgery.

- Helpful in specific situations: Imaging is valuable when:
  - The primary opening is hard to find.
  - There is a recurrent or persistent disease.
  - There are recurrent or multiple fistulas (to identify secondary tracts or missed primary openings) [18].

Available modalities:

- *Fistulography:* Injecting contrast into the fistula tract to visualize it on X-ray.
- *Ultrasonography (US):* Using ultrasound waves to create images of the fistula.
- *Magnetic resonance imaging (MRI):* Detailed images using magnetic fields and radio waves.
- *Computed tomography (CT):* Cross-sectional images using X-rays.
- *Barium enema:* Visualizing the large intestine with barium contrast (may be less helpful for fistulas specifically).
- *Small-bowel series:* Visualizing the small intestine with barium contrast (may be less helpful for fistulas specifically).

In short: While surgery often provides the necessary information, radiologic studies are useful in complex or recurrent cases to map the fistula tract(s) and identify any missed connections. MRI is often preferred for its detailed visualization of soft tissues.

2.2 Fistulography

- Contrast dye is injected through the *internal* opening of the fistula.
- X-ray images (anteroposterior, lateral, and oblique views) are taken to visualize the fistula tract.

Limitations and considerations:

- *Pain:* Injection can be painful.
- *Internal opening visualization:* Requires the ability to identify the internal opening.
- *Accuracy:* Accuracy is questionable, with reported rates ranging from only 16 to 48% [19].
- *Limited use:* Due to these limitations, fistulography is mainly used when there is concern about connections between the rectum and adjacent organs (e.g., bladder), where it *might* offer slightly more information than examination under anesthesia.

Key takeaway: While fistulography can help visualize the fistula tract, its accuracy is questionable, and it can be painful. Therefore, it is reserved for specific situations where other methods are insufficient, particularly when assessing potential connections to internal organs.

2.3 Endoanal or endorectal ultrasonography

This text describes the use of Endoanal Ultrasound (EAUS) or Endorectal Ultrasound (ERUS) in evaluating fistula-in-ano:
Technique:

- A 7- or 10-MHz ultrasound transducer is inserted into the anal canal.
- This helps visualize the muscular anatomy and distinguish between intersphincteric and transsphincteric fistulas.
- A water-filled balloon transducer can aid in evaluating the rectal wall for suprasphincteric extension.
- Injecting hydrogen peroxide through the external opening can help outline the fistula tract and identify missed internal openings.

Benefits and Limitations:

- Improved internal opening detection: EAUS/ERUS is reportedly 50% better than physical examination alone in finding difficult-to-locate internal openings.
- Not widely used: Despite its benefits, it is not routinely used for fistula evaluation [20].
- Pre- and postoperative use in LIFT: A study by Murad-Regadas et al. found 3D anorectal US helpful in LIFT procedures (ligation of the intersphincteric fistula tract) both preoperatively (to determine the muscle to be transected) and postoperatively (to assess healing, failure, or recurrence) [21].

Key takeaway: EAUS/ERUS is a valuable tool for visualizing fistula tracts and identifying internal openings, especially when physical examination is inconclusive. While not yet a standard practice for all fistula evaluations, it can be particularly useful in specific situations, such as pre- and postoperative assessments of complex procedures like LIFT.

2.4 Magnetic resonance imaging

It is:

- *High concordance:* MRI findings show an 80-90% match with what is found during surgery when looking at the primary fistula tract and any secondary extensions.
- *Study of choice:* MRI is increasingly preferred for evaluating complex and recurrent fistulas.

- *Reduced recurrence:* MRI helps reduce recurrence rates by revealing previously unknown extensions of the fistula tract [22, 23].

In short: MRI is a valuable tool for visualizing complex and recurrent fistulas, allowing surgeons to identify all extensions and plan a more effective surgical approach, ultimately leading to better outcomes and lower recurrence rates.

2.5 Computed tomography

It is:

- *Better for inflammatory disease:* CT scans are more useful for visualizing perirectal inflammatory disease than for small fistulas.

- *Fluid pockets:* CT excels at identifying and delineating fluid collections (abscesses) that require drainage.

- *Small fistulas:* CT is not as effective in visualizing the fine details of small fistula tracts.

- *Contrast needed:* CT requires the administration of both oral and rectal contrast to optimize visualization.

- *Muscle detail:* CT does *not* provide good visualization of the muscular anatomy, which is crucial for classifying fistulas (e.g., intersphincteric vs. transsphincteric) [22, 23].

In short: CT scans are a valuable tool for identifying and characterizing abscesses and other fluid collections in the perirectal region. However, due to its limitations in visualizing small fistula tracts and its poor delineation of muscle anatomy, it is not the ideal imaging modality for evaluating fistulas specifically. Other modalities like MRI are generally preferred for detailed fistula assessment.

2.6 Barium enema/small-bowel series

Mainly to ruling out IBD:

- In patients with multiple or recurrent fistulas, these studies can be helpful in ruling out inflammatory bowel disease (IBD), such as Crohn's disease [24, 25].

In short: Imaging is not just for visualizing the fistula tract itself. It can also provide information about the surrounding tissues and help determine if there is an underlying condition, like IBD, that might be contributing to the fistula(s) or affecting treatment choices.

1. Routine blood tests to assess the general condition of the patient and exclude other medical problems that could be related, like inflammatory bowel disease, malignancy, and TB.
   Treatment and management:
   General approach:

- *Symptomatic patients:* Treatment is indicated for those experiencing symptoms, typically recurrent anorectal sepsis. Abscesses can form if the external opening seals.

- *Asymptomatic patients:* If a fistula is found incidentally and the patient has no symptoms, no treatment is needed.

Crohn's Disease Considerations:

- *Complex fistulas:* Crohn's disease with multiple, complex fistulas requires careful surgical management.

- *Acute abscess:* Incision and drainage are needed for acute perianal abscesses.

- *Definitive repair:* Fistula repair should be done when intra-abdominal Crohn's is controlled with medication.

- *Infliximab:* Infliximab therapy has shown 50-60% response rates for Crohn's-related fistulas [24, 25].

- *Stem-cell therapy:* Adipose-derived stem-cell therapy is under investigation for Crohn's and other complex fistulas [26, 27].

- *Recurrent disease:* Pan proctocolectomy may be considered for recurrent disease with persistent sepsis.

Abscess management:

- *Acute phase:* Surgery for definitive fistula repair is *not* recommended during an acute abscess. Simple incision and drainage are sufficient [28].

- *Fistula development:* Only 7-40% of abscess patients develop a fistula.

- *Recurrence risk:* Recurrent sepsis and fistula formation are higher in younger patients (<40 years) and nondiabetics.

Preoperative considerations:

- *Bowel prep:* Rectal irrigation with enemas on the morning of surgery.

- *Anesthesia:* General, local with IV sedation, or regional block.

- *Antibiotics:* Preoperative antibiotics should be administered.

- *Positioning:* Prone jackknife position with buttocks apart is preferred.

Intraoperative considerations:

- *Examination under anesthesia:* To confirm the extent of the fistula.

- *Internal opening identification:* Crucial to prevent recurrence.

- *Local anesthetic:* Provides postoperative analgesia.

Historical note:

Past belief: Historically, surgery was believed to be the only treatment for fistula-in-ano [29].

Surgical treatment.

2.6.1 Fistulotomy

Indications:

- Fistulotomy is appropriate for 85-95% of primary fistulas, specifically those that are:

    o Submucosal

    o Intersphincteric

    o Low transsphincteric [30–33]

Procedure:

1. Probe insertion: A probe is carefully passed through the fistula tract, entering through the external opening and exiting through the internal opening.

2. Tract division: The tissue overlying the probe, including skin, subcutaneous tissue, and the internal sphincter muscle, is cut open using a knife or electrocautery. This lays the entire fistula tract open.

3. Sphincter division: In low-level fistulas, the internal sphincter and the subcutaneous part of the external sphincter can be safely divided without affecting continence (except when the fistulotomy is performed anteriorly in women).

4. Seton placement: If the fistula tract extends higher into the sphincter mechanism, a seton should be placed instead of dividing the sphincter.

5. Curettage: Granulation tissue within the opened fistula tract is removed using a curette.

6. Wound management:

    - The skin at the end of the wound is opened further (1-2 cm) to allow internal healing to begin before the external wound closes.

    - Some surgeons advocate for marsupialization (suturing the edges of the wound open) to potentially speed healing.

7. Biopsy: Any suspicious tissue encountered during the procedure should be biopsied.

Important Note:

- Fistulectomy vs. fistulotomy: Complete removal of the fistula tract (fistulectomy) creates a larger wound that takes longer to heal and does *not* offer any advantage in preventing recurrence compared to fistulotomy.

In essence: Fistulotomy is a common and effective procedure for many primary anal fistulas. It involves laying open the fistula tract to allow it to heal from the inside out. Care is taken to avoid compromising continence by not dividing too much of the sphincter muscle in higher tracts or in specific locations (anterior in women).

2.6.2 Setons

Seton can be utilized alone, alongside fistulotomy, or in a staged approach, particularly for complex (e.g., high transsphincteric, supra-sphincteric, extra-sphincteric), multiple, or recurrent fistulas; anterior fistulas in women; patients with weak preoperative sphincter pressures, Crohn disease, or immunosuppression [34, 35]. Setons serve to visualize involved sphincter muscle, facilitate drainage, promote fibrosis, and gradually divide the fistula tract. Materials include silk suture, Silastic vessel markers, or rubber bands.

2.7 Single-stage cutting seton placement

The seton is threaded through the opened fistula tract, encircling the deep external sphincter, then tightened and secured. Fibrosis develops above the seton as it slowly divides the sphincter, effectively exteriorizing the tract. The seton is progressively tightened until it pulls through (6-8 weeks). Cutting setons can be used independently of fistulotomy. Recurrence and incontinence are key considerations. While success rates range from 82 to 100%, incontinence may exceed 30% [36–38].

2.8 Two-stage seton (draining/fibrosing)

1. Initial placement:

    - After opening the skin, subcutaneous tissue, internal sphincter, and subcutaneous external sphincter, the seton is placed loosely around the deep portion of the external sphincter.

2. Purpose:

    - Unlike a cutting seton (which is tightened), this loose seton is meant for:

        o Drainage of the intersphincteric space.

        o Promoting fibrosis in the deep sphincter muscle.

3. Second stage:

    - After the superficial wound heals (2-3 months), the seton-bound sphincter muscle is divided.

4. Alternative approach (Studies with 0 Nylon Seton):

    - Two studies (involving 74 patients) used a 0 nylon seton in a two-stage approach [39, 40].

- After wound healing, the seton was removed without dividing the remaining encircled deep external sphincter muscle.

- This resulted in fistula eradication in 60-78% of cases.

Key takeaway: The two-stage seton technique prioritizes drainage and fibrosis in the first stage, followed by division of the sphincter in the second. An alternative approach, supported by some studies, involves simply removing the seton after healing, potentially avoiding sphincter division altogether in select cases.

3. Advanced procedures

3.1 Ligation of the intersphincteric fistula tract (LIFT)

LIFT procedure:

- *Introduction:* Introduced in 2007 [39].

- *Indication:* Primarily for complex or recurrent transsphincteric fistulas.

- *Technique:* Involves closure of the internal and external openings of the fistula tract and removal of infected cryptoglandular tissue.

Comparative studies:

- *LIFT vs. flap procedures:* A randomized trial showed LIFT had a higher success rate and faster return to work, but a higher recurrence rate and similar incontinence scores compared to flap procedures [40].

- *LIFT vs. conventional fistulotomy:* Another trial found LIFT to be effective (80% success rate) with lower incontinence and shorter healing time compared to open fistulotomy [41].

Overall assessment:

- *Potential:* LIFT shows promise for complex perianal fistulas, with a satisfactory success rate (75-87.5%) and low complication rates, especially incontinence [42–45].

- *Secondary success:* Repeat LIFT or other repair procedures after initial LIFT failure have shown acceptable results (80-86%) [46–48].

- *Crohn's disease:* LIFT has demonstrated good outcomes in patients with Crohn's-related fistulas [49–51].

In summary: LIFT is a sphincter-sparing technique that offers a promising alternative for complex transsphincteric fistulas, particularly in terms of healing time and incontinence rates. While recurrence is a concern, repeat procedures can still achieve good results. It is also a viable option for patients with Crohn's disease.

3.2 Fistula laser closure (FiLaCTM)

- *Technique:* Involves closing the internal opening of the fistula and then using a laser fiber (1470 nm wavelength) to deliver energy into the fistula tract *via* a catheter [52].

Effectiveness:

- *Success rate:* Reported short-term and long-term success rates range from 64.1 to 81.1% [53–55]. A meta-analysis estimated an overall success rate of about 63% [56, 57].

- *High-risk patients:* In patients with a high risk of incontinence after fistulotomy, the healing rate was 45.6%, with significant healing observed in those with high transsphincteric fistulas and age over 50 [55–57].

Incontinence:

- *Rate:* Reported incontinence rates after FiLaCTM range from 1.7 to 9.6% in studies with larger patient populations [53, 57].

Key takeaway: FiLaCTM is a minimally invasive, sphincter-saving option for anal fistula treatment with promising success rates and low incontinence rates. It may be particularly beneficial for patients at high risk for incontinence. However, its effectiveness might be lower in certain subgroups, and further research is needed to fully understand its long-term outcomes and compare it to other established techniques (**Figures 5–7**).

3.3 Over-the-scope clip system (OTSC)

- *Description:* A "bear claw" Nitinol clip originally designed for hemostasis in gastrointestinal endoscopy [58].

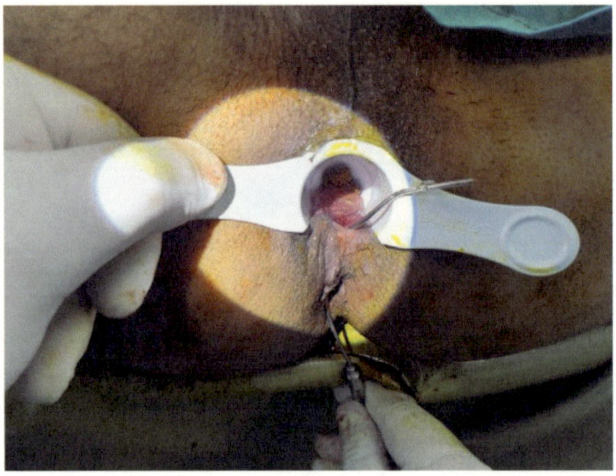

Figure 5.
Fistula laser closure (FiLaCTM). Showing different stages of the procedure. Images by Dr. Modhar AlOmary FIBMS, FACS.

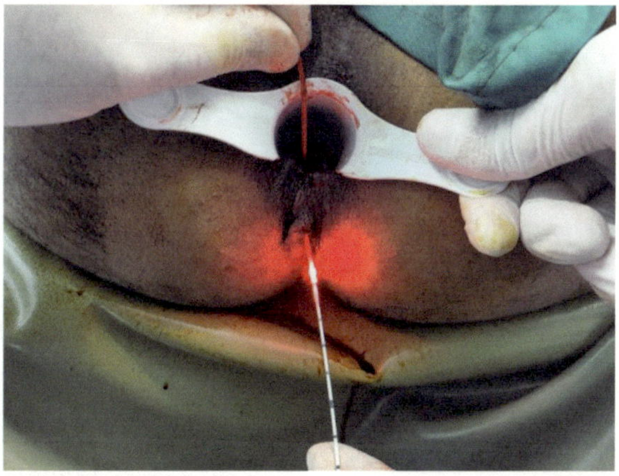

Figure 6.
Fistula laser closure (FiLaCTM). AlSalam Teaching hospital, Mosul, Iraq.

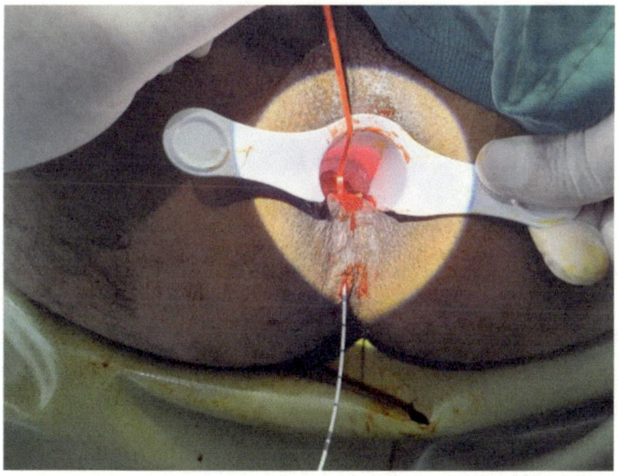

Figure 7.
Fistula laser closure (FiLaCTM).

- *Application:* Used to treat perianal fistulas by applying the clip to the internal opening [59].

Effectiveness:

- *Success rate:* Reported success rates for treating both complex and simple perianal fistulas range from 60 to 93.3% [60].

- *Comparison to fistulectomy:* Studies have shown a *higher* success rate with OTSC compared to standard fistulectomy.

- *Postoperative course:* OTSC is associated with shorter postoperative stays (1.3 days) and healing times (3.2 days) compared to fistulectomy [60].

In summary: The Over-The-Scope Clip (OTSC) system offers a minimally invasive endoscopic approach to fistula treatment with promising results, including high success rates and faster recovery compared to traditional surgery.

3.4 Anal fistula plug (AFP)

AFP technique:

- *Goal:* Primarily aims to close the internal opening of the fistula [61].
- *Procedure:* Involves inserting a biologic or synthetic plug into the internal opening of the fistula tract, secured with a suture [62, 63].
- *Advantages:* Simple, minimally invasive, and relatively quick [61, 64].

Effectiveness:

- *Healing rate:* Studies have shown variable healing rates, ranging from 54 to 80%, with shorter follow-up periods showing higher healing rates [65, 66].
- *Nasseri et al.'s review:* A review of 12 studies (84 Crohn's patients) concluded that AFP is safe, with low incontinence and morbidity risks. The mean healing rate was about 60%, and the recurrence rate was 13.6% [67].
- *GORE BIO-A plug:* Another review of 187 patients treated with GORE BIO-A plugs reported healing rates from 15.8 to 72.7%, with follow-up periods from 2 to 19 months.

Key takeaway: Anal fistula plugs offer a minimally invasive, sphincter-sparing option for fistula treatment. While healing rates vary, they appear to be a safe approach with low risks of incontinence and complications. However, long-term data is needed to fully assess their effectiveness and durability, especially considering the wide range of reported success rates.

3.5 Video-assisted anal fistula treatment (VAAFT)

VAAFT procedure:

- *Description:* A novel sphincter-saving method (**Figure 8**) [67].
- *Combination therapy:* Zhang et al. found satisfactory results combining VAAFT with an anal fistula plug [68].
- *Healing time:* The mean wound healing time was 46 days in the combined VAAFT and plug approach, with no sphincter function impairment [68].

Comparative studies:

- *VAAFT vs. Fistulotomy + Seton:* While both VAAFT and fistulotomy with seton placement yielded satisfactory results, VAAFT showed:

  o Significantly shorter healing time.

  o Minor postoperative incontinence scores (Wexner scale) [69, 70].

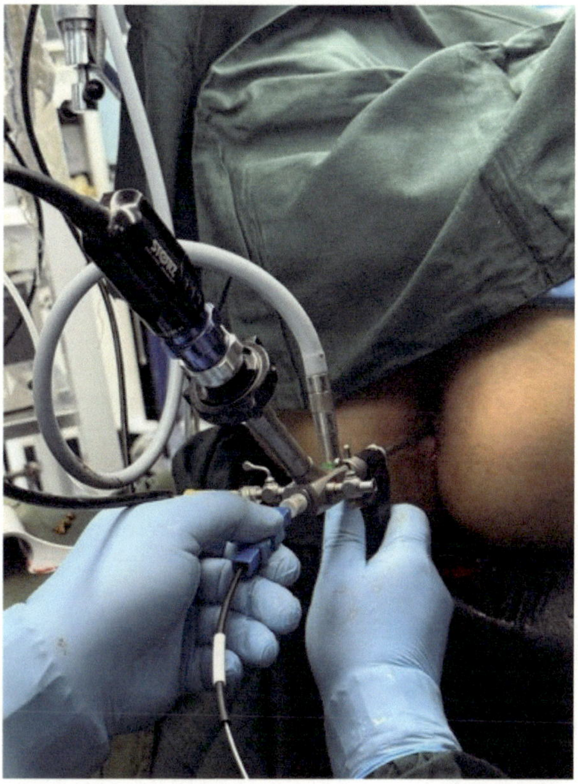

Figure 8.
Video-assisted anal fistula treatment (VAAFT) Images by Dr. Modhar AlOmary FIBMS, FACS AlSalam Teaching hospital, Mosul, Iraq.

Reported success rates:

- *Complex fistulas:* 71.2–87.1% [71–78].
- *Crohn's-related fistulas:* 82–84% [79].

In summary: VAAFT is a promising, minimally invasive, sphincter-preserving technique with shorter healing times and potentially lower incontinence rates compared to traditional methods. It has shown good results in both complex and Crohn's-associated anal fistulas.

3.6 Rectal advancement flap (RAF)

- *Technique:* A sphincter-preserving technique with a 66-87% healing rate, potentially optimal for complex cryptoglandular fistulas [11]. A trans anal approach is used to lift and advance the rectal flap without disturbing the sphincter [80].
- *Soltani & Kaiser review:* Had assessed 1654 patients with Crohn's or cryptoglandular fistulas who underwent RAF. Healing/incontinence rates were 80.8/13.2% for Crohn's and 64/9.4% for cryptoglandular fistulas, respectively [81].

- *Recurrence in Crohn's:* Mean recurrence rate after RAF for Crohn's-related anorectal fistulas is around 30% [82].

- *Comparison to LIFT:* While healing and recurrence rates may be similar between LIFT and RAF for both cryptoglandular and Crohn's fistulas, incontinence may be higher after RAF [82].

- *Comparison to collagen paste:* RAF showed better healing rates than Permacol collagen paste and lower incontinence than porcine collagen paste [83].

3.7 PERFACT procedure

1. *Description:* Proximal superficial cauterization, emptying regularly fistula tracts, and curettage of tracts (PERFACT) is another novel procedure for complex anorectal fistulas, targeting both the internal opening and the tract [84, 85].

2. *Results:* Reported healing rate of 80% and recurrence rate of 20% [84, 85].

Comparative analysis:

- *Need for multidimensional analysis:* The text emphasizes the need for comprehensive studies to compare the effectiveness of different fistula treatment techniques.

- *Lin et al.'s study:* It compared RAF and AFP (anal fistula plug), finding that RAF had better heal and recurrence rates, but no significant difference in complications. RAF may be a better choice for complex cryptoglandular fistulas, while AFP is less invasive and more comfortable [86].

- *RAF vs. Seton:* RAF may have lower recurrence and complication rates than seton placement in this patient group [87].

In summary: The Rectal Advancement Flap (RAF) is a promising sphincter-preserving technique with good healing rates but with the potential for higher incontinence compared to LIFT. It may be a preferred option for complex cryptoglandular fistulas compared to AFP and seton placement, but more research is needed to solidify these findings. The PERFACT procedure is another emerging option with favorable results. Direct comparative studies are crucial to guide clinical decision-making.

Now, because most surgeons use the setons in treating the perianal fistula, I believe that we need to speak in detail about the seton techniques.

Seton placement techniques for the treatment of perianal fistula:

The use of setons for perianal fistula treatment dates to Hippocrates, who first described the technique using horsehair wrapped around a lint thread [88]. Generally, a seton is a looped material that passes through the external and internal openings of the fistula tract, promoting abscess drainage and inducing a localized inflammatory response that leads to granulation tissue formation and fibrosis [35]. Seton placement is often the initial treatment for perianal fistulas, as it facilitates drainage of the fistula tract and any associated abscesses [89]. Antibiotics, typically metronidazole or ciprofloxacin, may be administered as an adjunct therapy to further encourage healing

[90]. Various materials, such as silk, wire, elastic bands, Penrose drains, and nylon, have been employed as setons [91]. Setons are classified as cutting, non-cutting, loose, or chemical, each of which will be discussed in detail below. While seton placement may appear straightforward initially, it requires careful consideration and should be performed by surgeons with extensive knowledge of perianal anatomy to ensure optimal quality of life following fistula healing.

There are multiple types of setons:

3.8 Cutting setons

Cutting setons, used for fistulas involving substantial sphincter muscle, are a common surgical technique [92]. They gradually divide the sphincters, minimizing damage compared to a fistulotomy [91]. The suture or band is passed through the tract, tightened around the sphincter, and progressively tightened every 1-2 weeks until complete division [29]. Alternatively, a two-stage fistulotomy involves seton placement for 6-8 weeks followed by fistulotomy [93, 94], though this increases incontinence risk, especially with multiple tracts [94].

Cutting setons demonstrate high efficacy and low recurrence for high perianal fistulas [95–99], comparable to mucosal advancement flaps (though healing may be longer and require more procedures) [63, 100, 101] and LIFT procedures (approximately 40% primary success, 75% subsequently) [102]. However, previous surgeries can complicate these techniques, making seton drainage a reasonable option to prevent recurrent abscesses [91], and the fibrosis around the seton during sphincter division prevents sphincter retraction.

Incontinence rates for cutting setons range from 3.2 to 30%, averaging 12% [103, 104]. Due to higher incontinence with high transsphincteric and supra-sphincteric fistulas, some suggest cutting setons for low transsphincteric fistulas where minor incontinence (gas or minor stool) is acceptable [105]. Recurrence rates range from 5 to 29%, typically below 10% [92, 93, 106–108], varying due to fistula anatomy, prior surgeries, follow-up, and healing factors.

Incontinence is a major complication. While some studies report high healing rates with no incontinence [109, 110], others report high incontinence rates [111, 112]. A systematic review of 18 studies showed 5% recurrence with internal anal sphincter preservation and 3% with division, with fecal incontinence rates of 5.6 and 25.2%, respectively [59]. Thus, routine seton use for all high fistulas is not necessarily safe.

There is no difference in incontinence between cutting seton and fistulotomy for low superficial fistulas. Acute perianal abscesses are typically drained first, with fistula treatment postponed for accurate assessment. Patients with major incontinence should not undergo cutting seton placement. Cutting setons are suitable for complex fistulas, but non-cutting setons may be considered for women and those with prior perianal surgery.

Cariati et al. proposed criteria for fistulotomy and seton insertion [72]. They recommend complete fistulotomy for subcutaneous, low intersphincteric, or very low transsphincteric fistulas (<10% external sphincter involvement) and cutting seton (with partial fistulectomy/fistulotomy) for transsphincteric fistulas (>10% involvement). This reportedly reduces sphincter cutting by 20%, with 100% healing, 11.5% transient soiling, and 6.5% recurrence. While steel wires were previously used [71, 113], they are now less common. Different seton types are discussed below.

3.9 Rubber band setons

First documented as a treatment for anal fistulas in 1966 [72, 73], they have been used for deep anterior space abscess/anal fistula and chronic perianal fistula. A study comparing rubber band setons and echelon sutures found complete healing in all patients within three months, with 7.5 and 2.5% recurrence rates, respectively [90]. Rubber setons are considered a cost-effective and well-tolerated option with lower pain scores [74, 90]. Compared to nylon ligation, rubber setons offered similar functionality, shorter hospital stays, fewer complications, and effective drainage in extra-sphincteric and transsphincteric fistulas [74].

3.10 Polypropylene (Prolene) setons

Made from a chemically resistant thermoplastic polymer, they are a potential option for perianal fistula treatment. However, patient dissatisfaction with the material and knot has limited their popularity [74, 96]. A comparison of silk and polypropylene setons showed shorter recovery times and higher pain scores in the polypropylene group, with no difference in recurrence or incontinence [75]. Local infection requiring fistulotomy was more common with silk setons, while pain was greater with polypropylene [76]. An animal study comparing fistulotomy, polypropylene, and polydioxanone wire found no difference in fibrosis, concluding that none were superior to fistulotomy [77].

3.11 Silk setons

A common nonabsorbable suture material used worldwide [74, 75, 78], they are susceptible to bacterial colonization and therefore not recommended for contaminated environments or prolonged use [114]. Silk sutures can function as both cutting [34] and non-cutting setons [115], demonstrating healing rates of 96 and 75%, respectively. Studies report recurrence rates between 2.4 and 9.8%, with 8-15.7% incontinence to flatus and no fecal incontinence [34, 74, 91].

3.12 Polyester setons

Also known as ETHIBOND EXCEL®, they are a nonabsorbable option made of polyethylene terephthalate. They are reported to cause less inflammation and discomfort than monofilament polypropylene sutures [64], making them potentially suitable for inflammatory conditions like Crohn's disease-related perianal sepsis or for long-term use [116, 117].

3.13 Loose setons

Loose setons involve passing a thread or band through the fistula tract, forming a loop tied around the sphincter without tension [118]. This avoids the constant pain associated with cutting setons and prevents sphincter injury [119]. However, healing is prolonged due to slow drainage and palliation [103, 120]. These "long-term setons" are intended to prevent abscess formation and perianal sepsis in chronic cases. Some surgeons believe loose setons can gradually divide tissue while preserving the sphincter, recommending them over cutting setons to avoid complications [120]. While some advocate for daily thread pulling to accelerate granulation [121], this is often painful and unreliable due to varying pressure and compliance. Loose setons are preferred when continence is a concern, such as in complex, previously operated fistulas or in inflammatory conditions like Crohn's disease [122–124].

4. Tissue engineering and stem cell therapy

Tissue engineering and stem cell therapy offer novel approaches for perianal fistula treatment, particularly in patients with Crohn's disease and other IBDs [124–127]. Tissue engineering, utilizing stem cells [128], scaffolds [79], and signaling molecules [129], aims to repair and restore damaged tissues, including fistula tracts. This interdisciplinary field, incorporating nanotechnology [130], micro/nanofabrication [131], biomaterials [131], and molecular medicine [132], can enhance seton-based therapies.

Bacterial infections, a major challenge in fistula treatment, can be addressed with antibacterial setons [133, 134]. Antibacterial agents, such as conventional antibiotics, metallic nanoparticles (silver [135], zinc [60], copper [136]), and naturally antibacterial polymers like chitosan [137], can be integrated into seton structures. Blaker et al. created porous spherical microscale scaffolds with silver-doped phosphate glass, demonstrating silver ion release and bacterial colonization reduction in a rodent wound model [138]. Silver nanoparticle incorporation into scaffolds enhances antibacterial, antiviral, and mechanical properties [139], with silver ions disrupting bacterial viability [140], making them valuable in wound healing and bone regeneration. Silver nanoparticles also exhibit anti-inflammatory effects in chronic digestive diseases like colitis [141], and silver nanoparticle-coated sutures improve antibacterial and mechanical properties, reduce inflammation, and enhance intestinal anastomosis healing in mice [142]. Incorporating antibacterial nanoparticles into setons can improve their efficacy in IBD-related fistulas.

Seton removal can be difficult if they become trapped. Biodegradable setons, manufactured using tissue engineering [143] with various degradable polymers optimized for different fistula types [144], offer a solution. Polyglycolic acid and trimethylene carbonate have shown promise in early studies [145, 146]. Pramudiati loaded the immunosuppressant polyphenol into PLGA films for biodegradable setons [147]. Biodegradable setons are advantageous in preventing foreign body granulomatous reactions in anal fistula treatment.

Injectable polymers like Salvecoll-E® gel show promise for anal fistula treatment. Drug-eluting setons, incorporating antibiotics, antibacterial agents, or anti-inflammatories like curcumin and 5-aminosalicylic acid [148, 149], offer sustained release and improved healing. Anti-TNF drugs like infliximab may also be incorporated [150–152].

Smart biomaterials offer further advancements. Responsive, self-healing, and shape-memory polymers can create smart scaffolds and nanodrugs that react to environmental stimuli [153–157]. 4D bioprinting allows for complex micro/nanostructures that adapt to fill tissue defects [158–160].

Setons also function as scaffolds for stem cell-based therapies [145]. These scaffolds mimic the natural tissue microenvironment [159–162], supporting cell proliferation and differentiation. Mesenchymal stem cells (MSCs), known for immunomodulatory properties [163]. Pre-seton placement before MSC infusion appears safe and effective for closing external openings [164–168].

5. Conclusion and future directions

Traditional perianal fistula treatments, fistulotomy and seton placement, have limitations [86]. While setons are commonly used for complex fistulas [74], healing is slow and faecal incontinence is a concern [168]. Regenerative medicine approaches, like tissue engineering and stem cell therapies, offer potential improvements by preserving sphincter health, reducing side effects, and accelerating healing [158, 159]. Advanced fabrication methods can enhance seton properties [138, 139], enabling them to serve as stem cell vectors and drug delivery systems [138, 142, 149]. However, research in this area is limited, and several challenges remain.

Few biomaterials have been used in setons, and clinical studies are scarce [146, 147]. Mechanical properties of scaffold setons, both cutting and non-cutting, require further investigation. Ideal scaffolds should be elastic, flexible, knot-able, and formable into small tubes [73, 169], with optimized degradation and drug release profiles. Biomaterial source (natural, synthetic, or hybrid) should align with FDA approvals [170, 171].

Scaffolds should mimic the fistula tissue microenvironment, loading cells and biomolecules necessary for tissue formation [172, 173]. Incorporating growth factors, anti-inflammatory agents, drugs, and antibiotics can enhance regeneration [174, 175], but release profiles and cytotoxicity must be investigated. Immune regulators like exosomes may also be beneficial [176]. Stem cell source (MSCs, hiPSCs, ESCs), population, and density are critical parameters [125, 177, 178]. Stem cell viability within setons is another crucial factor [179].

Developing setons as tissue engineering scaffolds for perianal fistula requires collaboration between surgeons, scientists, engineers, and clinicians. Addressing challenges in stem cell sourcing (GMP grade), biomaterials, manufacturing, and surgical procedures will enable wider clinical application of this promising bottom-up tissue regeneration approach [159].

Acknowledgements

To the talent colleague surgeon Hatim Ahmed, who drew the figures using digital art.

I acknowledge the use of Grammarly AI writing assistant to identify improvements in the writing style and correct the grammar errors.

Conflict of interest

I do not have any conflict of interest.

Dedication, thanks:

To **Allah** who enlightens my path,
To my **parents**, the greatest gift in life,
To my sole love, **Alyaa**.
To my daughters, **Ola** and **Sama**, who never stop believing in me and to the sweet **Misk** who gives the great taste of life.

Acronyms and abbreviations

CPT Coding	the Current Procedural Terminology (CPT) coding
IBD	inflammatory bowel disease
HIV	human immune deficiency virus
DRE	digital rectal examination
EAUS	endoanal ultrasound
ERUS	endorectal ultrasound
LIFT	ligation of the intersphincteric fistula tract
FiLaCTM	fistula laser closure
OTSC	over-the-scope clip system
AFP	anal fistula plug
VAAFT	video-assisted anal fistula treatment
RAF	rectal advancement flap
PERFACT	proximal superficial cauterization, emptying regularly fistula tracts, and curettage of tracts
MSCs	mesenchymal stem cells

Author details

Omar Alhafidh
Royal Bolton Hospital, Greater Manchester, United Kingdom

*Address all correspondence to: omaralhafidh.oa@gmail.com

References

[1] Fazio VW. Anal fistula. In: Corman ML, Bergamaschi RCM, Nicholls RJ, Fazio VW, editors. Corman's Colon and Rectal Surgery. 6th ed. Philadelphia: Lippincott Williams & Wilkins; 2013. pp. 384-427

[2] Manwaring ML. Anal fistula. In: Fazio VW, Church JM, Delaney CP, Kiran RP, editors. Current Therapy in Colon and Rectal Surgery. 3rd ed. Philadelphia: Elsevier; 2017. pp. 24-29

[3] Parks AG, Gordon PH, Hardcastle JD. A classification of fistula-in-ano. The British Journal of Surgery. 1976;**63**(1):1-12

[4] Phillips J, Lees N, Arnall F. Current management of fistula-in-ano. British Journal of Hospital Medicine (London, England). 2015;**76(3)**:142, 144-147

[5] Johnson EK, Bernier G. Cryptoglandular abscess and fistula. In: Steele SR, Hull TL, Hyman N, Maykel JA, Read TE, Whitlow CB, editors. The ASCRS Textbook of Colon and Rectal Surgery. 4th ed. Vol. 1. Cham, Switzerland: Springer; 2022. pp. 249-270

[6] Williams G, Williams A, Tozer P, Phillips R, Ahmad A, Jayne D, et al. The treatment of anal fistula: Second ACPGBI position statement – 2018. Colorectal Disease. 2018;**20**(Suppl 3):5-31

[7] Pirie E, Rosen L. Anorectal abscess-fistulae. The Surgical Clinics of North America. 1994;**74**(6):1293-1308

[8] Sneider EB, Maykel JA. Anal abscess and fistula. Gastroenterology Clinics of North America. 2013;**42**(4):773-784

[9] Cheung XC, Fahey T, Rogers AC, Pemberton JH, D.O. KavanaghSurgical management of idiopathic perianal fistulas: A systematic review and meta-analysis. Digestive Surgery. 2021;**38**:1-16

[10] Kelly ME, Heneghan HM, McDermott FD, Nason GJ, Freeman C, Martin ST, et al. The role of loose seton in the management of anal fistula: A multicenter study of 200 patients. Techniques in Coloproctology. 2014;**18**(10):915-919

[11] Vogel JD, Johnson EK, Morris AM, Paquette IM, Saclarides TJ, Feingold DL, et al. Clinical practice guideline for the management of anorectal abscess, fistula-in-ano, and rectovaginal fistula. Diseases of the Colon and Rectum. 2016;**59**(12):1117-1133

[12] Held D, Khubchandani I, Sheets J, Stasik J, Rosen L, Riether R. Management of anorectal horseshoe abscess and fistula. Diseases of the Colon and Rectum. 1986;**29**(12):793

[13] Litta F, Parello A, Ferri L, Torrecilla NO, Marra AA, Orefice R, et al. Simple fistula-in-ano: Is it all simple? A systematic review. Techniques in Coloproctology. 2021;**25**(4):385-399

[14] Gaillard F. Perianal fistula. Radiopaedia [Internet]. 2023. Available from: https://radiopaedia.org/articles/perianal-fistula [Accessed: 30 July 2025]

[15] Xiao J, Santos E, Bonsu NY, Kim W, Eisenberg M, Cusick M, et al. Anal fistula: From diagnosis and classification to surgical management. In: Vannelli A, editor. Anorectal Disorders - From Diagnosis to Treatment [Internet]. IntechOpen; 2024. Available from: https://www.intechopen.com/chapters/1153426 [Accessed: 30 July 2025]

[16] Buchanan G, Owen H, Torkington J, Lunniss P, Nicholls R, C. Cohen long-term outcome following loose-seton technique for external sphincter preservation in complex anal fistula. The British Journal of Surgery. 2004;**91**(4):476-480

[17] Sainio P. Fistula-in-ano in a defined population. Incidence and epidemiological aspects. Annales Chirurgiae et Gynaecologiae. 1984;**73**(4):219-224

[18] Sun MR, Smith MP, Kane RA. Current techniques in imaging of fistula in ano: Three-dimensional endoanal ultrasound and magnetic resonance imaging. Seminars in Ultrasound, CT, and MR. 2008;**29**(6):454-471

[19] Weisman RI, Orsay CP, Pearl RK, Abcarian H. The role of fistulography in fistula-in-ano. Report of five cases. Diseases of the Colon and Rectum. 1991;**34**(2):181-184

[20] Nevler A, Beer-Gabel M, Lebedyev A, Soffer A, Gutman M, Carter D, et al. Transperineal ultrasonography in perianal Crohn's disease and recurrent cryptogenic fistula-in-ano. Colorectal Disease. 2013;**15**(8):1011-1018. DOI: 10.1111/codi.12204

[21] Murad-Regadas SM, Regadas FSP, Regadas Filho FSP, Nogueira FR, Holanda EC, Dias Mont'Alverne RE, et al. Use of 3D anorectal ultrasonography in the preoperative assessment of complex anal fistulas and patterns of healing, failure, and recurrence after ligation of the Intersphincteric fistula tract (LIFT). Journal of Ultrasound in Medicine. 2024

[22] Beckingham IJ, Spencer JA, Ward J, Dyke GW, Adams C, Ambrose NS. Prospective evaluation of dynamic contrast enhanced magnetic resonance imaging in the evaluation of fistula in ano. The British Journal of Surgery. 1996;**83**(10):1396-1398

[23] Buchanan GN, Halligan S, Williams AB, Cohen CR, Tarroni D, Phillips RK, et al. Magnetic resonance imaging for primary fistula in ano. The British Journal of Surgery. 2003;**90**(7):877-881

[24] Seow-Choen F, Nicholls RJ. Anal fistula. The British Journal of Surgery. 1992;**79**(3):197-205

[25] Present DH, Rutgeerts P, Targan S, Hanauer SB, Mayer L, van Hogezand RA, et al. Infliximab for the treatment of fistulas in patients with Crohn's disease. The New England Journal of Medicine. 1999;**340**(18):1398-1405

[26] Cho YB, Park KJ, Yoon SN, Song KH, do S K, Jung SH, et al. Long-term results of adipose-derived stem cell therapy for the treatment of Crohn's fistula. Stem Cells Translational Medicine. 2015;**4**(5):532-537

[27] Garcia-Olmo D, Guadalajara H, Rubio-Perez I, Herreros MD, de la Quintana P, Garcia-Arranz M. Recurrent anal fistulae: Limited surgery supported by stem cells. World Journal of Gastroenterology. 2015;**21**(11):3330-3336

[28] Afşarlar CE, Karaman A, Tanır G, Karaman I, Yılmaz E, Erdoğan D, et al. Perianal abscess and fistula-in-ano in children: Clinical characteristic, management and outcome. Pediatric Surgery International. 2011;**27**(10):1063-1068

[29] Feroz SH, Ahmed A, Muralidharan A, Thirunavukarasu P. Comparison of the efficacy of the various treatment modalities in the Management of Perianal Crohn's fistula: A review. Cureus. 2020;**12**(12):e11882. DOI: 10.7759/cureus.11882

[30] Gaertner WB, Burgess PL, Davids JS, Lightner AL, Shogan BD, Sun MY, et al. The American Society of Colon and Rectal Surgeons clinical practice guidelines for the Management of Anorectal Abscess, fistula-in-Ano, and rectovaginal fistula. Diseases of the Colon and Rectum. 2022;**65**(8):964-985

[31] Ho YH, Tan M, Leong AF, Seow-Choen F. Marsupialization of fistulotomy wounds improves healing: A randomized controlled trial. The British Journal of Surgery. 1998;**85**(1):105-107

[32] Sangwan YP, Rosen L, Riether RD, Stasik JJ, Sheets JA, Khubchandani IT. Is simple fistula-in-ano simple? Diseases of the Colon and Rectum. 1994;**37**(9):885-889

[33] Blumetti J, Abcarian A, Quinteros F, Chaudhry V, Prasad L, Abcarian H. Evolution of treatment of fistula in ano. World Journal of Surgery. 2012;**36**(5):1162-1167

[34] McCourtney JS, Finlay IG. Setons in the surgical management of fistula in ano. The British Journal of Surgery. 1995;**82**(4):448-452

[35] Memon AA, Murtaza G, Azami R, Zafar H, Chawla T, Laghari AA. Treatment of complex fistula in ano with cable-tie seton: A prospective case series. International Scholarly Research Notices. 2011;**2011**:636952

[36] Cox SW, Senagore AJ, Luchtefeld MA, Mazier WP. Outcome after incision and drainage with fistulotomy for ischiorectal abscess. The American Surgeon. 1997;**63**(8):686-689

[37] Hammond TM, Knowles CH, Porrett T, Lunniss PJ. The snug Seton: Short and medium term results of slow fistulotomy for idiopathic anal fistulae. Colorectal Disease. 2006;**8**(4):328-337

[38] Dziki A, Bartos M. Seton treatment of anal fistula: Experience with a new modification. The European Journal of Surgery. 1998;**164**(7):543-548

[39] Mushaya C, Bartlett L, Schulze B, Ho YH. Ligation of intersphincteric fistula tract compared with advancement flap for complex anorectal fistulas requiring initial seton drainage Am. Journal of Surgery. 2012;**204**(3):283-289

[40] Al Sebai OI, Ammar MS, Mohamed SH, El Balshy MA. Comparative study between intersphinecteric ligation of perianal fistula versus conventional fistulotomy with or without seton in the treatment of perianal fistula: A prospective randomized controlled trial. Annals of Medicine and Surgery. 2021;**61**:180-184

[41] Tsang JS, Chan TY, Cheung HH, Wei R, Foo CC, Lo OSH. Porcine dermal collagen mesh (Permacol™) as a bioprosthesis in the ligation of intersphincteric tract (BioLIFT) procedure. Techniques in Coloproctology. 2020;**24**(12):1277-1283

[42] Wen K, Gu YF, Sun XL, Wang XP, Yan S, He ZQ, et al. Long-term outcomes of ligation of intersphincteric fistula tract for complex fistula-in-ano: Modified operative procedure experience. ABCD. Arquivos Brasileiros de Cirurgia Digestiva (São Paulo). 2018;**31**(4):e1404

[43] Kang WH, Yang HK, Chang HJ, Ko YT, Yoo BE, Lim CH, et al. High ligation of the anal fistula tract by lateral approach: A prospective cohort study on a modification of the ligation of the intersphincteric fistula tract (LIFT) technique. International Journal of Surgery. 2018;**60**:9-14

[44] Lau YC, Brown KGM, Cheong J, Byrne C, Lee PJ. LIFT and BioLIFT: A

10-year single-Centre experience of treating complex fistula-in-ano with ligation of intersphincteric fistula tract procedure with or without bio-prosthetic reinforcement (BioLIFT). Journal of Gastrointestinal Surgery. 2020;**24**(3):671-676

[45] Osterkamp J, Gocht-Jensen P, Hougaard K, Nordentoft T. Long-term outcomes in patients after ligation of the intersphincteric fistula tract Dan. Medizinhistorisches Journal. 2019;**66**(4):1-6

[46] Kamiński JP, Zaghiyan K, Fleshner P. Increasing experience of ligation of the intersphincteric fistula tract for patients with Crohn's disease: What have we learned? Colorectal Disease. 2017;**19**(8):750-755

[47] Rojanasakul A, Pattanaarun J, Sahakitrungruang C, Tantiphlachiva K. Repeat ligation of intersphincteric fistula tract (LIFT) after failed initial LIFT for complex anal fistula. Techniques in Coloproctology. 2017;**21**(12):969-973. DOI: 10.1007/s10151-017-1726-1

[48] Tan K-Y, Tan Y-M, Lim JF, et al. Repeat ligation of intersphincteric fistula tract (LIFT) for recurrent anal fistula: Is it worthwhile? International Journal of Colorectal Disease. 2013;**28**(6):761-765. DOI: 10.1007/s00384-013-1652-3

[49] Wood T, Truong A, Mujukian A, Zaghiyan K, Fleshner P. Increasing experience with the LIFT procedure in Crohn's disease patients with complex anal fistula. Techniques in Coloproctology. 2022;**26**:205-212. DOI: 10.1007/s10151-022-02582-4

[50] van Praag EM, Stellingwerf ME, van der Bilt JDW, Bemelman WA, Gecse KB, Buskens CJ. Ligation of the intersphincteric fistula tract and endorectal advancement flap for high perianal fistulas in Crohn's disease: A retrospective cohort study. The Journal of Crohn's and Colitis. 2020;**14**(6):757-763

[51] Mujukian A, Truong A, Fleshner P, Zaghiyan K. Long-term healing after complex anal fistula repair in patients with Crohn's disease. Techniques in Coloproctology. 2020;**24**(8):833-841

[52] Wilhelm A. A new technique for sphincter-preserving anal fistula repair using a novel radial emitting laser probe. Techniques in Coloproctology. 2011;**15**(4):445-449

[53] Wilhelm A, Fiebig A, Krawczak M. Five years of experience with the FiLaCTM laser for fistula-in-ano management: Long-term follow-up from a single institution. Techniques in Coloproctology. 2017;**21**(4):269-276

[54] Giamundo P, Esercizio L, Geraci M, Tibaldi L, Valente M. Fistula-tract laser closure (FiLaCTM): Long-term results and new operative strategies. Techniques in Coloproctology. 2015;**19**(8):449-453

[55] Giamundo P, Geraci M, Tibaldi L, Valente M. Closure of fistula-in-ano with laser–FiLaCTM: An effective novel sphincter-saving procedure for complex disease. Colorectal Disease. 2014;**16**(2):110-115

[56] Wolicki A, Jäger P, Deska T, Senkal M. Sphincter-saving therapy for fistula-in-ano: Long-term follow-up after FiLaC(®). Techniques in Coloproctology. 2021;**25**(2):177-184

[57] Frountzas M, Stergios K, Nikolaou C, Bellos I, Schizas D, Linardoutsos D, et al. Could FiLaCTM be effective in the treatment of anal fistulas? A systematic review of observational studies and proportional meta-analysis. Colorectal Disease. 2020;**22**:1874-1884

[58] Kirschniak A, Kratt T, Stüker D, Braun A, Schurr MO, Königsrainer A. A new endoscopic over-the-scope clip system for treatment of lesions and bleeding in the GI tract: First clinical experiences. Gastrointestinal Endoscopy. 2007;**66**(1):162-167

[59] Prosst RL, Herold A, Joos AK, Bussen D, Wehrmann M, Gottwald T, et al. The anal fistula claw: The OTSC clip for anal fistula closure. Colorectal Disease. 2012;**14**(9):1112-1117. DOI: 10.1111/j.1463-1318.2012.03013.x

[60] Mascagni D, Pironi D, Grimaldi G, Romani AM, La Torre G, Eberspacher C, et al. OTSC® proctology vs. fistulectomy and primary sphincter reconstruction as a treatment for low trans-sphincteric anal fistula in a randomized controlled pilot trial. Minerva Chirurgica. 2019;**74**(1):1-6

[61] O'Connor L, Champagne BJ, Ferguson MA, Orangio GR, Schertzer ME, Armstrong DN. Efficacy of anal fistula plug in closure of Crohn's anorectal fistulas. Diseases of the Colon and Rectum. 2006;**49**(10):1569-1573

[62] van Koperen PJ, D'Hoore A, Wolthuis AM, Bemelman WA, Slors JFM. Anal fistula plug for closure of difficult anorectal fistula: A prospective study. Diseases of the Colon and Rectum. 2007;**50**(12):2168-2172

[63] Champagne BJ, O'Connor LM, Ferguson M, Orangio GR, Schertzer ME, Armstrong DN. Efficacy of anal fistula plug in closure of cryptoglandular fistulas: Long-term follow-up. Diseases of the Colon & Rectum. 2006;**49**(12):1817-1821

[64] Schwandner O, Stadler F, Dietl O, Wirsching R, Fuerst A. Initial experience on efficacy in closure of cryptoglandular and Crohn's transsphincteric fistulas by the use of the anal fistula plug. International Journal of Colorectal Disease. 2008;**23**(3):319-324

[65] Ky AJ, Sylla P, Steinhagen R, Steinhagen E, Khaitov S, Ly EK. Collagen fistula plug for the treatment of anal fistulas. Diseases of the Colon and Rectum. 2008;**51**(6):838-843. DOI: 10.1007/s10350-007-9191-2

[66] Narang SK, Jones C, Alam NN, Daniels IR, Smart NJ. Delayed absorbable synthetic plug (GORE® BIO-A®) for the treatment of fistula-in-ano: A systematic review. Colorectal Disease. 2016;**18**(1):37-44

[67] Meinero P, Mori L. Video-assisted anal fistula treatment (VAAFT): A novel sphincter-saving procedure for treating complex anal fistulas. Techniques in Coloproctology. 2011;**15**(4):417-422

[68] Zhang Y, Li F, Zhao T, Cao F, Zheng Y, Li A. Treatment of complex anal fistula by video-assisted anal fistula treatment combined with anal fistula plug: A single-center study. Surgical Innovation. 2021:1553350621992924

[69] Zhang Y, Li F, Zhao T, Cao F, Zheng Y, Li A. Efficacy of video-assisted anal fistula treatment combined with closure of the internal opening using a stapler for parks II anal fistula. The Annals of Translational Medicine's. 2020;**8**(22):1517

[70] Meinero P, Mori L. Video-assisted anal fistula treatment (VAAFT): A novel sphincter-saving procedure for treating complex a nal fistulas. Techniques in Coloproctology. 2011;**15**(4):417-422

[71] Hyman C. Use of braided wire seton for two-stage anorectal fistula operation: Preliminary report. A.M.A. Archives of Surgery. 1955;**71**(6):890-891

[72] Cariati A. Fistulotomy or seton in anal fistula: A decisional

algorithm. Updates in Surgery. 2013;**65**(3):201-205

[73] Karpukhin OY, Sakulin K. Use of rubber seton in the treatment of anorectal. Kazan Medical Journal. 2018;**99**(2):326-329

[74] Shirah BH, Shirah HA. The impact of the outcome of treating a high anal fistula by using a cutting seton and staged fistulotomy on Saudi Arabian patients. Annals of Coloproctology. 2018;**34**(5):234-240

[75] Celik Y, Buldanli MZ. Comparison of loose silk and tightenable polypropylene seton placement in treatment of complex anal fistula. Age. 2021;**42**(12.1):43.00

[76] Akici M, Ersen O. The effect of suture selection in complex anal fistulas on the success of cutting seton placement and patient comfort. Pakistan Journal of Medical Sciences. 2020;**36**(4):816

[77] Tanus OAV, Santos C, Dourado DM, Conde AL, Giuncanse F, Souza IF, et al. Primary sphincteroplasty comparing two different stitches in anal fistula treatment: Experimental study in rats. ABCD - Brazilian Archives of Digestive Surgery. 2019;**32**(3):e1459

[78] Al-Wadees A, Al-Hakkak S, Akool M. Two staged operations using loose thick seton suture in the treatment of high type fistula in ano stimulate rapid healing and lower recurrence rate. Prensa Médica Argentina. 2020;**106**:6

[79] Schwandner O. Video-assisted anal fistula treatment (VAAFT) combined with advancement flap repair in Crohn's disease. Techniques in Coloproctology. 2013;**17**(2):221-225

[80] Jones IT, Fazio VW, Jagelman DG. The use of transanal rectal advancement flaps in the management of fistulas involving the anorectum. Diseases of the Colon and Rectum. 1987;**30**(12):919-923

[81] Soltani A, Kaiser AM. Endorectal advancement flap for cryptoglandular or Crohn's fistula-in-ano. Diseases of the Colon and Rectum. 2010;**53**(4):486-495

[82] Rozalén V, Parés D, Sanchez E, Troya J, Vela S, Pacha M, et al. Advancement flap technique for anal fistula in patients with crohn's disease: A systematic review of the literature. Cirugía Española. 2017;**95**(10):558-565

[83] Schiano di Visconte M, Bellio G. Comparison of porcine collagen paste injection and rectal advancement flap for the treatment of complex cryptoglandular anal fistulas: A 2-year follow-up study. International Journal of Colorectal Disease. 2018;**33**(12):1723-1731

[84] Garg P. PERFACT procedure to treat supralevator fistula-in-ano: A novel single-stage sphincter sparing procedure. World Journal of Gastrointestinal Surgery;**8**(4):326

[85] Garg P, Garg M. PERFACT procedure: A new concept to treat highly complex anal fistula. World Journal of Gastroenterology. 2015;**21**(13):4020-4029

[86] Lin H, Jin Z, Zhu Y, Diao M, Hu W. Anal fistula plug vs rectal advancement flap for the treatment of complex cryptoglandular anal fistulas: A systematic review and meta-analysis of studies with long-term follow-up. Colorectal Disease. 2019;**21**(5):502-515

[87] Jafarzadeh J, Najibpoor N, Salmasi A. A comparative study on the effectiveness of rectal advancement flap and seton placement surgeries in patients with anal fistula on the rate of recurrence, incontinence and infection. Journal of

Family Medicine and Primary Care. 2019;**8**(11):3591-3594

[88] Stellingwerf ME, Bak MTJ, de Groof EJ, Buskens CJ, Molenaar CBH, Gecse KB, et al. Knotless seton for perianal fistulas: Feasibility and effect on perianal disease activity. Scientific Reports. 2020;**10**(1):1-8

[89] Panés J, Rimola J. Perianal fistulizing Crohn's disease: Pathogenesis, diagnosis and therapy. Nature Reviews. Gastroenterology & Hepatology. 2017;**14**(11):652

[90] Mehanna M, Ahmed AM. Comparison between rubber band and Ethelon suture as a cutting seton in perianal fistula. Egyptian Journal of Hospital Medicine. 2018;**71**(4):3032-3038

[91] Raslan SM, Aladwani M, Alsanea N. Evaluation of the cutting seton as a method of treatment for perianal fistula. Annals of Saudi Medicine. 2016;**36**(3):210-215

[92] Goldberg S, Shelton A. Cutting Seton for anal fistulas-high risk of minor control defects. Williams & Wilkins. 1997:21201-22436

[93] Ramanujam PS, Prasad ML, Abcarian H, Tan AB. Perianal abscesses and fistulas. Diseases of the Colon and Rectum. 1984;**27**(9):593-597

[94] Garcia-Aguilar J, Belmonte C, Wong DW, Goldberg SM, Madoff RD. Cutting seton versus two-stage seton fistulotomy in the surgical management of high anal fistula. The British Journal of Surgery. 1998;**85**(2):243-245

[95] Vavricka SR, Rogler G. Fistula treatment: The unresolved challenge. Digestive Diseases. 2010;**28**(3):556-564

[96] Isbister WH, Al Sanea N. The cutting seton: An experience at king faisal specialist hospital. Diseases of the Colon and Rectum. 2001;**44**(5):722-727

[97] Ji L, Zhang Y, Xu L, Wei J, Weng L, Jiang J. Advances in the treatment of anal fistula: A mini-review of recent five-year clinical studies. Frontiers in Surgery. 2021;7:586891. Available from: https://www.frontiersin.org/articles/10.3389/fsurg.2020.586891/full [Accessed: 30 July 2025]

[98] Rosen DR, Kaiser AM. Definitive seton management for transsphincteric fistula-in-ano: Harm or charm? Colorectal Disease. 2016;**18**(5):488-495

[99] Motamedi MAK, Serahati S, Rajendran L, Brown CJ, Raval MJ, Karimuddin A, et al. Long-term outcomes after seton placement for perianal fistulae with and without Crohn's disease. Colorectal Disease. 2022;**23**:2407-2415

[100] van der Hagen SJ, Baeten CG, Soeters PB, van Gemert WG. Long-term outcome following mucosal advancement flap for high perianal fistulas and fistulotomy for low perianal fistulas. International Journal of Colorectal Disease. 2006;**21**(8):784-790

[101] Schouten WR, Zimmerman DD, Briel JW. Transanal advancement flap repair of transsphincteric fistulas. Diseases of the Colon and Rectum. 1999;**42**(11):22-23 1419-22; discussion

[102] Vander Mijnsbrugge G, Felt-Bersma R, Ho D, Molenaar C. Perianal fistulas and the lift procedure: Results, predictive factors for success, and long-term results with subsequent treatment. Techniques in Coloproctology. 2019;**23**(7):639-647

[103] Emile SH, Elfeki H, Thabet W, Sakr A, Magdy A, Abd El-Hamed TM, et al. Predictive factors for recurrence of high transsphincteric anal fistula

after placement of seton. The Journal of Surgical Research. 2017;**213**:261-268

[104] Ritchie R, Sackier J, Hodde J. Incontinence rates after cutting seton treatment for anal fistula. Colorectal Disease. 2009;**11**(6):564-571

[105] Gülmez S. An 8 years' experience in surgical treatment of anal fistula. Annals of Medical Research. 2020;**27**(8):2031-2035. DOI: 10.5455/annalsmedres.2020.07.707

[106] Lykke A, Steendahl J, Wille-Jørgensen PA. Treating high anal fistulae with slow cutting seton. Ugeskrift for Laeger. 2010;**172**(7):516-519

[107] Vial M, Parés D, Pera M, Grande L. Faecal incontinence after seton treatment for anal fistulae with and without surgical division of internal anal sphincter: A systematic review. Colorectal Disease. 2010;**12**(3):172-178

[108] Hasegawa H, Radley S, Keighley MR. Long-term results of cutting seton fistulotomy. Acta Chirurgica Iugoslavica. 2000;**47**(4):19-21

[109] Mentes BB, Öktemer S, Tezcaner T, Azılı C, Leventoğlu S, M. OğuzElastic one-stage cutting seton for the treatment of high anal fistulas: Preliminary results. Techniques in Coloproctology. 2004;**8**(3):159-162

[110] Munir A, Falah SQ. Management of high fistula in ano with cutting seton. Gomal Journal of Medical Sciences. 2014;**12**(4):210-212

[111] Zhang JF. Records of bizarre Jurassic brachycerans in the Daohugou biota, China (Diptera, brachycera, archisargidae and rhagionemestriidae). Palaeontology. 2010;**53**(2):307-317

[112] Äinen KPJHÄ, Sainio AP. Cutting seton for anal fistulas. Diseases of the Colon and Rectum. 1997;**40**(12):1443-1447

[113] Misra MC, Kapur BML. A new non-operative approach to fistula in ano. The British Journal of Surgery. 1988;**75**(11):1093-1094. DOI: 10.1002/bjs.1800751114

[114] Burkhardt R, Lang NP. Influence of suturing on wound healing. Periodontology 2000. 2015;**68**(1):270-281

[115] Subhas G, Gupta A, Balaraman S, Mittal VK, Pearlman R. Non-cutting setons for progressive migration of complex fistula tracts: A new spin on an old technique. International Journal of Colorectal Disease. 2011;**26**(6):793-798

[116] Thornton M, Solomon MJ. Long-term indwelling seton for complex anal fistulas in Crohn's disease. Diseases of the Colon and Rectum. 2005;**48**(3):459-463

[117] White RA, Eisenstat TE, Rubin RJ, Salvati EP. Seton management of complex anorectal fistulas in patients with Crohn's disease. Diseases of the Colon and Rectum. 1990;**33**(7):587-589

[118] Verkade C, Zimmerman DDE, Wasowicz DK, Polle SW, de Vries HS. Loss of seton in patients with complex anal fistula: A retrospective comparison of conventional knotted loose seton and knot-free seton. Techniques in Coloproctology. 2020;**24**(10):1043-1046

[119] Galis-Rozen E, Tulchinsky H, Rosen A, Eldar S, Rabau M, Stepanski A, et al. Long-term outcome of loose seton for complex anal fistula: A two-Centre study of patients with and without Crohn's disease. Colorectal Disease. 2010;**12**(4):358-362. DOI: 10.1111/j.1463-1318.2009.01796.x

[120] Sungurtekin U, Ozban M, Erbis H, Birsen O. Loose seton: A misnomer

of cutting seton. Surgical Science. 2016;**07**:219-225

[121] Bakhtawar N, Usman M. Factors increasing the risk of recurrence in fistula-in-ano. Cureus. 2019;**11**(3):e4200

[122] Atkin G, Martins J, Tozer P, Ranchod P, Phillips R. For many high anal fistulas, lay open is still a good option. Techniques in Coloproctology. 2011;**15**(2):143-150

[123] Papaconstantinou I, Kontis E, Koutoulidis V, Mantzaris G, Vassiliou I. Surgical management of fistula-in-ano among patients with Crohn's disease: Analysis of outcomes after fistulotomy or seton placement—Single-center experience. Scandinavian Journal of Surgery. 2017;**106**(3):211-215

[124] Mujukian A, Zaghiyan K, Banayan E, Fleshner P. Outcomes of definitive draining seton placement for complex anal fistula in crohn's disease. The American Surgeon. 2020;**86**:0003134820964462

[125] Herreros M, Garcia-Olmo D, Guadalajara H, Georgiev-Hristov T, Brandariz L, Garcia-Arranz M. Stem cell therapy: A compassionate use program in perianal fistula. Stem Cells International. 2019;**2019**:1-6. DOI: 10.1155/2019/6132340

[126] Giarratano G, Shalaby M, Toscana C, Sileri P. Video-assisted anal fistula treatment for complex anal fistula: A long-term follow-up study. Colorectal Disease. 2020;**22**(8):939-944. DOI: 10.1111/codi.15005

[127] Regusci L, Fasolini F, Meinero P, Caccia G, Ruggeri G, Serati M, et al. Video-assisted anal fistula treatment (VAAFT) for complex anorectal fistula: Efficacy and risk factors for failure at 3-year follow-up. Techniques in Coloproctology. 2020;**24**(7):741-746

[128] Zelić M, Karlović D, Kršul D, Bačić Đ, Warusavitarne J. Video-assisted anal fistula treatment for treatment of complex cryptoglandular anal fistulas with 2 years follow-up period: Our experience. Journal of Laparoendoscopic & Advanced Surgical Techniques. Part A. 2020;**30**(12):1329-1333

[129] Adegbola SO, Sahnan K, Tozer PJ, Strouhal R, Hart AL, Lung PFC, et al. Symptom amelioration in Crohn's perianal fistulas using video-assisted anal fistula treatment (VAAFT). Journal of Crohn's & Colitis. 2018;**12**(9):1067-1072

[130] Yao YB, Xiao CF, Wang QT, Zhou H, Dong QJ, Cao YQ, et al. VAAFT plus FiLaC™: A combined procedure for complex anal fistula. Techniques in Coloproctology. 2021;**25**:977-979. DOI: 10.1007/s10151-021-02411-0

[131] Zhang Y, Li F, Zhao T, Cao F, Zheng Y, Li A. Video-assisted anal fistula treatment combined with anal fistula plug for treatment of horseshoe anal fistula. The Journal of International Medical Research. 2021;**49**(1):300060520980525

[132] La Torre M, Lisi G, D'Agostino E, Boccuzzi M, Campanelli M, Varriale M, et al. Lift and VAAFT for high trans-sphincteric anal fistula: A single center retrospective analysis. International Journal of Colorectal Disease. 2020;**35**(6):1149-1153

[133] Tozer P, Sahnan K, Adegbola S, Shaikh S, Lung P. Video-assisted anal fistula treatment (VAAFT) assisted seton placement - a video vignette. Colorectal Disease. 2019;**21**(12):1462

[134] Zheng L, Lu J, Pu Y, Xing C, Zhao K. Comparative study of clinical efficacy between video-assisted anal fistula treatment and traditional fistula resection plus seton in treatment

of complex anal fistula Zhonghua wei chang Wai ke za zhi. Chinese Journal of Gastrointestinal Surgery. 2018;**21**(7):793-797

[135] Romaniszyn M, Walega P. Video-assisted anal fistula treatment: Pros and cons of this minimally invasive method for treatment of perianal fistulas. Gastroenterology Research and Practice. 2017;**2017**:9518310

[136] Raffi M, Mehrwan S, Bhatti TM, Akhter JI, Hameed A, Yawar W, et al. Investigations into the antibacterial behavior of copper nanoparticles against Escherichia coli. Annals of Microbiology. 2010;**60**(1):75-80. DOI: 10.1007/s13213-010-0015-6

[137] Wiarachai O, Thongchul N, Kiatkamjornwong S, Hoven VP. Surface-quaternized chitosan particles as an alternative and effective organic antibacterial material. Colloids and Surfaces, B: Biointerfaces. 2012;**92**:121-129

[138] Blaker JJ, Pratten J, Ready D, Knowles JC, Forbes A, Day RM. Assessment of antimicrobial microspheres as a prospective novel treatment targeted towards the repair of perianal fistulae. Alimentary Pharmacology & Therapeutics. 2008;**28**(5):614-622

[139] Paladini F, Pollini M. Antimicrobial silver nanoparticles for wound healing application: Progress and future trends. Materials. 2019;**12**(16):2540

[140] Yin IX, Zhang J, Zhao IS, Mei ML, Li Q, Chu CH. The antibacterial mechanism of silver nanoparticles and its application in dentistry. International Journal of Nanomedicine. 2020;**15**:2555

[141] Krajewska JB, Długosz O, Sałaga M, Banach M, Fichna J. Silver nanoparticles based on blackcurrant extract show potent anti-inflammatory effect in vitro and in DSS-induced colitis in mice. International Journal of Pharmaceutics. 2020;**585**:119549

[142] Zhang S, Liu X, Wang H, Peng J, Wong KK. Silver nanoparticle-coated suture effectively reduces inflammation and improves mechanical strength at intestinal anastomosis in mice. Journal of Pediatric Surgery. 2014;**49**(4):606-613

[143] Maternini M, Guttadauro A, Mascagni D, Milito G, Stuto A, Renzi A, et al. Non cross-linked equine collagen (Salvecoll-E gel) for treatment of complex ano-rectal fistula. Asian Journal of Surgery. 2020;**43**(2):401-404

[144] Williams DF. Biocompatibility pathways: Biomaterials-induced sterile inflammation, mechanotransduction, and principles of biocompatibility control. ACS Biomaterials Science & Engineering. 2017;**3**(1):2-35. DOI: 10.1021/acsbiomaterials.6b00607

[145] Dozois EJ, Lightner AL, Mathis KL, Chua HK, Kelley SR, Fletcher JG, et al. Early results of a phase I trial using an adipose-derived mesenchymal stem cell-coated fistula plug for the treatment of transsphincteric cryptoglandular fistulas. Diseases of the Colon and Rectum. 2019;**62**(5):615-622. DOI: 10.1097/DCR.0000000000001333

[146] Dietz AB, Dozois EJ, Fletcher JG, Butler GW, Radel D, Lightner AL, et al. Autologous mesenchymal stem cells, applied in a bioabsorbable matrix, for treatment of perianal fistulas in patients with Crohn's disease. Gastroenterology. 2017;**153**(1):59-62e2

[147] Pramudiati C. The study of PLGA drug delivery systems: Implications for management of Crohn's disease. Kaleidoscope. 2015;**5**(1):11

[148] Li H, Jiang B, Yan J, Yang Z, Chen Y, Zhang W, et al. A drug-laden elastomer for surgical treatment of anal fistula. Drug Delivery and Translational Research. 2011;**1**(6):439-447

[149] Xie X, Liu L, Zheng Z, Han Z, Zhi M, Kaplan DL, et al. Silk fibroin-based fibrous anal fistula plug with drug delivery function. Macromolecular Bioscience. 2018;**18**(3):e1700302

[150] Zhang L, Wang J, Xu A, Zhong C, Lu W, Deng L, et al. A rationally designed TNF-α epitope-scaffold immunogen induces sustained antibody response and alleviates collagen-induced arthritis in mice. PLoS One. 2016;**11**(9):e0163080

[151] Zhao Y, Gao C, Liu H, Liu H, Feng Y, Li Z, et al. Infliximab-based self-healing hydrogel composite scaffold enhances stem cell survival, engraftment, and function in rheumatoid arthritis treatment. Acta Biomaterialia. 2020;**121**:653-664. DOI: 10.1016/j.actbio.2020.12.005

[152] Zhao Y, Gao C, Liu H, Liu H, Feng Y, Li Z, et al. Infliximab-based self-healing hydrogel composite scaffold enhances stem cell survival, engraftment, and function in rheumatoid arthritis treatment. Acta Biomaterialia. 2021;**121**:653-664

[153] Mantha S, Pillai S, Khayambashi P, Upadhyay A, Zhang Y, Tao O, et al. Smart hydrogels in tissue engineering and regenerative medicine. Materials. 2019;**12**(20):3323. DOI: 10.3390/ma12203323

[154] Zhang K, Wang S, Zhou C, Cheng L, Gao X, Xie X, et al. Advanced smart biomaterials and constructs for hard tissue engineering and regeneration. Bone Research. 2018;**6**(1):1-15

[155] Mao Q, Hoffmann O, Yu K, Lu F, Lan G, Dai F, et al. Self-contracting oxidized starch/gelatin hydrogel for noninvasive wound closure and wound healing. Materials and Design. 2020;**194**:108916

[156] Zhao X, Wu H, Guo B, Dong R, Qiu Y, Ma PX. Antibacterial anti-oxidant electroactive injectable hydrogel as self-healing wound dressing with hemostasis and adhesiveness for cutaneous wound healing. Biomaterials. 2017;**122**:34-47

[157] Li G, Wang Y, Wang S, Liu Z, Liu Z, Jiang J. A thermo- and moisture-responsive zwitterionic shape memory polymer for novel self-healable wound dressing applications. Macromolecular Materials and Engineering. 2019;**304**(3):1800603. DOI: 10.1002/mame.201800603

[158] Joshi S, Rawat K, Karunakaran C, Rajamohan V, Mathew AT, Koziol K, et al. 4D printing of materials for the future: Opportunities and challenges. Applied Materials Today. 2020;**18**:100490

[159] Champeau M, Heinze DA, Viana TN, de Souza ER, Chinellato AC, Titotto S. 4D printing of hydrogels: A review. Advanced Functional Materials. 2020;**30**(31):1910606

[160] Norman JJ, Desai TA. Methods for fabrication of nanoscale topography for tissue engineering scaffolds. Annals of Biomedical Engineering. 2006;**34**(1):89-101

[161] Lanza R, Langer R, Vacanti JP, Atala A. Principles of Tissue Engineering. Academic Press; 2020

[162] Khademhosseini A, Langer R, Borenstein J, Vacanti JP. Microscale technologies for tissue engineering and biology. Proceedings of the National Academy of Sciences. 2006;**103**(8):2480-2487

[163] Aggarwal S, Pittenger MF. Human mesenchymal stem cells modulate allogeneic immune cell responses. Blood. 2005;**105**(4):1815-1822

[164] Panes J, Garcia-Olmo D, Van Assche G, Colombel JF, Reinisch W, Baumgart DC, et al. Expanded allogeneic adipose-derived mesenchymal stem cells (Cx601) for complex perianal fistulas in Crohn's disease: A phase 3 randomised, double-blind controlled trial. Lancet. 2016;**388**(10051):1281-1290

[165] Panes J, Garcia-Olmo D, Van Assche G, Colombel JF, Reinisch W, Baumgart DC, et al. Long-term efficacy and safety of stem cell therapy (Cx601) for complex perianal fistulas in patients with Crohn's disease. Gastroenterology. 2018;**154**(5):1334-1342e4

[166] Philandrianos C, Serrero M, Grimaud F, Magalon J, Visee C, Velier M, et al. First clinical case report of local microinjection of autologous fat and adipose-derived stromal vascular fraction for perianal fistula in Crohn's disease. Stem Cell Research & Therapy. 2018;**9**(1):4

[167] Wainstein C, Quera R, Fluxa D, Kronberg U, Conejero A, Lopez-Kostner F, et al. Stem cell therapy in refractory perineal Crohn's disease: Long-term follow-up. Colorectal Disease. 2018;**20**:68-75. DOI: 10.1111/codi.14002

[168] El Mohamady MS. Cutting seton in management of complex perianal fistula–is it a safe procedure? Menoufia Medical Journal. 2018;**31**(3):867

[169] Al-Marzooq TJ, Hassan QA, Alnaser MK, Al-Edani MS. Treatment of fistula-in-ano with tight (cutting) seton: Analysis of outcomes and efficacy assessment. Journal of Clinical and Diagnostic Research. 2017;**11**(11)

[170] Szymczyk-Ziółkowska P, Łabowska MB, Detyna J, Michalak I, Gruber P. A review of fabrication polymer scaffolds for biomedical applications using additive manufacturing techniques. Biocybernetics and Biomedical Engineering. 2020;**40**(2):624-638

[171] Khalil H, Jummaat F, Yahya EB, Olaiya N, Adnan A, Abdat M, et al. A review on micro-to nanocellulose biopolymer scaffold forming for tissue engineering applications. Polymers. 2020;**12**(9):2043

[172] Jang M, Bae S, Jung Y, Kim J, Kim J, Park S, et al. Enhanced wound healing using a 3D printed VEGF-mimicking peptide incorporated hydrogel patch in a pig model. Biomedical Materials. 2021;**16**(4):045013

[173] Da Silva K, Kumar P, Choonara YE, du Toit LC, Pillay V. Three-dimensional printing of extracellular matrix (ECM)-mimicking scaffolds: A critical review of the current ECM materials. Journal of Biomedical Materials Research. Part A. 2020;**108**(12):2324-2350

[174] Kowalczewski CJ, Saul JM. Biomaterials for the delivery of growth factors and other therapeutic agents in tissue engineering approaches to bone regeneration. Frontiers in Pharmacology. 2018;**9**:513

[175] Ye K, Kuang H, You Z, Morsi Y, Mo X. Electrospun nanofibers for tissue engineering with drug loading and release. Pharmaceutics. 2019;**11**(4):182

[176] Ocansey DK, Zhang L, Wang Y, Yan Y, Qian H, Zhang X, et al. Exosome-mediated effects and applications in inflammatory bowel disease. Biological Reviews. 2020;**95**(5):1287-1307

[177] Cao Y, Su Q, Zhang B, Shen F, Li S. Efficacy of stem cells therapy for Crohn's fistula: A meta-analysis and systematic review. Stem Cell Research & Therapy. 2021;**12**(1):1-11

[178] Jiang Z, Liu G, Meng F, Wang W, Hao P, Xiang Y, et al. Paracrine effects of mesenchymal stem cells on the activation of keratocytes. The British Journal of Ophthalmology. 2017;**101**(11):1583-1590

[179] Mohamed MG, Ambhorkar P, Samanipour R, Yang A, Ghafoor A, Kim K. Microfluidics-based fabrication of cell-laden. Microgels Biomicrofluidics. 2020;**14**(2):021501

Chapter 3

Solitary Rectal Ulcer Syndrome in Children

Sabina Więcek and Dagmara Adamska-Tomaszewska

Abstract

Solitary rectal ulcer syndrome is a condition of unexplained cause, in which there is an ulcer in the rectal wall – single or multiple. The suspected cause of this disease is defecation disorders – strenuous, ineffective pushing causes folding of the rectal wall, gradual thickening and reconstruction of the wall at the place of greatest pressure. Local ischaemia caused by pressure can eventually lead to ulceration and symptoms. The exact incidence of this disease, especially in the paediatric population, is unknown, as in many cases it is asymptomatic. It is estimated that 1–3 people per 100,000 adults develop it annually. The most common symptoms are rectal bleeding and the presence of mucus in the stool. There may also be pain in the anal area, lower abdomen, a feeling of incomplete bowel movements, varying degrees of faecal incontinence and constipation. Sometimes the course is asymptomatic. The diagnosis is made on the basis of clinical picture, endoscopic and histopathological examination. The basic therapy is diet modification and special training (biofeedback rehabilitation) to facilitate bowel movements and avoid excessive pushing. Infusions with substances with a local healing effect are also used. In rare cases, surgical treatment is necessary – removal of the lesion with electrocoagulation, laser or surgical excision. The aim of the study is to analyse the causes, clinical course, diagnostic and therapeutic management in paediatric patients diagnosed with solitary rectal ulcer syndrome.

Keywords: solitary rectal ulcer syndrome, children, pathophysiology, diagnostic and therapeutic management, complications

1. Introduction

Solitary rectal ulcer syndrome (SRUS) is a mild, chronic inflammatory condition of not fully understood etiopathology, rarely occurring in the paediatric population. It is often linked with abnormalities in stool passing and in the motor activity [1–8]. Solitary rectal ulcer syndrome was first described by Cruveilhier in 1829 and involved the description of four cases of SRUS [9]. The name "solitary rectal ulcer syndrome" was regularly used by Lloyd-Davis by the end of the 30s in the twentieth century and in 1969 the diseases became commonly recognisable after the review of 68 cases by Madigan et al. [7]. A few years later, in 1975, Rutter and Riddell described the probably etiopathogenesis of the condition [10]. Since then, solitary rectal ulcer syndrome has developed a few synonyms such as enterogenous cyst of the rectum, colitis cystica profunda, and hamartomatous inverted polyp of the rectum. Solitary rectal ulcer is a confusing name because the ulcerations are observed in 40% of patients, with only 20% of patients having a single ulcer. The lesions seen in the remaining percentage of patients are uncharacteristic and differ in shape and size or are sometimes characteristic of erythematous mucosa of the rectum or sessile polyps [1–4, 11, 12].

2. Epidemiology

SRUS is a rare, not diagnosed or misdiagnosed disorder with the incidence rate of 1–3/100000 people/year – which is underestimated due to the uncharacteristic clinical and endoscopic picture. Solitary rectal ulcer syndrome is most commonly diagnosed in patients aged 30–40, proportionally infrequently in children. In adult patients, men and women are equally affected by this condition, with a marginal domination in female patients but 75–80% of children diagnosed with SRUS are boys [1, 2, 5, 6, 11]. Suresh et al. assessed 325 children below the age of 18 hospitalised for gastrointestinal bleeding - 22 (6,8%) patients were diagnosed with SRUS, the children were aged from 18 months to 18 years (the median: 10 years), with 18/325 (81.8%) $\geq$ 8 years old. The male to female ratio in this group was 1.4:1 [13]. The youngest patient with SRUS so far was 1.5 years old. Gabra et al. also described two boys with SRUS aged 2 and 3 [14]. The average time since the onset of symptoms to the diagnosis of solitary rectal ulcer syndrome is from 3 months to 30 years (about 5 years for adults) and for paediatric patients from 1,2 to 5,5 years (mean age 3.2 years) [1, 3, 10, 11] Similar results were presented by Malik et al. in 2023- out of 310 children presented with haematochezia, 4,5% were diagnosed with SRUS [15]. *Etiopathogenesis.* The pathophysiology of SRUS is not fully known; however, the oversensitivity of the rectum leading to persistent tenesmus and the need for defecation as well as the feeling of incomplete defecation may play an important role. Local trauma due to repeated self-digitation as a result of chronic constipation may also play a role in SRUS pathogenesis [16].

a. *Fuctional and anatomic theory.* Some importance is also given to the abnormal contraction of the puborectalis muscle and rectal prolapse. In some patients, especially in children, injuries to the rectal/perirectal area and/or bowel wall ischaemia are said to play a part [5, 10, 17–20]. An injury to the rectal/perirectal area results in focal ischaemia and ulceration, disorders within the pelvic floor, mucosal prolapse and/or systemic inflammatory process [6, 19–22]. Rectal prolapse may be an especially important part of SRUS pathogenesis in anorectic patients, as a result of perivisceral adipose tissue degeneration and prolapse in consequence of morphological changes in the pelvic floor. This group of patients sometimes needs surgical intervention, which may be exceptionally hard to perform due to malnutrition and tissue weakness [23].

Rectal intussusception may lead to local vascular damage and, as a result, to a single ulcer. In his study involving 256 children who underwent endoscopic assessment of recurrent lower-GI bleeding, Dehghani diagnosed solitary rectal ulcer syndrome in 4.7% [4]. It has been suggested that descent of the perineum and abnormal contraction of the puborectalis muscle during straining on defecation, or defecation in the squatting position, result in trauma and compression of the anterior rectal wall on the upper anal canal, and internal intussusceptions or prolapsed rectum. Mucosal prolapse, occult or overt, is the most common pathogenetic mechanism underlying the condition. The ischaemia may also be linked to the fibroblasts replacing the blood vessels and the pressure caused by the anal sphincter. Anorectal physiology studies have shown that 25–82% of patients with SRUS may have dyssynergia with paradoxical anal contraction. According to a study conducted by Womack et al., the average contraction of the anal sphincter was 24% greater in patients with SRUS compared to the control group ($p < 0.02$) and the average pressure in the rectum in patients with SRUS was 74 mmHg compared to 44 mmHg in the control group ($p < 0,02$) [19]. This is why it is believed that patients with overactive anal sphincters and SRUS benefit from biofeedback therapy as a way to correct paradoxical external sphincter contraction. In children, paradoxical contraction of the pelvic floor muscles and external sphincter contributes to constipation, rectal prolapse, ischaemia and finally rectal ulcers. Morio and his colleagues found that SRUS patients, compared with three control groups (dyssynergic defecation alone, rectal prolapse with or without mucosal changes), had more frequent increases in anal pressure and paradoxical puborectalis contraction during strain.

b. *Psychiatric problems.* Gouriou et al. highlighted in a study published in 2021 the importance of psychiatric issues coexisting with SRUS in one-third of examined patients. The same study showed significance in IBS diagnosis in patients suffering from SRUS [24].

c. *Mechanic damage of rectum.* There are studies indicating the correlation between the use of electric, high-pressure bidets and solitary rectal ulcer, rectal prolapse and inflammation of the large intestine [25]

In 2023, Cheng-cheng et al. published a case study that presented two patients- mother and son- with inherited CHECK2 p.H371Y mutation, which may play a role in SRUS development and prognosis. Further studies on genetic tendencies in SRUS development may shed light on the issue in future [26].

Clinical symptoms. Solitary rectal ulcer syndrome is a spectrum of disorders with a confusing name, as not all the lesions are ulcers, not all affect the rectum and vary in terms of size, shape and look, from simple erythematous patches to polyp-like or multiple ulcerating lesions.

The clinical picture is dominated by:

a. *Lower gastrointestinal bleeding* – blood and mucous in stool. The volume of blood in stool ranges from a small amount of fresh blood to significant haemorrhage, leading to severe anaemia and the need for blood transfusion. It has been suggested that haematochezia may be more likely to occur in groups of older patients due to age-related vascular fragility and comorbid conditions, which increase the risk of bleeding [20].

b. *Problems with defecation* – the sensation of incomplete defecation and tenesmus

c. *Pain in the abdominal and genital area*

d. *Diarrhoea.* Some children experience apparent diarrhoea (due to long-lasting visits to the toilet), lower gastrointestinal bleeding related to it, abdominal pain and need to defecate, which may lead clinicians to believe that there is an Inflammatory Bowel disease [3, 11, 14, 27–30].

e. *Incontinence of stool*. Seventeen per cent of adult patients reported faecal incontinence, probably associated with mucus discharge (**Table 1**) [24].

f. *Asymptomatic course.* As many as 26% of patients with solitary rectal ulcer syndrome have no clinical manifestations.

There are few studies describing coexisting anal fistula which would prompt the exclusion of Crohn's disease. A misdiagnosis may put the patients at risk of steroid- and immunotherapy and may also lead to serious side effects of the treatment [30].

Diagnostics. Diagnosing solitary rectal ulcer syndrome in children is very often challenging and equally often leads to misdiagnosis. The following should be considered during analysis:

a. Thoroughly conducted medical history

b. Results of the laboratory tests (CRP, Hb, Hct, WBC, PLT, TSH, calprotectin in stool, and bacteriological stool test). In some patients: IgA + tTGIgA, hydrogen breath test).

c. Results of the endoscopic examination. Endoscopic lesions may include:

Symptom	Differential diagnosis	Examinations
Bleeding from the lower alimentary tract: • Bloody stools • Anaemia	• Fissure ani • Varices ani • Perianal fistula • Rectal polyps/tumours • Inflammatory bowel disease • Sexual harassment	• Physical examination • Colonoscopy/rectoscopy
Pain in abdomen/rectal area	• Fissure ani • Varices ani • Sexual harassment	• Physical examination • Colonoscopy/rectoscopy • Manometry • Defecography • Psychological consultation
Constipation/problem with defecation	• Functional defecation • Abnormal/restricted diet • Endocrinological problems (hypothyroidism, hypercalcaemia)	• Anorectal manometry • Defecography • Anorectal usg • Laboratory test • Dietetic consultation
Diarrhoea	• Bacterial/viral infection • Inflammatory bowel disease • Celiac disease • Small intestinal overgrowth • Intolerance to lactose/fructose	• Blood/stool test • Calprotectin in stool • Colonoscopy/rectoscopy • IgA+ tTGIgA • Hydrogen breath test

Table 1.
Symptoms and differential diagnosis of SRUS.

- erythematous rectal mucosa,
- ulceration of the anus, ranging from a few millimetres to a few centimetres,
- various size polyp-like lesions (hyperplastic polyps and telangiectasias).

Rectal ulcerations are reported in 40% of patients, with 20% having a single ulcer, and the remaining lesions varying in shape and size. The macroscopic picture of SRUS in the endoscopic examination most often shows ulcerations on the erythematous surrounding mucosa, most often on the anterior wall of the rectum, 5–10 cm from the anal sphincter. The ulcerations may range from 0.5 to 10 cm in diameter but are usually between 1 and 1.5 cm [5, 30]. The polypoid variant of SRUS is very rare in children and may be confused with rectal malignant or inflammatory conditions [31]. Some available data indicate the sigmoid as the location of the lesions related to solitary rectal ulcer syndrome. Magnification in NBI and chromoendoscopy are useful, and histopathological examination should be performed to confirm the diagnosis [32, 33].

a. *Histopathological examination*. Histopathological assessment of the biopsy is indispensable for the diagnostic confirmation of SRUS. Histological diagnostic criteria for solitary rectal ulcer syndrome involve:

    - the obliteration of fibromuscular tissue in the lamina propria,
    - the proliferation of fibroblasts and muscle fibres between the crypts,
    - the thickening of the muscularis mucosa,
    - the presence of branched and distorted glandular crypts,
    - mucous cell proliferation, mucosal gland distortion,
    - diffuse collagen infiltration of the lamina propria,
    - thickening mucosal layer [4, 11, 32–34].

b. Due to the wide spectrum of the endoscopic lesions of SRUS and the fact that the condition may remain undiagnosed or, more often, misdiagnosed, it is crucial to collect biopsy specimens from the affected areas to confirm the diagnosis and exclude other conditions such as cancer [18, 32]. It is important to mention that histological examination may be useful in the SRUS diagnostic path, giving the answer even in lack of ulcer occurrence in endoscopy [35]. It has also been highlighted that an insufficient depth of biopsy sample may lead to difficulties with diagnosis, and in such cases, repeating the diagnosis with deeper sections should be recommended [36].

c. Knowing the importance of observation of fibromuscular tissue in histopathological examination, it has been reported that, in case of doubt, immunohistochemistry for small muscle actin (SMA) and staining with Masson Trichrome may be useful to highlight fibromuscular areas [37].

d. Histopathological examination may also be useful in differential diagnosis—a case of a 3-year-old patient with gastric heterotropia mimicking SRUS has been reported by Abdulrahman et al. [38].

e. *Defecography.* Defecography is a useful method to detect intussusception or external or internal rectal prolapse, and may detect occult anal sphincter atrophy as well as nonrelaxing puborectalis muscle and incomplete or delayed emptying of the rectum [39]. Temiz et al. recommended that routine defecography and anorectal manometry be performed in all children with SRUS to determine the primary pathophysiological abnormalities and select the best treatment protocol. Sphincter atrophy may be occult, and defecography may help to diagnose it [40]. Use of MR defecography in the SRUS diagnostic path may provide insight into many different pelvic floor abnormalities, such as bladder, vaginal and bowel opacification, leading to improvement of treatment results [41].

f. *Anorectal manometry*. Anorectal manometry and electromyography provide useful information about anorectal inhibitory reflex, pressure profiles, defecation dynamics, and rectal compliance and sensory thresholds.

g. *Anorectal ultrasound.* Latest studies have shown that anorectal ultrasound is useful for the assessment of the thickness of the internal anal sphincter, which, as has been proven, is increased in patients with solitary rectal ulcer syndrome.

h. *Dynamic magnetic resonance imaging.* Current studies highlight the importance of this examination for the modern diagnostics of gastrointestinal motor activity disorders.

i. However, it has been reported that SRUS may be falsely diagnosed as cancer in typical ultrasound and MR methods; therefore, clinical judgement and biopsies should always remain the gold standard [42].

The differential diagnostics should involve:

a. Inflammatory bowel diseases,

b. Amoebiasis,

c. Lymphatic granuloma,

d. Chronic ischaemic colitis,

e. Endometriosis,

f. Rectal fissure,

g. Rectal polyps,

h. Rectal tumours,

i. Mechanical damage including sexual assault,

j. Occult rectal mucosa prolapse,

k. Health-related anxiety, obsessive-compulsive disorders,

l. Pelvic dyssynergia.

Obstructing anal symptoms (anismus) in children may be interpreted by parents as constipation. The co-occurring lower gastrointestinal bleeding may be misinterpreted as originating from the anal fissure caused by constipation or other causes, for example, juvenile polyps [1, 2, 11, 31, 32, 43, 44].

Treatment. The treatment of solitary rectal ulcer syndrome is often very complex and ineffective. There are no robust guidelines for the medical treatment of SRUS. Patients are advised of the following line of treatment:

a. *Prevention/treatment of constipation*. Macrogol and lactulose are often the first-line therapy

b. *The topical use of sucralfate* may be effective in the treatment of SRUS in some patients

Many drugs beneficial in the treatment of patients with non-specific inflammatory bowel diseases (sulfasalazine, corticoids) have been used in patients with SRUS; however, there is no data confirming their effectiveness [5, 44]. AlGhulayqah et al. observed a significant improvement in 85% of patients with SRUS treated with mesalazine and a fibre-rich diet [2]. Uygur concluded the total withdrawal of symptoms over a six-month observation period in 82.6% of patients after the per rectum application of mesalazine, which would confirm its therapeutic effectiveness [20]. In 2023, Shafiq published a study that confirmed 61% and 46% response rates in patients who received mesalazine and budesonide enemas (7A). Studies and case reports on the paediatric population seem to support the thesis of the validity of using hydrocortisone enemas in children with SRUS as a part of first-line treatment [35, 45].

c. *Biofeedback*. Biofeedback therapies, aimed at training the intestines by techniques such as the time spent in the toilet, the coordination of the pelvic floor and abdominal muscles to improve their function, or additional use of the Valsalva techniques, among others, improve the healing of solitary rectal ulcers in as many as 75% of patients [46]. Derya et al. in 2022 suggested that biofeedback should be considered especially for patients with dyssynergic defecation, as this group is typically observed as non-responders to typical treatment [47]. Results of a study performed on a group of 140 children with SRUS confirmed that behavioural modification combined with laxative and topical steroids provides a good clinical response [35]. It was, however, highlighted that biofeedback itself results in less satisfactory effects than biofeedback combined with rectal therapies such as sulfasalazine enema [48]

Biofeedback may also play a significant role in eliminating feelings of faecal incontinence reported by 17% adult patients with SRUS, probably associated rather with mucus discharge than defecation by itself [24].

d. *Surgical treatment.* The surgical treatment of SRUS involves rectopexy, excision and the Delorme procedure. The choice of procedure will depend on the intensity of the symptoms and whether there has been rectal prolapse or not. Sclerotherapy injection into the submucosa or retrorectal space with 5% phenol, 30% hypertonic saline or 25% glucose and perianal cerclage is effective in treating rectal prolapse. Local excision of polypoid rectal ulcer and rectopexy for overt rectal prolapse, however, have a higher long-term cure rate. However, as highlighted in 2023 by Zhand et al. in case report presenting a 14-year-old patient that underwent transanal resection of rectal lesions in SRUS, postoperative monitoring is extremely important, as the recurrence of SRUS may happen [49]. Proctectomy may be required in patients with intractable rectal pain and bleeding, who have not responded to other surgical treatments [3, 28, 29, 31, 32, 44, 50–54] Gaj and colleagues in meta-analysis in 2024 suggested a SRUS treatment flow-chart, that could play useful role in decision making process in SRUS treatment, allowing to choose between mucosal resection and proctectomy in patients with external prolapse, endoscopic local treatment and biofeedback in case of lack of prolapse and rectopexy or anterior rectal resection treating internal prolapse in case of lack of improvement after typical interventions as patient education, medical treatment and biofeedback [55].

e. *Botulinum toxin*. The therapeutic aspect of injecting botulinum toxin into the external anal sphincter to treat SRUS and dyssynergic defecation-linked constipation has been described by Keshtgar et al. [56]. The botulinum toxin's action lasts around 3 months, which may be more beneficial than biofeedback therapy.

f. *Endoscopic treatment*. Some studies have indicated that new therapies such as argon plasma coagulation (APC) are useful, especially in the treatment of bleeding ulcers when compared to conservative treatment options [2, 57, 58]. Shah et al. confirmed 100% control over bleeding and a 71% success rate in the healing of ulcers in patients with treatment-resistant SRUS treated with APC. They have suggested that the combination of mesalazine and APC may have the dual benefit of using mesalazine to reduce the inflammation and APC for the instant control of bleeding [59]. Another possible treatment path could be reported by Gagliardi et al. in 2021, a successful case of Purastat application. Purastat is defined as a self-assembling peptide with haemostatic effect, which, due to its nanostructure, may improve the proliferation process in treated tissue [60]. Endoscopic procedures may also become a promising treatment path for patients with polypoid SRUS (P-SRUS), as was reported in 2024 by Forootan et al. in a study presenting results of snare-assisted mucosal and fibrosis resection [61].

g. *Diet therapy*. A diet rich in fibre. Blackburn et al. reported that behavioural therapy, high-fibre diet, and lactase therapy resulted in remission in seven out of eight children and in 18 of 24 children [3].

h. *Psychological care*. Simple behavioural modifications yield positive outcomes in the treatment of SRUS in childhood, probably due to the short span of the disease compared to adult patients.

Methods of therapy for solitary rectal ulcer syndrome are shown in **Table 2**.

Proper treatment and adherence to medical advice in children may prevent the condition from progressing and from unsatisfactory response to treatment, which is sometimes observed in adult patients [3]. The treatment recommended by Abbas et al.

Pharmacological therapy	*Treatment of constipation:* • Macrogol • Lactulose *Local therapy* - sucralfate rectal enemas, mesalazine enemas/suppositories Corticoid enemas/suppositories
Endoscopic treatment	Argon plasma coagulation Sclerotherapy Purastat application Botulin toxin injection
Surgical treatment	Transanal resection Rectopexy, excision The Delorme procedure Botulin toxin injection
Biofeedback therapies	Training the intestines by techniques such as the time spent in the toilet, the coordination of the pelvic floor and abdominal muscles
Psychological care	
Dietary treatment	Fibre-rich diet

Table 2.
Therapy of solitary rectal ulcer syndrome.

is initially conservative, and in the case of failure, it should be followed by transanal resection and then by fibre-rich diet [1]. Conservative treatment, including behavioural modifications and reducing the amount of time they strain for while defecating, has been claimed to be an effective method of treatment [3, 46]. It is important to highlight that even though the local treatment, such as APC or enemas, may result in short-term improvement, they fail to treat the underlying aetiology of SRUS; therefore, interventions that lead to improvement of the anorectal function and reduction of pathological behaviour should be considered as the most important in long-term treatment [55].

3. Complications

Relapse caused by not following the medical advice is an important risk, and children with confirmed solitary rectal ulcer syndrome should be monitored regularly and long-term in specialist outpatient surgeries. SRUS is considered an element of a longer disease process which encompasses polyp-type inflammatory lesions and vascular ectasia. In reality, all those syndromes show the same histopathological features. A prolonged diagnostic period and/or misdiagnosis may have serious consequences such as ischaemia and/or heavy bleeding from the lower gastrointestinal tract, weak appetite/lack of increase in the body weight in growing children, pain and worse quality of life [37, 62]. In 2022, Abdolreza et al. reported a case of a 15-year-old child with previously reported SRUS, which developed into cap polyposis determined by colonoscopy and histologic findings. This case highlights the importance of reassessment of the patient in the event of the progression of symptoms or lack of response to SRUS treatments [63]. Moreover, a case of a 29-year-old patient with SRUS, who suffered cancerous transformation into mucinous carcinoma has been reported, which highlights the importance of regular monitoring and diagnosis reassessment in SRUS patients, especially in case of treatment failure [64]. However, it is important

Alimentary tract	Massive, chronic bleeding from alimentary tract Painful ailments Habitual constipation associated with pain during defecation
Systemic symptoms	Anaemia - weakness, poor exercise tolerance, fatigue Decreased quality of life Decreased appetite- > lost body mass Deficiency pf growth

Table 3.
The most often complications of solitary rectal ulcer syndrome.

to highlight that there are no recommendations to repeat endoscopy or biopsies in patients with good response to treatment—such interventions should only be taken into consideration in case of treatment failure or change of clinical symptoms [65].

Complications of treatment itself should also be monitored and reassessed during the child's development after the treatment, as we take the organism that is constantly changing into consideration. It is worth mentioning that members of medical teams taking care of patients during and after the treatment should remember about possible complications of surgical treatment, such as sexual dysfunction, impotence or stricture formation [66].

The most common complications of solitary rectal ulcer are presented in **Table 3**.

4. Conclusions

Solitary rectal ulcer syndrome is a benign disorder of defecation, characterised by lower gastrointestinal bleeding, constipation/problems passing stool and/or abdominal discomfort. It occurs in the paediatric population too.

In the diagnosis of SRUS, the dominant role is played by endoscopic examination with histopathology of specimens.

It requires a complex diagnostic and therapeutic approach, which also includes the conservative treatment—pharmacology and biofeedback, as well as endoscopic and/or surgical procedures. This prevents serious complications from occurring.

Author details

Sabina Więcek[1*] and Dagmara Adamska-Tomaszewska[2]

1 Department of Paediatrics, Medical University of Silesia, Katowice, Poland

2 Doctoral School, Medical University of Silesia, Katowice, Poland

*Address all correspondence to: sabinawk@wp.pl

References

[1] Abbas T, Ismail A, Abdulrahman H, Ali M, et al. Solitary rectal ulcer syndrome, a Pediatric problem: Case report. Oman Medical Journal. 2011;**26**(5):e024. DOI: 10.5001/omj.2011.98

[2] AlGhulayqah A, Abu-Farhaneh E, AlSohaibani F, Almadi M, et. Solitary rectal ulcer syndrome: A single-center case series. Saudi Journal of Gastroenterology. 2016;**22**(6):456-460. DOI: 10.4103/1319-3767.195555

[3] Blackburn C, McDermott M, Bourke B. Clinical presentation of and outcome for solitary rectal ulcer syndrome in children. Journal of Pediatric Gastroenterology and Nutrition. 2012;**54**:263-265. DOI: 10.1097/MPG.0b013e31823014c0

[4] Dehghani S, Haghighat M, Imanieh M, Geramizadeh B. Solitary rectal ulcer syndrome in children: A prospective study of cases from southern Iran. European Journal of Gastroenterology & Hepatology. 2008;**20**:93-95 16. DOI: 10.1097/MEG.0b013e3282f1cbb6

[5] Dehghani S, Malekpour A, Highighat M. Solitary rectal ulcer syndrome in children: A literature review. World Journal of Gastroenterology. 2012;**18**(45):6541-6545. DOI: 10.3748/wzjg.v.18.i45.6541

[6] Felt-Bersma R, Cuesta M. Rectal prolapse, rectal intussception, rectocele, and solitary rectal ulcer syndrome. Gastroenterology Clinics of North America. 2001;**30**:199-222. DOI: 10.1016/j.gtc.2008.06.001

[7] Madigan M, Morson B. Solitary ulcer of the rectum. Gut. 1969;**10**:871-881. DOI: 10.1136/gut.10.11.871

[8] Haray P, Morris-Stiff G, Foster M. Solitary rectal ulcer syndrome–An underdiagnosed condition. International Journal of Colorectal Disease. 1997;**12**:313-315. DOI: 10.1007/s003840050113

[9] Cruveilhier J. Ulcere chronique du rectum. In: Bailliere JB, editor. Anatomie Pathologique du Corps Human. Paris; 1829

[10] Rutter K, Riddell R. The solitary ulcer syndrome of the rectum. Clinics in Gastroenterology. 1975;**4**:505-530

[11] Ford M, Anderson J, Gilmour H, Holt S, Sircus W. Clinical spectrum of "solitary ulcer" of the rectum. Gastroenterology. 1983;**84**:1533-1540

[12] Gopal D, Young C, Katon R. Solitary rectal ulcer syndrome presenting with rectal prolapse, severe mucorrhea and eroded polypoid hyperplasia: Case report and review of the literature. Canadian Journal of Gastroenterology. 2001;**15**:479-483. DOI: 10.1155/2001/145041

[13] Suresh N, Ganesh R, Sathiyasekaran M. Solitary rectal ulcer syndrome: A case series. Indian Pediatrics. 2010;**47**:1059-1061. DOI: 10.4103/1319-3767.195555

[14] Gabra H, Roberts J, Variend S, Shawis R. Solitary rectal ulcer syndrome in children. A report of three cases. European Journal of Pediatric Surgery. 2005;**15**:213-216. DOI: 10.1055/s-2004-821180

[15] Malik I, Sami A, Waseem YW. Etiological profile of lower gastrointestinal bleeding in children and adolescents from Kashmir; A

tale of 5 years. Middle East Journal of Digestive Diseases. 2023;**15**(3):180-184. DOI: 10.34172/mejdd.2023.341

[16] Zhu Q, Shen R, Qin H. Solitary rectal ulcer syndrome: Clinical features, pathophysiology, diagnosis and treatment strategies. World Journal of Gastroenterology. 2014;**20**(3):738-744. DOI: 10.3748/wjg.v20.i3.738

[17] Halligan S, Nicholls R, Bartram C. Evacuation proctography in patients with solitary rectal ulcer syndrome: Anatomic abnormalities and frequency of impaired emptying and prolapse. AJR. American Journal of Roentgenology. 1995;**164**:91-95. DOI: 10.2214/ajr.164.1.7998576

[18] Pai R, Mathai A, Magar D, Tantry B. Solitary rectal ulcer syndrome in childhood. Tropical Gastroenterology. 2008;**29**:177-178

[19] Womack N, Williams N, Holmfield J, Morrison J. Pressure and prolapse–The cause of solitary rectal ulceration. Gut. 1987;**28**:1228-1233. DOI: 10.1136/gut.28.10.1228

[20] Uygur F, Goktepe M, Aydm G, Agiirman E, et al. Clinical and laboratory characteristics of solitary rectal ulcer syndrome: A rectospective analysis of 36 case. Scientific Reports. 2025;**15**(1):2122. DOI: 10.1038/s41598-025-86324-0

[21] Tandon R, Atmakuri S, Mehra N, Malaviya A, et al. Is solitary rectal ulcer a manifestation of a systemic disease? Journal of Clinical Gastroenterology. 1990;**12**:286-290. DOI: 10.1097/00004836-199006000-00010

[22] Thirumal P, Sumathi B, Nirmala D. A clinical entity often missed-solitary rectal ulcer syndrome in children. Frontiers in Pediatrics. 2020;**8**:1-8. DOI: 10.3389/fped.2020.03396

[23] Vescovo M, Pesci L, Lapenna L. Severe rectal prolapse and solitary rectal ulcer in a young anorectic woman with myxoid degeneration of visceral adipose tissue. Pathologica. 2021;**113**(6):475-480. DOI: 10.32074/1591-951X-253

[24] Gouriou C, Siproudhis L, Chambaz M. Solitary rectal ulcer syndrome in 102 patients: Do different phenotypes make sense? Digestive and Liver Disease. 2021;**53**(2):190-195. DOI: 10.1016/j.dld.2020.10.041

[25] Nishiwaki T, Nakachi K, Inoue S, Ashikawa T, et al. Severe circumferential rectal ulcer associated with electric bidet toilet use. DEN Open. 2024;**4**(1):e347. DOI: 10.1002/deo2.347

[26] He C, Wag S, Zhou P. Inherited CHEK2 p.H371Y mutation in solitary rectal ulcer syndrome among familial patients: A case report. World Journal of Gastroenterology. 2023;**29**(31):4809-4814. DOI: 10.3748/wjg.v29.i31.4809

[27] Ejaz Z, Khan S, Rehman R, Jibran M. Solitary rectal ulcer syndrome in patients presenting with lower gastrointestinal bleeding: A tertiary-care hospital experience. Cureus. 2023;**15**(2):e35247. DOI: 10.7759/cureus.35247

[28] Marchal F, Bresler L, Brunaud L, Adler S, et al. Solitary rectal ulcer syndrome: A series of 13 patients operated with a mean follow-up of 4.5 years. International Journal of Colorectal Disease. 2001;**16**:228-233. DOI: 10.1007/s003840100303

[29] Martin C, Parks T, Biggart J. Solitary rectal ulcer syndrome in Northern Ireland. 1971-1980. The British Journal of Surgery. 1981;**68**:744-747. DOI: 10.1002/bjs.1800681021

[30] Powell C, Lawson J, Lindholm P. Solitary rectal ulcer syndrome mimicking

perianal Crohn's disease. Cureus. 2022;**14**(4):e23733. DOI: 10.7759/cureus.23733

[31] Saadah O, Al-Hubayshi M, Ghanem A. Solitary rectal ulcer syndrome presenting as polypoid mass lesions in a young girl. World Journal of Gastrointestinal Oncology. 2010;**2**(8):332-334. DOI: 10.4251/wzgo.v2.i8.332

[32] Sharara AI, Azar C, Amr S, Haddad M, Eloubeidi M. Solitary rectal ulcer syndrome: Endoscopic spectrum and review of the literature. Gastrointestinal Endoscopy. 2005;**62**:755-762. DOI: 10.1016/j.gie.2005.07.016

[33] Abusharifah O, Bokhary R, Mosil M, Saadah O. Solitary rectal ulcer syndrome in children and adolescents: A descriptive clinicopathologic study. International Journal of Clinical and Experimental Pathology. 2021;**14**(4):399-407

[34] Tjandra J, Fazio V, Church J, Lavery I, Oakley J, et al. Clinical conundrum of solitary rectal ulcer. Diseases of the Colon and Rectum. 1992;**35**:227-234. DOI: 10.1007/BF02051012

[35] Poddar U, Yachha S, Krishnani N. Solitary rectal ulcer syndrome in children: A report of 140 cases. Journal of Pediatric Gastroenterology and Nutrition. 2020;**71**(1):29-33. DOI: 10.1097/MPG.0000000000002680

[36] Wong Y, Kabincong C, Jabar M. Rectal polyposis in mucosal prolapse syndrome. Diagnostics (Basel). 2022;**12**(4):966. DOI: 10.3390/diagnostics12040966

[37] Sawhney M, Madan J, Nath D, et al. Solitary rectal ulcer syndrome- A rare entity in the pediatric population. Türk Patoloji Dergisi. 2025;**41**:16-20. DOI: 10.5146/tjpath.2025.13667

[38] Al-Hussaini A, Lone K, Al-Soyfani M. Gastric heterotopia of rectum in a child: A mimicker of solitary rectal ulcer syndrome. Annals of Saudi Medicine. 2014;**34**(3):245-249. DOI: 10.5144/0256-4947.2014.245

[39] Goei R, Baeten C, Arends J. Solitary rectal ulcer syndrome: Findings at barium enema study and defecography. Radiology. 1988;**168**:303-306. DOI: 10.1148/radiology.168.2.3393650

[40] Temiz A, Tander B, Temiz M, Barış S, Arıtürk E. A rare cause of chronic rectal bleeding in children; solitary rectal ulcer: Case report. Ulusal Travma ve Acil Cerrahi Dergisi. 2011;**17**:173-176

[41] Abdelatty M, Halligan S, Sayed R. Solitary rectal ulcer syndrome (SRUS): Observational case series findings on MR defecography. European Radiology. 2021;**31**(11):8597-8605. DOI: 10.1007/s00330-021-08075-6

[42] Blanco F, Frasson M, Flor-Lorente B. Solitary rectal ulcer ultrasonographic and magnetic resonance imaging patterns mimicking rectal cancer. European Journal of Gastroenterology & Hepatology. 2011;**23**(12):1262-1266. DOI: 10.1097/MEG.0b013e32834b0dee

[43] Daya D, O'Connell G, DeNardi F. Rectal endometriosis mimicking solitary rectal ulcer syndrome. Modern Pathology. 1995;**8**:599-602

[44] Kennedy D, Hughes E, Masterton J. The natural history of benign ulcer of the rectum. Surgery, Gynecology & Obstetrics. 1977;**144**:718-720

[45] Kowalska-Duplaga K, Lazowska-PrzeorekI,Karolewksa-BochenekK. Solitary rectal ulcer syndrome in children: A case series study. Advances in Experimental Medicine

and Biology. 2017;**1020**:105-112. DOI: 10.1007/5584_2017_2

[46] Jarrett M, Emmanuel A, Vaizey C, Kamm M. Behavioural therapy (biofeedback) for solitary rectal ulcer syndrome improves symptoms and mucosal blood flow. Gut. 2004;**53**:368-370. DOI: 10.1136/gut.2003.025643

[47] Ari D, Öztürk Ö, Özin Y. The efficacy of biofeedback therapy in patients with solitary rectal ulcer and dyssynergic defecation. Digestive Diseases. 2022;**40**(6):728-733. DOI: 10.1159/000522180

[48] Abdi S, Tavakolikia N, Yamini M. Solitary rectal ulcer syndrome: Addition of rectal therapies to biofeedback is more effective than biofeedback alone. Gastroenterology and Hepatology from Bed to Bench. 2019;**12**(3):197-202

[49] Zhan Y, Tian F, Li H. Solitary rectal ulcer syndrome coexisting with colitis Cystica Profunda—Is mucosal resection radical or not? Inflammatory Bowel Diseases. 2023;**29**(6):1008-1009. DOI: 10.1093/ibd/izac232

[50] Ashcraft K, Garred J, Holder T, Amoury R, et al. Rectal prolapse: 17-year experience with the posterior repair and suspension. Journal of Pediatric Surgery. 1990;**25**:992-994; discussion 994-995. DOI: 10.1016/0022-3468(90)90245-5

[51] Kargar S, Salmanroughani H, Binesh F, Taghipoor S. Laparoscopic rectopexy in solitary rectal ulcer. Acta Medica Iranica. 2011;**49**:810-813

[52] Nicholls R, Simson J. Anteroposterior rectopexy in the treatment of solitary rectal ulcer syndrome without overt rectal prolapse. The British Journal of Surgery. 1986;**73**:222-224. DOI: 10.1002/bjs.1800730324

[53] Sitzler P, Kamm M, Nicholls R, McKee R. Long-term clinical outcome of surgery for solitary rectal ulcer syndrome. The British Journal of Surgery. 1998;**85**:1246-1250. DOI: 10.1046/j.1365-2168.1998.00854.x

[54] Ihre T, Seligson U. Intussusception of the rectum-internal procidentia: Treatment and results in 90 patients. Diseases of the Colon and Rectum. 1975;**18**:391-396. DOI: 10.1007/BF02587429

[55] Gaj F, Lai Q, Gelormini E. Efficacy of surgical treatments for the management of solitary rectal ulcer syndrome: A network meta-analysis. Colorectal Disease. 2024;**26**(8):1515-1534. DOI: 10.1111/codi.17080

[56] Keshtgar A, Ward H, Sanei A, Clayden G. Botulinum toxin, a new treatment modality for chronic idiopathic constipation in children: Long-term follow-up of a double-blind randomized trial. Journal of Pediatric Surgery. 2007;**42**:672-680. DOI: 10.1016/j.jpedsurg.2006.12.045

[57] Somani S, Ghosh A, Avasthi G, Goyal R, et al. Healing of solitary rectal ulcers with multiple sessions of argon plasma coagulation. Digestive Endoscopy. 2010;**22**:107-111. DOI: 10.1111/j.1443-1661.2010.00941

[58] Zergani F, Shaiesthe A, Hajiani E, et al. Evaluation of argon plasma coagulation in healing of a solitary rectal ulcer in comparison with conventional therapy: A randomised controlled trial. Przegląd Gastroenterologiczny. 2017;**12**:128-134. DOI: 10.5114/pg.2016.64846

[59] Shah A, Bohra S, Desai S. Argon plasma coagulation-an effective treatment for solitary rectal ulcer syndrome: A single-center experience

from western India. Indian Journal of Gastroenterology. 2021;**40**(1):35-40. DOI: 10.1007/s12664-020-01089-w

[60] Gagliardi M, Sica M, Oliviero G. Endoscopic application of Purastat® in the treatment of solitary rectal ulcer syndrome. Journal of Gastrointestinal and Liver Diseases. 10 Aug 2021. DOI: 10.15403/jgld-3680. Online ahead of print

[61] Forootan M, Repici A, Rajabnia M. Endoscopic resection of polypoid solitary rectal ulcer: A novel first-line therapeutic strategy using snare-assisted mucosal and fibrosis resection. DEN Open. 2025;**6**(1):e70108. DOI: 10.1002/deo2.70108

[62] Alexander-Williams J. Solitary-ulcer syndrome of the rec tum. Its association with occult rectal prolapse. Lancet. 1977;**1**:170-171. DOI: 10.1016/s0140-6736(77)91766-4

[63] Emami A, Shrivani J, Hosseini A. Solitary rectal ulcer transformation to cap polyposis in a 15-year-old child. BMC Gastroenterology. 2022;**22**:104. DOI: 10.1186/s12876-022-02122-2

[64] Tan Q, Zhou J, Zhao K. A rare case report of mucinous adenocarcinoma exacerbated by long-standing solitary rectal ulcer syndrome. AME Case Reports. 2024;**8**:63. DOI: 10.21037/acr-23-207

[65] Gouriou C, Chambaz M, Ropert A. Management of solitary rectal ulcer syndome: Results of a French National Survey Société Nationale Française de Coloproctologie SNFCP, France. Digestive and Liver Disease. 2020;**52**(8):885-888. DOI: 10.1016/j.dld.2020.05.013

[66] Jha A, Purkayastha S, Mohan V. Endoscopic mucosectomy: A novel technique for Management of Polypoidal Solitary Rectal Ulcer Syndrome. ACG Case Reports Journal. 2021;**8**(4):e00563. DOI: 10.14309/crj.0000000000000563

Section 2

Hemorrhoids: Evidence-Based and Special Settings

Chapter 4

Clinical Guidelines for the Treatment of Hemorrhoids with Traditional Chinese Medicine

Yongfeng Liu, Di Qiu, Tingyu Wang, Jinhuan Zhang, Xingxian Huang and Haibo Yu

Abstract

This manuscript provides a comprehensive overview of traditional Chinese medicine (TCM) approaches for the treatment of hemorrhoids. Hemorrhoids, referred to as "zhì" in TCM, are categorized under anal diseases and have been documented in ancient texts such as the Huangdi Neijing. The etiology and pathogenesis of hemorrhoids in TCM are attributed to prolonged sitting or standing, improper diet, chronic diarrhea or constipation, and fatigue, leading to disharmony of qi and blood in the anal region. The manuscript discusses various TCM treatment strategies, including internal medication tailored to different syndromes (e.g., wind damaging the intestinal network, damp-heat descending, qi stagnation and blood stasis, and spleen deficiency with qi sinking), external therapies such as fumigation and sitz baths, topical applications, suppositories, and herbal enemas. Additionally, it explores acupuncture and moxibustion therapies, auricular therapy, acupoint embedding, fire needle therapy, and cupping therapy. The use of TCM patent medicines like Zhiran Xiao Tablets and Lianzhi San Ointment is also highlighted. The manuscript further addresses common postoperative reactions and their management, emphasizing pain relief, urinary retention, bleeding, and edema. Clinical observations and studies are cited to support the efficacy of these TCM interventions in treating hemorrhoids and improving patient outcomes.

Keywords: traditional Chinese medicine (TCM), hemorrhoids, internal medication, external therapies, acupuncture and moxibustion, etiology and pathogenesis, clinical efficacy

1. Introduction

In traditional Chinese medicine (TCM), hemorrhoids fall under the category of "anal diseases" and are referred to as "zhì" (痔), "cháng pì" (肠澼), "xià xuè" (下血), etc. [1]. These conditions have been documented in classic texts such as Huangdi Neijing (The Yellow Emperor's Inner Canon) and Yizong Jinjian (Golden Mirror of Medicine).

2. Etiology and pathogenesis

The diagnosis and treatment of hemorrhoids in traditional Chinese medicine originate from its holistic perspective and theory of dynamic equilibrium, identifying the condition as a manifestation of "local disharmony of qi and blood". The Huangdi Neijing (The Yellow Emperor's Inner Canon) states: "The transverse relaxation of sinews and vessels leads to hemorrhoidal disorders (intestinal afflictions manifest as hemorrhoids)", emphasizing the interplay between damp-heat stagnation and deficiency of vital qi (zhengqi). The Waike Zhengzong (Orthodox Manual of Surgery) further specifies that "hemorrhoids pertain to the Liver and Spleen meridians", deepening the pathological interpretation through visceral syndrome differentiation.

Hemorrhoids often arise from prolonged sitting or standing, carrying heavy loads over long distances; improper diet with a preference for spicy, sweet, and fatty foods; chronic diarrhea or long-term constipation; or fatigue and childbirth. These factors can lead to disharmony of qi and blood in the anal region, stasis of blood in the collaterals, and the accumulation of damp-heat, resulting in hemorrhoids [2].

3. Differential diagnosis and treatment

3.1 Internal medication

3.1.1 Wind damaging the intestinal network

Symptoms: Bleeding during bowel movements, dripping blood, or jet-like bleeding, with bright red blood, varying in amount, sometimes accompanied by anal itching, dry mouth and throat, and hard stools [3]. The tongue is red with a thin white or yellow coating, and the pulse is floating and rapid.

Analysis: Wind is characterized by its mobility and variability, often combined with heat. Wind heat damaging the intestinal network causes blood to deviate from its normal course, leading to bright red bleeding or sudden jet-like bleeding. Thirst, hard stools, red tongue with yellow coating, and rapid pulse indicate an excess of internal heat.

Treatment: Clear heat, cool blood, and dispel wind.

Formula: Modified Liangxue Dihuang Tang (Cooling Blood and Rehmannia Decoction) from Waike Dacheng (Great Compendium of Surgery).

Common ingredients: *Rehmannia glutinosa* (Shengdihuang), *Angelica sinensis* (Dangguiwei), *Sanguisorba officinalis* (Diyu), *Sophora japonica* (Huanglian), *Scutellaria baicalensis* (Huangqin), *Trichosanthes kirilowii* (Tianhuafen), *Cimicifuga racemosa* (Shengma), Aurantium (Zhike), *Schizonepeta tenuifolia* (Jingjie), *Paeonia lactiflora* (Chishao), *Glycyrrhiza uralensis* (Gancao). For elderly patients with physical weakness, Pseudostellariae Radix (Taizishen) may be added.

A domestic study indicated that for mixed hemorrhoids with wind damaging the intestinal network, Modified Liangxue Dihuang Tang was used: *Rehmannia glutinosa* 9 g, *Angelica sinensis* 6 g, Aurantium 3 g, *Paeonia lactiflora* 3 g, *Sanguisorba officinalis* (Diyuzhi) 3 g, *Schizonepeta tenuifolia* (Jingjie Zhi) 3 g, *Rheum palmatum* (Shengdahuang) 3 g (added last), *Trichosanthes kirilowii* 3 g, and *Glycyrrhiza uralensis* 1.5 g. If bowel movements are not smooth, add *Rheum palmatum* 3 g; if bleeding is jet-like, add *Platycladus orientalis* (Cebaiye) 10 g and increase the amount of *Sanguisorba officinalis* (Diyuzhi) to enhance hemostasis. After 1 week of treatment, the total effective rate of the internal medication group was as high as 95.35%, indicating that Modified Liangxue Dihuang Tang has a significant effect on treating hemorrhoids with wind damaging the intestinal network [4]. For strangulated internal hemorrhoids with edema, Liangxue Dihuang Tang (*Rehmannia glutinosa* 15 g, *Angelica sinensis* 15 g, *Paeonia lactiflora* 15 g, *Sanguisorba officinalis* (Diyuzhi) 15 g, *Sophora japonica* 15 g, *Trichosanthes kirilowii* 15 g, *Scutellaria baicalensis* 15 g, *Cimicifuga racemosa* 10 g, *Schizonepeta tenuifolia* 10 g, *Scutellaria baicalensis* 10 g, Aurantium 10 g, *Glycyrrhiza uralensis* 10 g) plus *Astragalus membranaceus* (Zhihuangqi) 25 g, *Atractylodes macrocephala* (Baizhu) 20 g, and sodium sulfate (Mangxiao) 10 g (added last) can be used. The decoction is boiled three times, with the first two for oral use and the third for fumigation and washing [5]. A double-blind trial study showed that Modified Liangxue Dihuang Tang (*Sophora japonica* 9 g, *Platycladus orientalis* 6 g, *Sanguisorba officinalis* 6 g, *Scutellaria baicalensis* 6 g, *Rehmannia glutinosa* 6 g, *Angelica sinensis* 4.5 g, Aurantium 3 g, *Scutellaria baicalensis* 3 g, *Paeonia lactiflora* 3 g, *Schizonepeta tenuifolia* 3 g, *Trichosanthes kirilowii* 2.4 g, *Cimicifuga racemosa* 1.5 g, and *Glycyrrhiza uralensis* 1.5 g) could effectively relieve bleeding in hemorrhoids [6].

3.1.2 Damp-heat descending

Symptoms: Bright red bleeding during bowel movements, with a significant amount of blood, anal burning, prolapsed anal mass that can retract spontaneously, hard or loose stools, and short, red urine. The tongue is red with yellow, greasy coating, and the pulse is string-like and rapid.

Analysis: This often results from improper diet and overconsumption of raw, cold, or fatty foods, which injure the spleen and stomach and generate internal dampness. Dampness combined with heat descends into the large intestine, causing disordered qi and blood in the anal region, leading to internal hemorrhoids. Excessive heat forces blood to flow erratically, resulting in bleeding; damp-heat descending into the large intestine causes intestinal qi stagnation and obstructed collaterals, leading to a prolapsed anal mass. Hard or loose stools, yellow urine, red tongue, yellow and greasy coating, and a slippery and rapid pulse indicate the presence of damp-heat.

Treatment: Clear heat, dry dampness, and stop bleeding.

Formula: Modified Zanglian Wan (Intestine-Connecting Pill) from Zhengzhi Zhunsheng (Standard Rules for Treatment). Common ingredients include *Coptis chinensis* (Huanglian) and pig large intestine. For significant bleeding, add *Sanguisorba officinalis* (Diyuzhi) and Herba Agrimoniae (Xianhecao); for severe burning, add *Pulsatilla chinensis* (Baitouweng) and *Gentiana macrophylla* (Qinjiao). For obese patients with a phlegm-dampness constitution, Atractylodis Rhizoma (Cangzhu) and Coicis Semen (Yiyiren) may be added to the formula.

For women with hemorrhoids during the perinatal period, who have bleeding from internal hemorrhoids or prolapsed hemorrhoidal nuclei that can retract, Compound Zanglian Wan can be used orally: *Sanguisorba officinalis* (Diyuzhi) 150 g, *Schizonepeta tenuifolia* (Jingjie Zhi) 150 g, *Scutellaria baicalensis* (Huangqin) 150 g, *Coptis chinensis* (Huanglian) 150 g, *Saposhnikovia divaricata* (Fangfeng) 150 g, *Rheum palmatum* (Shengjinwen) 150 g, *Sophora japonica* (Shenghuami) 250 g, *Cannabis sativa* (Huomaren) 250 g, *Rehmannia glutinosa* (Shengdihuang) 250 g, and pig large intestine five pieces. The herbs are ground into powder, mixed with honey to form pills, and taken for a 10-day course. If the hemorrhoidal nuclei cannot retract or are accompanied by anal fissures, a fumigation and washing formula can be added: *Lonicera japonica* (Jinyinhua) 30 g, *Sophora flavescens* (Kushenpian) 30 g, *Phellodendron chinense* (Chuanpo) 30 g, *Lactuca sativa* (Loulu) 30 g, and *Gossypium herbaceum* (Wahua) 30 g, plus sodium sulfate (Mangxiao) 15 g (dissolved separately). The herbs are boiled to extract the liquid, used for fumigation while hot, and then for sitting baths when warm, twice a day for 15 minutes each time [7]. If perianal eczema is present, add Cnidii Fructus (Shechuangzi) 15 g and Kochiae Fructus (Difuzi) 15 g to the fumigation and sitz bath formula to enhance the effects of drying dampness and relieving itching.

3.1.3 Qi stagnation and blood stasis

Symptoms: Prolapsed anal mass, sometimes with strangulation, anal sphincter contraction, a feeling of heaviness and swelling pain, and in severe cases, edema and thrombus formation around the anus, with significant tenderness upon touch; the tongue is red or dark red, with a white or yellow coating, and the pulse is thin, wiry, and choppy.

Analysis: Qi is the leader of blood; when qi flows smoothly, blood follows, but when qi is stagnant, blood becomes stagnant. Heat congeals in the intestines obstruct the flow of qi, leading to blood stasis at the anus. This causes the anal mass to protrude and cause swelling and pain. When qi flow is disrupted and unable to regulate blood, blood deviates from its normal course, leading to thrombus formation. A dark red tongue and a choppy pulse indicate the presence of internal blood stasis.

Treatment: Clear heat and dampness, dispel wind, and activate blood circulation.

Formula: Modified Zhitong Roushen Tang (Pain-Relieving and Marvelous Decoction) from Waike Qixuan (Mysteries of Surgery). Common ingredients include *Gentiana macrophylla* (Qinjiao), *Prunus persica* (Taoren), *Semen gleditsiae* (Zaojiazi), *Atractylodes lancea* (Cangzhu), *Saposhnikovia divaricata* (Fangfeng), *Phellodendron amurense* (Huangbai), *Angelica sinensis* (Dangguiwei), *Alisma plantago* (Zexie), *Areca catechu* (Binglang), and *Rheum palmatum* (Shudahuang).

Domestic research has shown that Modified Zhitong Roushen Tang is effective for bleeding from internal hemorrhoids with qi stagnation and blood stasis. The formula consists of *Gentiana macrophylla* 10 g, *Prunus persica* 6 g, *Sanguisorba officinalis* 15 g, *Sophora japonica* 10 g, *Atractylodes lancea* 10 g, *Saposhnikovia divaricata* 6 g, *Schizonepeta tenuifolia* 6 g, *Phellodendron amurense* 10 g, *Angelica sinensis* 10 g, *Alisma plantago* 10 g, *Areca catechu* 6 g, and *Rheum palmatum* 10 g. The herbs are boiled in water and taken hot on an empty stomach, twice a day. If there is anal dampness and itching, add *Stephania tetrandra* (Fangji) and *Notopterygium incisum* (Qianghuo); for swelling and pain, add *Citrus aurantium* (Qingpi) and *Corydalis yanhusuo* (Yanhusuo); for excessive bleeding, add *Rehmannia glutinosa* (Shengdihuang) and Moutan Cortex (Danshen) [8].

3.1.4 Spleen deficiency and Qi Sinking

Symptoms: Anal relaxation, prolapsed hemorrhoidal nuclei requiring manual repositioning, bright red or pale bleeding, pale complexion, fatigue, lack of energy, shortness of breath, poor appetite, and loose stools. The tongue is pale with a thin white coating, and the pulse is weak.

Analysis: This condition often occurs in the elderly with qi deficiency, women who have given birth frequently, or children with chronic diarrhea or dysentery. These factors lead to abnormal spleen and stomach functions, spleen deficiency with qi sinking, insufficient middle qi, and an inability to retain the hemorrhoidal nuclei. Qi deficiency impairs the production of blood and the regulation of blood flow, leading to pale bleeding. Spleen deficiency also causes poor nourishment of the skin and muscles, resulting in fatigue and a pale complexion. A pale tongue, white coating, and weak pulse indicate spleen qi deficiency.

Treatment: Tonify the spleen and boost qi.

Main formula: Modified Bu Zhong Yi Qi Tang (Tonify the Middle and Boost Qi Decoction) from Pi Wei Lun (Treatise on the Spleen and Stomach). Common ingredients include *Astragalus membranaceus* (Huangqi), *Panax ginseng* (Renshen), *Atractylodes macrocephala* (Baizhu), *Angelica sinensis* (Danggui), *Glycyrrhiza uralensis* (Zhi Gancao), *Cimicifuga racemosa* (Shengma), *Bupleurum chinense* (Chaihu), and *Citrus reticulata* (Chenpi). For slightly dry stools, add *Cistanche deserticola* (Roucongrong) and *Cannabis sativa* (Huomaren); for severe anemia, combine with Siwu Tang (Four-Ingredient Decoction). Common ready-made medicines include *Sophora japonica* (Huajiao) pills, *Sanguisorba officinalis* (Diyu) pills, Zanglian Wan (Intestine-Connecting pills), and Bu Zhong Yi Qi Wan (Tonify the Middle and Boost Qi pills), which are selected based on differential diagnosis.

"Chronic illness often leads to deficiency." Patients with hemorrhoids who have long-term bleeding are bound to consume qi and injure blood, often worsening with fatigue and showing signs of insufficient middle qi. Following the principles of "warming the exhausted" and "tonifying the damaged," Modified Bu Zhong Yi Qi Tang can be used, with ingredients such as *Astragalus membranaceus* 30 g, *Codonopsis pilosula* (Dangshen), *Atractylodes macrocephala* (Baizhu), *Angelica sinensis* (Danggui), *Sanguisorba officinalis* (Diyuzhi), *Sophora japonica* (Huajiao Zhi), *Platycladus orientalis* (Cebai Zhi), *Lonicera japonica* (Jinyinhua) 10 g each, *Taraxacum mongolicum* (Pugongying) 15 g, *Bupleurum chinense* (Chaihu), *Cimicifuga racemosa* (Shengma), and *Glycyrrhiza uralensis* (Zhi Gancao) 6 g each, combined with heat-clearing and hemostatic herbs, which often show good results [9]. A large dose of Astragalus membranaceus helps alleviate the prolapse and swelling of the anus in patients with internal hemorrhoids (**Table 1**) [10].

3.2 External therapies

3.2.1 Fumigation and sitz bath

Herbs are boiled in water, and the steam is used to fumigate the affected area before washing or using a towel dipped in the hot herbal liquid for warm compresses. The water is replaced when it cools. Alternatively, a sitz bath can be taken in a warm herbal solution. The heat from the water dilates local blood vessels, promotes blood flow, enhances the absorption of medicinal properties, improves local circulation, and has effects such as activating blood circulation to relieve pain and reducing swelling. Common formulas include Modified Wubeizi Tang (Fivefold Powder Decoction) [*Galla chinensis* (Wubeizi), sodium sulfate (Mangxiao), *Taxillus chinensis* (Sangjisheng), *Lycopodium clavatum* (Zelan), *Schizonepeta tenuifolia* (Jingjie), *Nelumbo nucifera* (Lianfang) 30 g each, *Phellodendron amurense* (Huangbai), *Rheum palmatum* (Shudahuang), *Lonicera japonica* (Jinyinhua), *Lithospermum erythrorhizon* (Zicao), *Angelica dahurica* (Baizhi) 15 g each, *Angelica sinensis* (Danggui) 12 g, *Cimicifuga racemosa* (Shengma) 9 g [11] and Modified Ku Shen Tang (Sophora Decoction) [*Sophora flavescens* (Kushen), *Scutellaria baicalensis* (Huangqin), *Lonicera*

Differentiation criteria	Wind-damaging intestinal collaterals	Damp-heat descending	Qi stagnation and blood stasis	Spleen deficiency with qi sinking
Core pathogenesis	Wind-heat scorching collaterals	Damp-heat accumulation	Qi stagnation and blood stasis	Middle qi collapse
Tongue manifestation	Red tongue with yellow coating	Red tongue with yellow greasy coating	Dark purple tongue with ecchymosis	Pale, swollen tongue with tooth marks
Pulse characteristics	Floating and rapid	Slippery and rapid	Wiry and choppy	Thready and weak
Primary formula	Liangxue Dihuang Decoction (Cool Blood Rehmannia Decoction)	Zang Lian Pills (Visceral Coptis Pills)	Zhitong Rushen Decoction (Pain-Relieving Divine Decoction)	Buzhong Yiqi Decoction (Tonify the Middle, Boost Qi Decoction)
Modern pharmacological targets	Inhibits vascular permeability	Regulates intestinal flora balance	Improves microcirculatory disorders	Enhances smooth muscle tension

Table 1.
Hemorrhoid pattern differentiation in TCM.

japonica (Jinyinhua), *Schisandra chinensis* (Wuweizi), *Galla chinensis* (Wubeizi) 9 g each, and other herbs] [12].

3.2.2 Topical application

Medicines are applied directly to the affected area. This method has effects such as reducing swelling, relieving pain, stopping bleeding, and promoting tissue regeneration. For example, Jiuhua Ointment (Nine-Flower Ointment) [Talcum (Huaishi) 50 g, *Gypsum fibrosum* (Yueshi) 75 g, *Draconis ossifragium* (Longgu) 100 g, *Platycodon grandiflorus* (Jiegeng), *Borneolum syntheticum* (Bingpian), and Pearl (Zhenzhu) 15 g each, plus additional ingredients] can be applied to the affected area, 1–2 times a day, and is suitable for various anorectal diseases [13].

3.2.3 Suppositories

Medicines are formulated into suppositories and inserted into the anus. They have effects such as reducing swelling, relieving pain, and stopping bleeding. Pujixie Suppository is effective in improving pain, exudation, bleeding, and swelling after hemorrhoid surgery [14].

3.2.4 Herbal enema

Retention enema with traditional Chinese medicine can effectively reduce the feeling of anal fullness and the incidence of bleeding [15]. In patients with ulcerative colitis complicated by hemorrhoids, the use of shallow catheter retention enema has been shown to reduce discomfort and improve therapeutic efficacy [16].

3.3 Treatment with traditional chinese patent medicines

Commonly used medications include:

a. Zhiran Xiao Tablets (composed of 18 traditional Chinese medicinal herbs including frankincense, myrrh, *Rehmannia glutinosa*, *Codonopsis pilosula*, *Sophora japonica*, *Cynomorium songaricum*, *Astragalus membranaceus*, *Bupleurum chinense*, Typhae Pollen, and *Aurantium immaturum*. Oral administration: three times a day, three tablets each time) [17].

b. Lianzhi San Ointment (ingredients: *Coptis chinensis*, *Phellodendron amurense*, *Scutellaria baicalensis*, *Rheum palmatum*, *Borneolum syntheticum*, Sanguis Draconis, and *Lithospermum erythrorhizon*) [18].

c. Diyu Huajiao Pills.

d. Jingwanhong Ointment [19].

e. Ma Yinglong Musk Hemorrhoids Ointment, etc.

3.4 Acupuncture and moxibustion therapies

3.4.1 Theoretical foundation of TCM

TCM holds that the formation of hemorrhoids (Zhì) is closely related to the "blockage of the meridians and collaterals and the obstruction of qi and blood circulation". The Huangdi Neijing (Inner Canon of the Yellow Emperor) states that "The meridians are used to circulate qi and blood and nourish yin and yang." If one sits or stands for a long time or has an irregular diet, it can lead to the stagnation of qi and blood in the Bladder Meridian of Foot-Taiyang (which runs around the anus and rectum), and then hemorrhoid nuclei will develop.

"The unobstructed flow of qi and blood leads to no pain" is the core principle of acupuncture and moxibustion. By stimulating specific acupoints such as Changqiang (GV1) and Chengshan (BL57) [20], it can activate the meridian qi, dredge the stagnation around the anus and rectum, and achieve the effects of "promoting blood circulation, dissipating nodules, relieving pain and reducing swelling"[21].

4. Specific steps

4.1 Acupuncture

4.1.1 Principle of acupoint selection

See **Table 2** and **Figure 1** [22].

Primary points	**Changqiang (GV1) [2], Chengshan (BL57), Erbai (EX-UE2)**
syndrome of wind injuring the intestinal collaterals	Fengmen (BL12), Dachangshu (BL25), Kunlun (BL60)
Syndrome of downward flow of damp-heat	Yinlingquan (SP9), Dachangshu (BL25), Ciliao (BL32)
Syndrome of qi deficiency failing to control	Baihui (GV20), Pishu (BL20), Guanyuan Shu (BL26)
Syndrome of blood stasis blocking the collaterals	Qihai (CV6), Guanyuan (CV4), Xuehai (SP10)
Anal swelling and pain	Add Zhibian (BL54)
Constipation	Add Shangjuxu (ST37)

Table 2.
Table of acupoint selection based on syndrome differentiation.

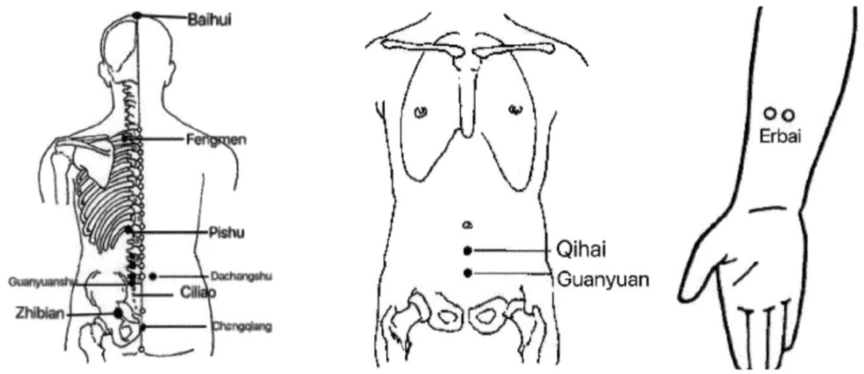

Figure 1.
Schematic diagram of main acupoints.

4.1.2 Operating methods

1. Body position: Prone or lateral position, exposing the anal area.
2. Needles: Select filiform needles with a diameter of 0.25–0.35 mm and a length of 25–50 mm, depending on the depth of the acupoints.
3. Local disinfection: Use 75% alcohol or iodine tincture to disinfect the needling area to prevent infection.
4. Specific acupuncture manipulation:

Changqiang (GV1): Located at the midpoint between the coccyx and the anus, below the end of the coccyx. Insert the needle vertically or at an angle, with a depth of about 1–1.5 transverse finger widths. The needle sensation should radiate to the perineum, and the needle is retained for 20 minutes.

Chengshan (BL57): Located on the posterior side of the lower leg, at the midpoint line between the heel and the popliteal fossa, below the gastrocnemius muscle. Insert the needle vertically for 1–1.5 transverse finger widths. After obtaining the Qi sensation, perform reinforcing or reducing techniques. For hemorrhoids with excess syndrome, use the reducing method with large amplitude lifting and thrusting and rapid twisting to enhance the needle sensation. For hemorrhoids with deficiency syndrome, use the reinforcing method with small amplitude lifting and thrusting and slow twisting to warm and tonify the meridian Qi.

Erbai (EX-UE2): Located on the anterior side of the forearm, four transverse finger widths above the wrist crease, on both sides of the tendon of the flexor carpi radialis, with one point on each side, totaling two points. Insert the needle vertically for 1–1.5 transverse finger widths, retain the needle for 15–20 minutes, and use the balanced reinforcing-reducing method.

5. Treatment course and precautions:

Mild hemorrhoids: Acupuncture treatment 2–3 times a week, with one treatment course consisting of 10–15 sessions.

Moderate to severe hemorrhoids: Three to four times a week. The treatment frequency can be appropriately increased in the early stage, and the treatment course can be extended to 20–30 sessions.

Interval between treatment courses: Take an interval of 3–5 days after each treatment course before starting the next one to consolidate the therapeutic effect.

Precautions:

1. For hemorrhoids with severe concurrent infection or necrosis, surgical treatment should be carried out first and then combined with acupuncture treatment.

2. Control of acupuncture depth: During the acupuncture process, the depth should be strictly mastered, especially for acupoints around the anus (such as Changqiang, etc.). Avoid inserting the needle too deeply. Inserting the needle too deeply may pierce the rectal wall, causing local injury or infection. The depth of insertion is generally preferably 0.5–1 cun. For some non-sensitive areas, attention should also be paid to the acupuncture depth. For example, for the Chengshan acupoint, it is recommended to insert the needle straight for 1–2 cun, and avoid inserting it deep into the gastrocnemius muscle to prevent damage to nerves and blood vessels.

3. Strictly adhere to the principle of aseptic operation: The skin should be fully disinfected before and after acupuncture, and disposable sterile needles should be used to avoid cross-infection.

4. During the acupuncture process, closely observe the patient's reaction and adjust the operation in a timely manner:

   It is a normal needling sensation for the patient to feel soreness, numbness, distension, and heaviness. If the patient experiences severe pain or an electric shock-like sensation, it may be that the nerve has been accidentally injured, and the acupuncture depth and angle should be adjusted immediately or the needle should be withdrawn.

   Some individual patients may experience syncope reactions during acupuncture, such as dizziness, sweating, palpitations, and nausea. Stop the acupuncture immediately, let the patient lie flat and rest, and give warm water or a small amount of sugar water.

5. Contraindications of acupuncture

Pregnant women: Especially in the early stage of pregnancy (within 3 months), it is prohibited to acupuncture the acupoints on the abdomen and lumbosacral region, such as Tianshu (ST25), Changqiang (GV1), and Yaoyan (EX-B7), to avoid inducing uterine contractions and leading to miscarriage.

Patients with coagulation disorders: If the patient has hemophilia or is taking anticoagulant drugs, there may be continuous bleeding or hematoma after acupuncture, so careful consideration should be given to whether acupuncture treatment is suitable.

Local skin infection or ulcer: If there is infection, ulcer, or acute inflammation on the skin around the anus, acupuncture at the affected area is prohibited to prevent the aggravation of the infection.

6. Precautions for acupuncture for special populations

Diabetic patients: Their skin has a weaker healing ability, and they are prone to infection or hematoma after acupuncture. More attention should be paid to aseptic operation during the operation, and thinner needles should be selected. Frequent acupuncture at the same site should be avoided.

Cardiac patients: If there is a cardiac pacemaker, avoid using electroacupuncture therapy to prevent interfering with the function of the pacemaker.

Elderly patients: The tissues of the elderly are fragile, and the meridian qi and blood are insufficient. The manipulation during acupuncture should be gentle and slow, the time should not be too long, and the depth should be controlled within the patient's tolerance range.

4.2 Picking therapy

Picking therapy is a form of traditional Chinese external treatment, evolved from the ancient "nine needles" technique known as "luo pricking" [23]. It primarily involves using a three-edged needle to prick hemorrhoid points on the back-shu acupoints or the Yintang (GV28) acupoint in the oral cavity to expel stagnant blood or metabolic waste. This method aims to unblock the meridians and harmonize the flow of Qi and blood. Picking therapy is particularly effective in treating hemorrhoids, especially internal and mixed hemorrhoids, by alleviating symptoms and reducing recurrence. The specific steps for treating hemorrhoids with picking therapy are as follows:

4.2.1 Preoperative preparation

- Patient assessment: Determine the type and stage of hemorrhoids. Picking therapy is suitable for early-stage internal and mixed hemorrhoids. For external hemorrhoids (e.g., thrombosed external hemorrhoids), it is only used after the condition has stabilized. Confirm whether the patient has contraindications such as coagulation disorders, local infections, or immune system diseases.

- Instrument and material preparation: Prepare a three-edged needle (strictly sterilized), alcohol, iodine tincture, cotton swabs, sterile gauze, hemostatic forceps, and other auxiliary tools.

- Environment and position: Maintain a sterile environment during treatment to avoid infection risks. The patient may assume a knee-chest position, prone position, or lateral position to fully expose the hemorrhoid area while ensuring the patient's comfort.

4.2.2 Operating steps

1. Disinfect the treatment area with 75% alcohol or iodine tincture to prevent bacterial infection.

2. Hemorrhoid point picking: Hemorrhoid points are typically located within the range of the two axillary posterior lines from the sides of the seventh thoracic vertebra to the second sacral bone. They appear papule-like shapes but do not protrude above the skin, are about the size of a large-headed pin, and are usually grayish-white, dark red, brownish, or light red in color. If the hemorrhoid points are not obvious, rub the waist and sacral area with a ginger block until the skin turns red, and carefully search for the points. If no distinct hemorrhoid points are found, select acupoints for picking therapy. Commonly used acupoints include Dachangshu (BL25), Xiaochangshu (BL27), Mingmen (GV4), Changqiang (GV1), Shangliao (BL31), Ciliao (BL32), Zhongliao (BL33), and Xialiao (BL34). Select 1–3 distinct hemorrhoid points for treatment each time, and it is ideal to cut through the subcutaneous white fibrous tissue during the procedure. Perform picking therapy once every 10 days, with three sessions constituting one course of treatment.

3. Gingtang (GV28) picking: The Gingtang acupoint is located at the frenulum of the upper lip. "Observing the lip frenulum for diagnosing internal hemorrhoids" is a method for examining and diagnosing anal and rectal diseases such as hemorrhoids and fistulas. In most hemorrhoid patients, one or more millet-sized papules can be observed at the Gingtang acupoint. A three-edged needle or a small scalpel needle can be used for picking and bloodletting therapy.

4.2.3 Postoperative management

- Wipe away any exudate or blood from the puncture site with sterile gauze and disinfect again with iodine tincture.

- Apply gentle pressure to the puncture site until bleeding stops, then cover the wound with sterile gauze to protect it.

4.2.4 Course of treatment and precautions

- Treat once a week, with two to four sessions constituting one course of treatment. Adjust the duration of the course based on the severity of the hemorrhoids and the patient's constitution.

- Maintain cleanliness around the anus after the procedure. Take a warm water sitz bath daily to prevent infection.
- If there is a significant increase in redness, swelling, heat, and pain at the site, seek medical attention promptly.
- Avoid excessive picking to prevent damage to normal tissue or bleeding.
- Do not use picking therapy in patients with infected hemorrhoids or a significant tendency to bleed.

4.3 Acupoint embedding therapy

Acupoint embedding is a minimally invasive technique in traditional Chinese acupuncture and moxibustion treatment [24]. It involves embedding absorbable medical protein threads into specific acupoints to provide continuous stimulation, thereby regulating the functions of the viscera, improving local circulation, and enhancing immunity. The specific steps for treating hemorrhoids with acupoint embedding are as follows:

4.3.1 Preoperative preparation

Collect medical history to confirm the type (internal, external, or mixed hemorrhoids) and stage of hemorrhoids and exclude contraindications for embedding, such as local infection or coagulation disorders.

Choose a sterile operating environment and prepare disposable medical embedding needles, absorbable protein threads (such as catgut or collagen threads), and disinfectants like alcohol or iodine tincture.

Have the patient assume a prone or lateral position, adjusting the position according to the specific location of the acupoints to fully expose the operating area.

4.3.2 Acupoint selection

Select specific acupoints related to hemorrhoids based on the principles of traditional Chinese medicine diagnosis and treatment. Refer to the acupoint selection in the acupuncture method mentioned above.

4.3.3 Operating steps

Disinfect the area around the acupoints three times with 75% alcohol or iodine tincture to ensure a sterile operating environment.

Use a disposable embedding needle and follow aseptic operating standards:

- Quickly insert the embedding needle into the marked acupoint and push the thread into the acupoint after reaching the optimal depth. Slowly withdraw the embedding needle, ensuring that the thread is completely retained within the acupoint without exposure or residue.
- Press the embedding site with a clean cotton swab to check for bleeding. If there is slight bleeding, apply pressure with sterile gauze to stop the bleeding.
- Cover the site with sterile dressing after disinfection to prevent infection.

4.3.4 Course of treatment and precautions

- Typically, embedding is performed every 2 weeks, with the course of treatment determined based on the severity of the hemorrhoids and the patient's constitution, usually requiring 3–5 sessions.
- Avoid contact with water at the embedding site to prevent infection.
- If local redness, pain, fever, or allergic reactions occur, discontinue treatment and manage the symptoms accordingly.

4.4 Fire needle therapy

Fire needle therapy is a form of traditional Chinese external treatment that involves using a red-hot needle to stimulate the affected area or specific acupoints to achieve the effects of clearing heat and detoxifying, reducing swelling and relieving pain, and promoting tissue regeneration [25]. Fire needle therapy is particularly effective in treating internal and mixed hemorrhoids. The specific steps for treating hemorrhoids with fire needle therapy are as follows:

4.4.1 Preoperative preparation

- Patient preparation:
    - Confirm the type (internal, external, or mixed hemorrhoids) and stage of hemorrhoids. This therapy is commonly used for patients with first- to second-degree internal hemorrhoids or mild to moderate mixed hemorrhoids.
    - Exclude contraindications such as severe infection at the site, local skin ulceration, coagulation disorders, or excessive fear of fire needle therapy.
    - Have the patient assume a knee-chest or lateral position to expose the anal area, ensuring stability and comfort during treatment.
- Instrument preparation: Select stainless steel medical fire needles with length and diameter adjusted according to the size of the patient's hemorrhoids (commonly used thick needles range from 0.8 mm to 1.5 mm). Prepare an alcohol lamp or a dedicated fire needle heating device, 75% alcohol, iodine tincture, sterile cotton swabs, hemostatic forceps, gauze, and sterile dressings.

4.4.2 Acupoint selection

Direct puncture of the lesion:

Internal hemorrhoids: Directly puncture the surface of the hemorrhoid nucleus, with 3–5 puncture points per nucleus, focusing on the central or most protruding part.

External hemorrhoids: Puncture the protruding part of the external hemorrhoid, avoiding excessive stimulation of the normal perianal skin.

Acupoints for syndrome differentiation and treatment: Refer to the acupoint selection in the acupuncture method mentioned above for systemic regulation.

4.4.3 Operating steps

Disinfect the perianal skin and the hemorrhoid area with 75% alcohol or iodine tincture, ensuring the disinfection area is slightly larger than the treatment area. Heat the fire needle in the flame of the alcohol lamp until it is uniformly red-hot (approximately 600–800°C).

Direct Puncture of the lesion: Quickly insert the red-hot fire needle into the surface of the hemorrhoid nucleus. Adjust the insertion depth according to the thickness of the nucleus, usually 0.5–2 mm, and withdraw the needle immediately after insertion. Ensure even distribution of puncture points and avoid repeated insertion into the same area. For larger hemorrhoids, increase the number of puncture points appropriately.

Superficial puncture of auxiliary acupoints: For acupoints used for systemic regulation (e.g., Changqiang [GV1] and Chengshan [BL57]), lightly puncture 1–2 mm to regulate the flow of Qi and blood and promote local recovery.

Postoperative management: Immediately press the puncture site with a sterile cotton swab to check for bleeding. After treatment, disinfect the area again with iodine tincture and cover with sterile gauze to prevent infection.

4.4.4 Course of treatment and precautions

- Treat once a week based on the severity of the condition, with four to six sessions constituting one course of treatment. After the hemorrhoids have significantly reduced in size, extend the interval between treatments to consolidate the therapeutic effect.

- Maintain cleanliness around the anus after the procedure. Take a warm saltwater sitz bath daily to promote local circulation and prevent infection.

- Local redness and pain are normal phenomena, usually lasting 1–3 days. Apply erythromycin ointment topically for anti-inflammatory effects. If there is a significant increase in redness, swelling, heat, and pain, seek medical attention promptly and consider anti-infective treatment.

4.5 Moxibustion

Moxibustion, a type of thermal therapy, involves burning moxa wool to warm and stimulate acupoints, thereby warming the meridians, dispersing cold, relieving pain, and promoting blood circulation [26]. It is a commonly used adjunctive therapy for hemorrhoids. The detailed steps for treating hemorrhoids with moxibustion are as follows:

- Suspended moxibustion: After acupuncture, moxibustion can be applied to acupoints such as Changqiang (GV1), Chengshan (BL57), Qihai (CV6), and Baihui (GV20) to warm the meridians and promote blood circulation. Light the moxa stick and hold it 3–5 cm away from the acupoint, performing suspended moxibustion for 10–15 minutes per point until the area feels warm but not painfully hot.

- Ginger-partition moxibustion: Suitable for hemorrhoids of the deficiency-cold type, this method has the effect of warming the meridians and dispersing cold. Cut fresh ginger slices about 0.2 cm thick and pierce several holes in the center. Place the ginger slice on the acupoint and place the ignited moxa cone on the ginger slice. Replace the moxa cone after it has burned out, performing this process three to five times.

4.6 Cupping therapy

Cupping therapy involves using negative pressure to stimulate local skin and acupoints, promoting blood circulation, reducing swelling, relieving pain, and warming the meridians [27]. It is used to treat hemorrhoids by improving blood circulation around the anus, reducing the size of the hemorrhoids, and alleviating local itching and pain.

4.6.1 Common cupping sites

Back bladder meridian: Dachangshu (BL25), Ciliao (BL32), Changqiang (GV1).
Local lesion sites:

- Perianal area around the hemorrhoids: Handle gently to avoid direct stimulation of the hemorrhoids.
- Limb meridian acupoints: Chengshan (BL57), Erbai (EX-UE2).
- Abdominal acupoints: Qihai (CV6), Zhongwan (CV12).

4.6.2 Operating steps

Cleaning and disinfection: Disinfect the treatment area with iodine tincture or alcohol swabs to maintain skin cleanliness.

Application of lubricant: Apply a small amount of lubricant to the cupping site to facilitate the adhesion of the cup to the skin and reduce discomfort.

Cupping method: Hold an ignited alcohol-soaked cotton ball with fire tongs, quickly burn it inside the cup, and immediately place the cup opening over the acupoint. Perform the operation quickly to ensure the formation of negative pressure and secure the adhesion of the cup to the skin.

Retention time: Retain the cup for 10–15 minutes, until the skin shows a slight redness or mild ecchymosis.

Removal of cup: Press one side of the cup opening with your hand and gently lift the cup to avoid pulling on the skin and causing pain.

4.6.3 Precautions

- Cupping is contraindicated in patients with local skin ulcers, infections, or bleeding tendencies.

- Patients with severe heart disease, anemia, or sensitive skin should use cupping with caution.

- During fire cupping, control the fire source to avoid burning the skin.

4.7 Auricular therapy

Auricular therapy involves stimulating specific acupoints in the ear to regulate the body's functions and treat hemorrhoids [28]. The dense distribution of ear acupoints is connected to the viscera and meridians throughout the body. Stimulating these points can clear heat and dampness, promote blood circulation, remove blood stasis, and relieve pain.

4.7.1 Common auricular acupoints and their locations

- Large intestine point: On the upper edge of the helix, below the stomach point.

- Rectum lower segment: At the recess on the lower edge of the helix.

- Anus point: On the outer side of the triangular fossa, near the root of the helix.

- Spleen point: In the lower part of the triangular fossa, below the stomach point.

- Endocrine point: In the central part of the earlobe.

- Shenmen point: In the lower part of the triangular fossa, near the lower edge of the helix.

4.7.2 Operating steps for auricular acupuncture or seed pressing

Ear disinfection: Clean the auricle with alcohol swabs or iodine tincture, especially the skin area around the selected acupoints.

Locating sensitive points: Use a probe to gently press the auricular acupoint area to find sensitive points that are tender to pressure or slightly hard in texture. These points are the target sites for acupuncture or seed pressing.

Acupuncture operation:

- Needle insertion: Hold the auricle with the left hand and insert the needle with the right hand. Insert the needle quickly into the auricular acupoint to a depth of about 1–2 mm, with a slight inward angle to avoid over-penetration.

- Needling technique:

  a. For deficiency-type hemorrhoids, use the tonifying method: Gently lift and thrust or slowly twist the needle for about 1 minute.

  b. For excess-heat type hemorrhoids, use the reducing method: Quickly lift and thrust and twist the needle for 1–2 minutes to enhance the stimulation.

- Retention time: Retain the needle for 20–30 minutes, and intermittently twist the needle during retention to enhance the stimulation effect.

Seed pressing:

- Apply Vaccaria seeds to the sensitive points found. Gently press the auricular acupoints 3–5 times a day for 1–2 minutes each time. Each application lasts 3–5 days. Clean the auricle before reapplying and observe for any local irritation or skin discomfort. If redness or allergic reactions occur, discontinue use until the skin recovers and then resume application.

4.8 Acupoint injection therapy

Acupoint injection is a therapeutic method that combines traditional Chinese acupuncture with modern medicine [29]. It involves injecting medication into specific acupoints to regulate the meridians, improve local blood circulation, and reduce inflammatory responses. This therapy is effective in treating early-stage internal and mixed hemorrhoids, alleviating symptoms, reducing the size of hemorrhoids, and preventing recurrence. The specific steps and precautions for treating hemorrhoids with acupoint injection are as follows:

4.8.1 Indications and contraindications

- Indications:
    - Internal hemorrhoids (mainly grades I-III), mixed hemorrhoids, and acute or chronic simple external hemorrhoids. Symptoms include bleeding during defecation, pain, and prolapse of hemorrhoids.
- Contraindications:
    - Severe local infection or purulent inflammation.
    - Patients with significant bleeding tendencies (e.g., coagulation disorders).
    - Allergy to the injected medication.
    - Pregnant women or patients with special constitutions should use it with caution.

4.8.2 Preparation for operation

- Instruments: Sterile syringes (25 ml), needles (generally 27G–30G), and disinfectants such as 75% alcohol or iodine tincture.
- Common medications: Vitamin B1, Vitamin B12, Danshen injection, anti-inflammatory and analgesic drugs (e.g., dexamethasone), and compound matrine injection, etc.

4.8.3 Operating steps

Position: Common positions include lateral, knee-chest, or prone positions to fully expose the perianal area and selected acupoints.

Disinfection: Strictly disinfect the perianal area and selected acupoints with iodine tincture or 75% alcohol to prevent infection.

Acupoints: Chengshan (BL57), Erbai (EX-UE2), Changqiang (GV1), Dachangshu (BL25), Tianshu (ST25).

Injection operation:

- Draw the medication, confirm the dosage, and expel any air from the syringe to ensure no bubbles are present. Insert the sterile injection needle vertically or slightly angled into the subcutaneous tissue of the acupoint, with a depth generally of 0.5–1.0 cm. Slowly inject the medication, with 0.5–1 ml per acupoint. Monitor the patient's reaction during injection to avoid excessive pain or strong local reactions. After injection, press the needle site gently with a cotton swab for 1–2 minutes to prevent extravasation of the medication or bleeding. Cover the site with a sterile adhesive patch and instruct the patient to keep the injection site clean.

- Course of treatment: Treat 2–3 times per week, with 10 sessions constituting one course of treatment. Adjust the duration of the course based on the improvement of the patient's symptoms.

5. Postoperative management strategies integrating TCM and Western medicine

The postoperative management of hemorrhoids is a core link in ensuring the therapeutic effect and reducing the recurrence rate. Based on the principle of traditional Chinese medicine that "in case of an emergency, treat the symptoms first; when the condition is stable, address the root cause," and combined with the precise monitoring technology of modern medicine, this guideline proposes a phased and multidimensional postoperative management plan. It aims to optimize the patient's rehabilitation process through the synergistic effect of traditional Chinese medicine and Western medicine.

5.1 Postoperative management framework and principles

See **Table 3** and **Figure 2**.

Acute phase (0–72 hours after surgery):	The core focuses are analgesia, hemostasis, and anti-infection, with priority given to controlling complications.
Sub-acute phase (3–7 days after surgery):	Promote wound healing and relieve edema and urinary retention.
Recovery phase (1–4 weeks after surgery):	Focus on functional rehabilitation and prevent recurrence.

Table 3.
Postoperative management.

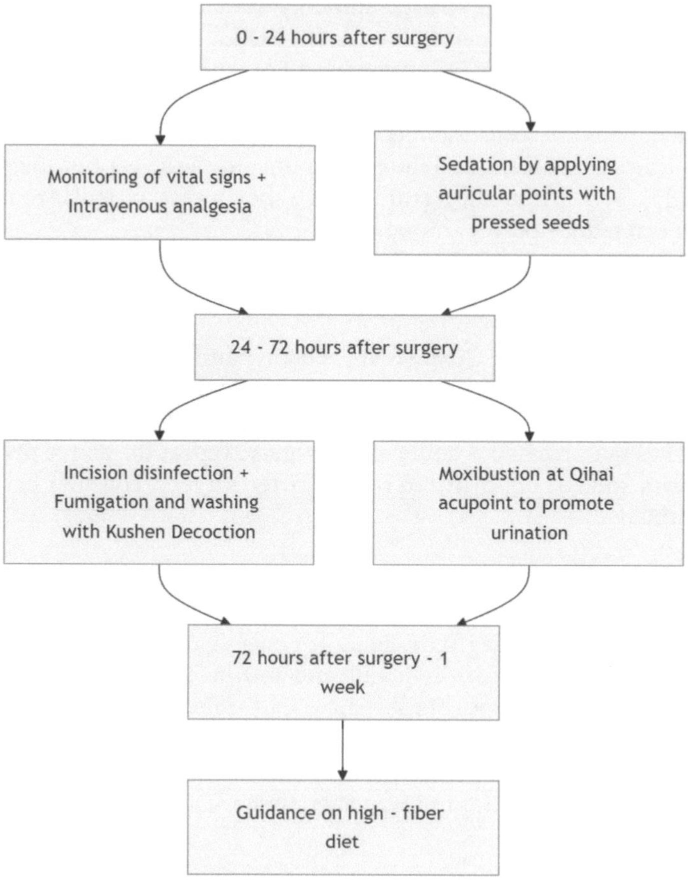

Figure 2.
Phased management path diagram.

5.2 Postoperative TCM management

1. Pain

- Herbal fumigation and washing: This method can activate blood circulation, reduce swelling, and relieve pain. A heat-clearing and stasis-eliminating formula can be used, with the following ingredients: 20 g each of *Sophora flavescens*, *Astragalus membranaceus*, *Phellodendron amurense*, Honeysuckle flower, *Chrysanthemum indicum*, and Dandelion; 15 g each of *Sophora japonica*, *Angelica sinensis*, *Lithospermum erythrorhizon*, and *Corydalis yanhusuo*. The patient should first fumigate the affected area with the herbal liquid, then wash it, ensuring the liquid completely covers the wound. This should be done twice a day for 10 minutes each time [30].

- Acupuncture therapy: The main acupoints used are bilateral Erbai (EX-UE2), with additional points such as Hegu (LI4) and Taichong (LR3). Electroacupuncture can also be applied to the *Baliao acupoints* [31]. Embedding therapy at Changqiang (GV1) is another option [32].

- Auricular therapy: This is also a commonly used method for pain relief. Acupoints such as Shenmen (TF4), Anus (HX5), Rectum Lower Segment (HX2), Large Intestine (CO6), Cortex (AT4), and Adrenal Gland (SP2) can be selected. Depending on the patient's condition, five to six acupoints are chosen each time, with the seeds retained for 1–3 days. Patients can press the acupoints several times a day for 3–5 minutes each time until the ear becomes flushed and warm [33]. Multiple medical studies have shown that auricular therapy before surgery can reduce postoperative pain.

2. Urinary retention

- Select acupoints such as Qihai (RN6), Guanyuan (RN4), Zhongji (RN3), and Sanyinjiao (SP6) [34, 35]. Use a moxa stick held 2–3 cm away from the skin for 15 minutes, until the surrounding skin of the acupoint becomes flushed. If the patient has not urinated 4 hours after surgery, repeat the above procedure. If the patient still has not urinated 6 hours after surgery, consider performing catheterization.

3. Bleeding

- Administer 10 ml of Kangfuxin liquid for enema at a depth of 5–7 cm, followed by the application of a pain-relieving and anti-inflammatory ointment on the external area, secured with sterile gauze [36]. Select auricular acupoints such as Kidney (CO10), Bladder (CO9), Shenmen (TF4), Cortex (AT4), Sympathetic (AH6a), and Anus (HX5). Apply the seeds for 3 days, pressing the acupoints several times a day for 3–5 minutes each time [37].

4. Edema

- Take 50 g each of Lithospermum erythrorhizon, Bletilla striata, Rheum palmatum, and Calcined Gypsum, and 2.5 g of Borneol. Grind them into a fine powder to make Zibai Powder, then mix with Vaseline (1:4) to create Zibai Ointment for external application on the wound, which can help reduce inflammation and swelling [38]. Alternatively, use a modified Sophora Decoction (*Sophora flavescens* 30 g, sodium sulfate 30 g, *Phellodendron amurense* 25 g, *Acorus tatarinowii*, *Kochia scoparia*, *Cnidium monnieri*, *Angelica dahurica* 15 g each, Dandelion, Honeysuckle flower, *Chrysanthemum indicum* 20 g each, *Atractylodes lancea*, Borneol 10 g each) for fumigation and washing, combined with acupoint patch application at the Baliao points to achieve the effect of reducing swelling [39].

5.3 Synergistic management of common postoperative symptoms with TCM and Western medicine

1. Pain management.

   Western medicine approach:

   Stepwise analgesia: For mild pain (VAS $\leq$ 4), oral paracetamol is administered; for moderate to severe pain (VAS > 4), tramadol is combined.

Local treatment: Nitroglycerin ointment is used to relieve sphincter spasm.

TCM intervention:

Acupuncture analgesia: Select acupoints Erbai (EX-UE2) and Changqiang (GV1), stimulate with high-frequency electroacupuncture (2 Hz) for 20 minutes, once a day.

Auricular point pressing with seeds: Apply Vaccaria seeds on Shenmen (TF4) and Subcortex (AT3) auricular points. Patients press them by themselves three times a day, 1 minute each time.

2. Prevention and control of urinary retention

   Western medicine assessment: Monitor the residual urine volume in the bladder by ultrasound (catheterization is required if it is >100 ml).

   TCM approach:

   Moxibustion to promote urination: Suspend moxa sticks to moxibustion Qihai (CV6) and Zhongji (CV3) acupoints, keep a distance of 3 cm from the skin until the local area turns red, for 15 minutes each time.

   Hot compress with Chinese herbal medicine: Stir-fry 30 g of Fennel Fruit and 200 g of coarse salt until hot, wrap them in a cloth and apply them to the lower abdomen, two times a day.

3. Bleeding and wound repair

   Western medicine emergency treatment: For active bleeding, use an adrenaline-soaked cotton ball for compression or electrocoagulation hemostasis.

   TCM to promote healing:

   Enema with Chinese herbal medicine: Use 10 g of carbonized sanguisorba root, 5 g of Bletilla striata powder, and 1 g of Borneol. Decoct them into 50 ml of soup and retain the enema once a day for 5 consecutive days.

   Acupoint pricking treatment: Use a Sanleng needle to prick and release 3–5 drops of blood at Yinjiao (GV28) acupoint, two times a week.

4. Control of edema and inflammation

   Western medicine treatment: Wet compress with 50% magnesium sulfate solution, 20 minutes each time, three times a day.

   External treatment with TCM:

   Pricking and cupping: After disinfecting the skin around the hemorrhoid nucleus, tap gently with a plum blossom needle until there is slight bleeding, and perform flash cupping three to five times, once every other day.

   External application of Chinese herbal medicine: Boil 30 g of *Lithospermum erythrorhizon*, 15 g of *Phellodendron amurense*, and 200 ml of sesame oil to make lithospermum ointment. After refrigeration, apply it to the affected area.

6. Personalized care plans in traditional Chinese medicine (TCM)

In traditional Chinese medicine (TCM), the development of a personalized treatment plan is a meticulous process that takes into account the unique physiological, emotional, and environmental factors of each individual. After a thorough assessment—which includes diagnostic techniques such as pulse reading, tongue examination, and a detailed patient history—TCM practitioners craft a tailored approach to address the root cause of the condition and restore balance within the body. For conditions like hemorrhoids, this personalized treatment plan may include a combination of dietary recommendations and lifestyle modifications. Below is a detailed explanation of each component:

6.1 Dietary recommendations

Diet plays a crucial role in TCM, as it is believed to directly influence the balance of Qi and blood in the body. For hemorrhoid patients, dietary recommendations are tailored to address underlying issues such as poor digestion, heat accumulation, or blood stagnation. Common dietary advice includes:

- *Increasing fiber intake*: To soften stools and prevent constipation, a major contributor to hemorrhoids.
- *Avoiding spicy and greasy foods*: These are considered to generate "heat" in the body, which can exacerbate inflammation and bleeding.
- *Incorporating cooling foods*: Such as cucumbers, watermelon, and mung beans, to reduce internal heat.
- *Strengthening the spleen*: With foods like pumpkin, sweet potatoes, and oats, which are easy to digest and support digestive health.

The dietary plan is personalized based on the patient's constitution, age, and specific symptoms. For example, older patients with weaker digestion may be advised to consume smaller, more frequent meals, while younger patients with heat-related symptoms may focus on cooling foods.

6.2 Lifestyle modifications

Lifestyle adjustments are an integral part of TCM treatment plans, as they address habits and behaviors that may contribute to the condition. For hemorrhoids, lifestyle modifications may include:

- *Improving bowel habits*: Encouraging patients to avoid straining during bowel movements and to establish a regular bathroom routine.
- *Increasing physical activity*: Gentle exercises like Tai Chi or walking are recommended to improve circulation and prevent blood stagnation.
- *Stress management*: Techniques such as meditation, deep breathing, or Qi Gong are suggested to reduce stress, which can negatively impact digestion and exacerbate hemorrhoids.

- *Proper hydration*: Drinking adequate water to support digestion and prevent constipation.

These recommendations are tailored to the patient's daily routine, physical capabilities, and overall health. For instance, sedentary office workers may be advised to take frequent breaks to move around, while patients with mobility issues may focus on seated exercises.

7. Conclusion

This manuscript systematically evaluated the clinical value of comprehensive traditional Chinese medicine (TCM) therapies in the treatment of hemorrhoids and explored their synergistic potential when combined with Western medicine. The results show that TCM treatment can not only effectively relieve symptoms but also improve long-term prognosis through holistic regulation. However, there are still some limitations. Firstly, most TCM clinical trials have a relatively small sample size ($n < 200$) and lack long-term follow-up data for more than 5 years, which limits the universality of the conclusions. Secondly, the standardization of operations for therapies such as acupoint pricking and blood-letting is insufficient, and they rely on the experience of physicians, which may affect the reproducibility of the curative effect. Future research should focus on technology integration and interdisciplinary verification, promote the international formulation of the "Consensus on the Integrated Diagnosis and Treatment of Hemorrhoids with Traditional Chinese and Western Medicine", and incorporate TCM into the regulatory frameworks of the EMA/FDA, which is expected to further enhance its global influence.

In conclusion, TCM treatment for hemorrhoids has significant clinical value, especially in individualized treatment and improvement of long-term prognosis. Through the synergy of TCM and Western medicine, not only can the curative effect be optimized, but also a more comprehensive treatment plan can be provided for patients. Future research should be committed to addressing existing limitations, promoting the modernization and internationalization of TCM, and bringing more benefits to hemorrhoid patients worldwide.

Acknowledgements

The author acknowledges the use of an online translation tool for translating the manuscript from Chinese to English.

Funding

This research was funded by the "Sanming Project" of the China Academy of Chinese Medical Sciences, specifically the innovation and application team for clinical evaluation methods in traditional Chinese acupuncture and moxibustion led by Academician Liu Baoyan (Project No. SZZYSM202311002) and the Guangdong Province Famous Traditional Chinese Medicine Doctor's Studio (Yu Haibo) (Document No. Yue TCM Office [2023] No. 108).

Appendix

See **Table A1**.

Syndrome pattern	Chinese herbal medicine	Image	Efficacy	Notes
Wind Damaging the Intestinal Network	Rehmannia Root (Shengdihuang)	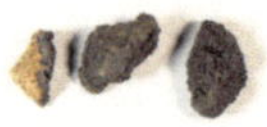	Clears heat, cools blood, nourishes yin, generates fluids	
	Garden Burnet Root (Diyu)	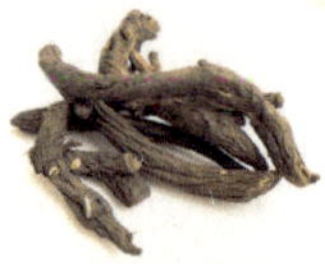	Cools blood, stops bleeding, detoxifies, heals sores	
	Chinese Angelica Root Tail (Dangguiwei)	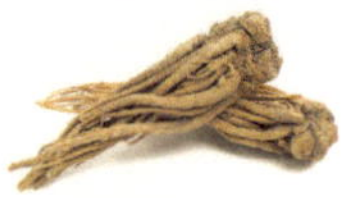	Promotes blood circulation, removes blood stasis, regulates menstruation, relieves pain	
	Coptis Root (Huanglian)	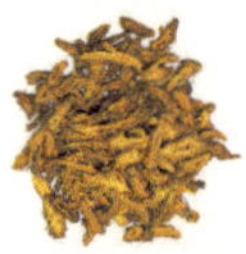	Clears heat, dries dampness, purges fire, detoxifies	
	Scutellaria Root (Huangqin)	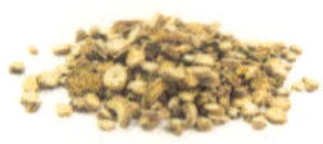	Clears heat, dries dampness, purges fire, detoxifies, calms the fetus	
	Trichosanthes Root (Tianhuafen)	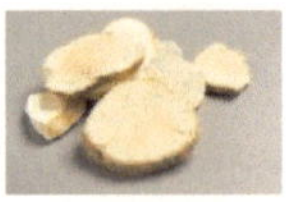	Clears heat, purges fire, generates fluids, relieves thirst, reduces swelling, discharges pus	
	Cimicifuga Rhizome (Shengma)	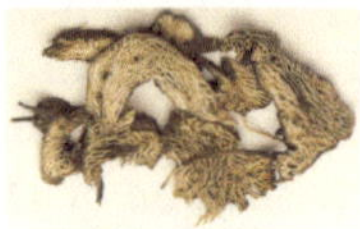	Releases the exterior, promotes rash eruption, clears heat, detoxifies, raises yang qi	
	Bitter Orange Peel (Zhiqiao)	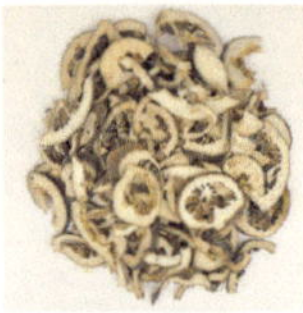	Regulates qi, soothes the middle, relieves stagnation, reduces distension	
	Schizonepeta Herb (Jingjie)	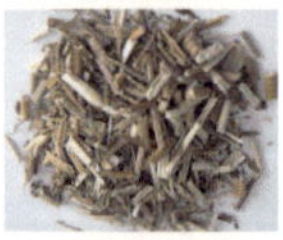	Releases the exterior, dispels wind, promotes rash eruption, relieves sores, stops bleeding	
	Red Peony Root (Chishao)	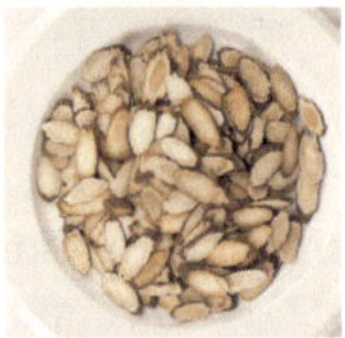	Clears heat, cools blood, disperses blood stasis, relieves pain	

Syndrome pattern	Chinese herbal medicine	Image	Efficacy	Notes
	Licorice Root (Gancao)	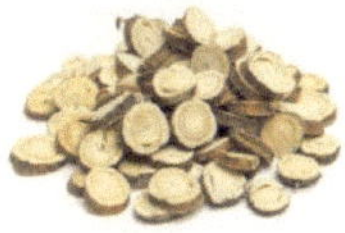	Tonifies the spleen, boosts qi, clears heat, detoxifies, harmonizes other herbs	
	Pseudostellaria Root (Taizishen)	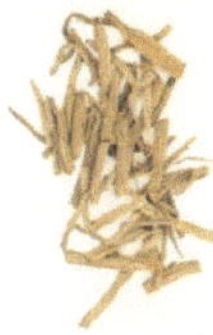	Tonifies qi, strengthens the spleen, generates fluids, moistens the lungs	
	Raw Rhubarb Root (Shengdahuang)	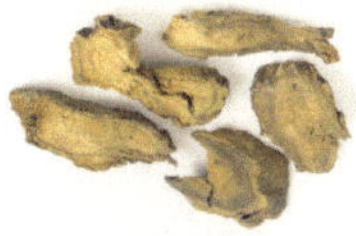	Purges accumulation, clears heat, purges fire, cools blood, detoxifies	Added Later
	Biota Tops (Cebaiye)	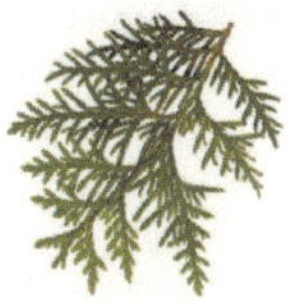	Cools blood, stops bleeding, resolves phlegm, relieves cough	
	Pagoda Tree Flower (Huaihua)	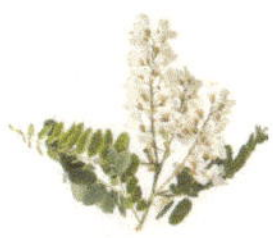	Cools blood, stops bleeding, clears liver fire	
	Honey-fried Astragalus Root (Zhihuangqi)	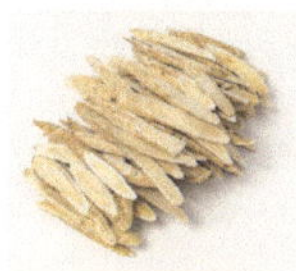	Tonifies qi, raises yang, secures the exterior, stops sweating, promotes urination, reduces swelling	
	Atractylodes Rhizome (Baizhu)	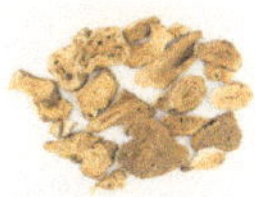	Strengthens the spleen, tonifies qi, dries dampness, promotes urination, stops sweating, calms the fetus	
	Mirabilite (Mangxiao)	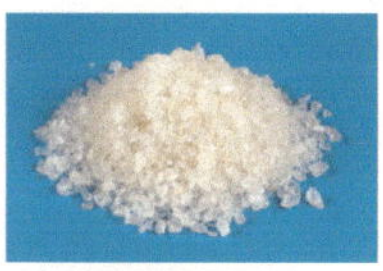	Purges accumulation, moistens dryness, softens hardness, clears heat, reduces swelling	Added Later
Damp-Heat Descending	Coptis Root (Huanglian)	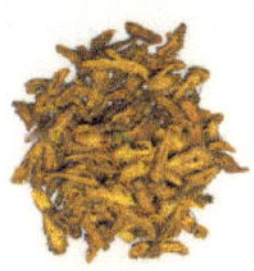	Clears heat, dries dampness, purges fire, detoxifies	
	Pig Large Intestine (Zhudachang)	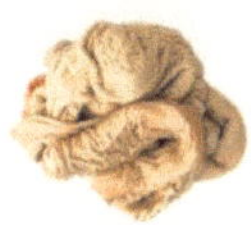	Moistens intestines, relieves constipation, tonifies deficiency	

Syndrome pattern	Chinese herbal medicine	Image	Efficacy	Notes
	Charred Garden Burnet Root (Diyutan)	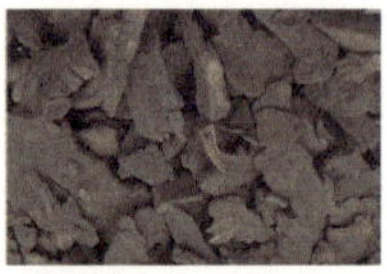	Astringes, stops bleeding, cools blood	
	Hairyvein Agrimonia Herb (Xianhecao)		Astringes, stops bleeding, detoxifies, reduces swelling	
	Pulsatilla Root (Baitouweng)	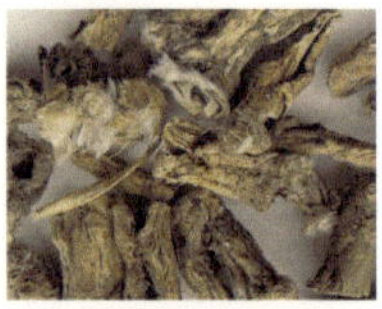	Clears heat, detoxifies, cools blood, stops dysentery	
	Largeleaf Gentian Root (Qinjiao)	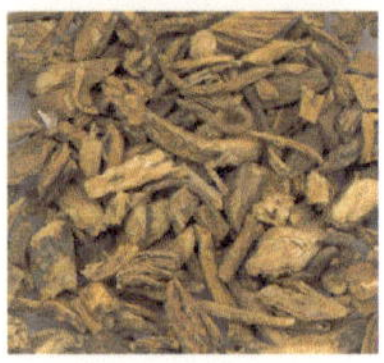	Dispels wind-damp, clears damp-heat, relieves pain	
	Atractylodes Rhizome (Cangzhu)	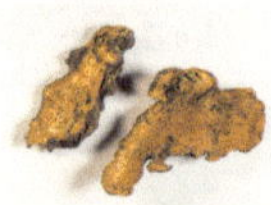	Dries dampness, strengthens the spleen, dispels wind, disperses cold	
	Coix Seed (Yiyiren)	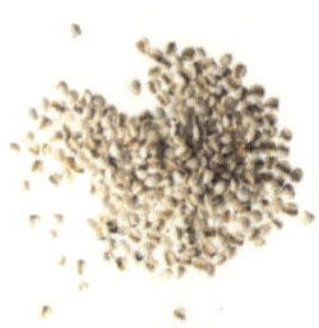	Strengthens the spleen, drains dampness, clears heat, discharges pus	
	Charred Schizonepeta Herb (Jingjietan)	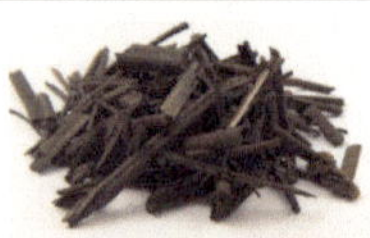	Astringes, stops bleeding, dispels wind, releases the exterior	
	Scutellaria Root (Huangqin)	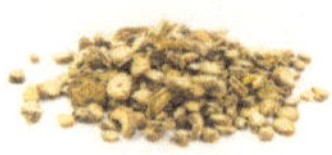	Clears heat, dries dampness, purges fire, detoxifies, calms the fetus	
	Saposhnikovia Root (Fangfeng)	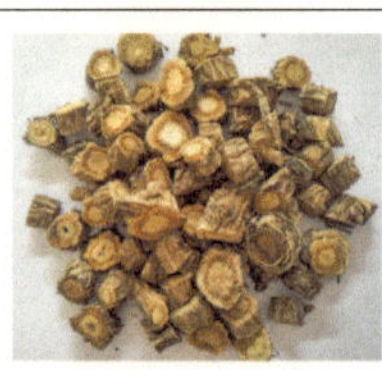	Dispels wind, releases the exterior, overcomes dampness, relieves pain	
	Raw Rhubarb Root (Shengjinwen)	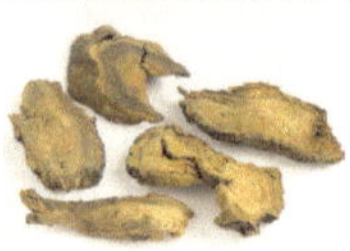	Purges accumulation, clears heat, purges fire	Also Known as Raw Rhubarb Root (Shengdahuan)

Syndrome pattern	Chinese herbal medicine	Image	Efficacy	Notes
	Raw Pagoda Tree Flower Bud (Shenghuaimi)	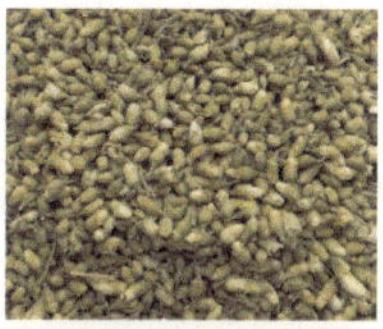	Cools blood, stops bleeding, clears liver fire	
	Hemp Seed (Huomaren)	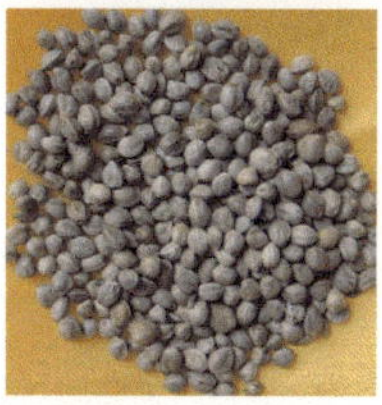	Moistens intestines, relieves constipation, nourishes deficiency	
	Rehmannia Root (Shengdihuang)	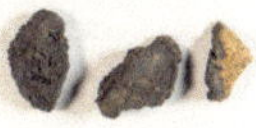	Clears heat, cools blood, nourishes yin, generates fluids	
	Honeysuckle Flower (Jinyinhua)	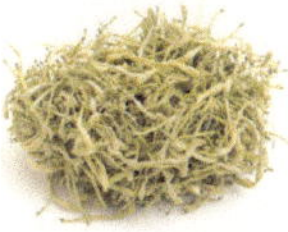	Clears heat, detoxifies, dispels wind-heat	
	Sophora Root (Kushenpian)	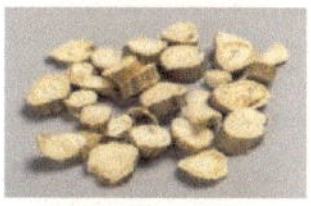	Clears heat, dries dampness, kills parasites, relieves itching	
	Fried Phellodendron Bark (Chaochuanbai)	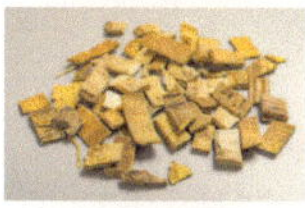	Clears heat, dries dampness, purges fire, detoxifies	
	Rhaponticum Root (Loulu)	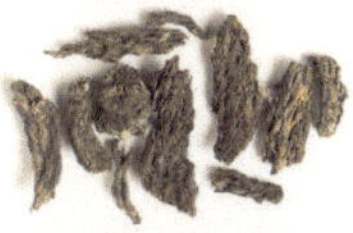	Clears heat, detoxifies, reduces swelling, discharges pus	
	Orostachys Herb (Wahua)	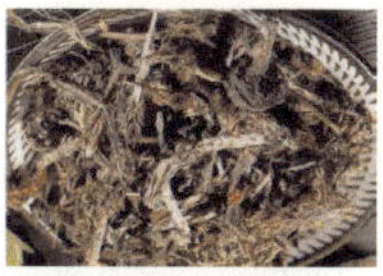	Clears heat, detoxifies, stops bleeding, reduces swelling	Also known as Orostachys Herb (Wasong)
	Mirabilite (Mangxiao)	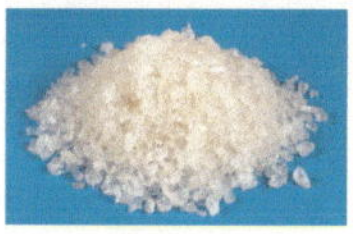	Purges accumulation, moistens dryness, softens hardness	
	Cnidium Seed (Shechuangzi)	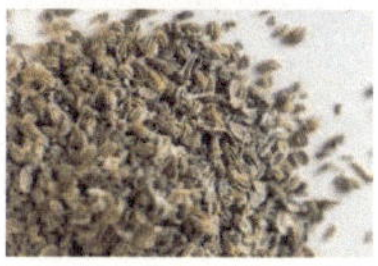	Dries dampness, kills parasites, warms the kidneys, strengthens yang	

Syndrome pattern	Chinese herbal medicine	Image	Efficacy	Notes
	Kochia Seed (Difuzi)		Clears heat, drains dampness, dispels wind, relieves itching	
Qi Stagnation and Blood Stasis	Largeleaf Gentian Root (Qinjiao)	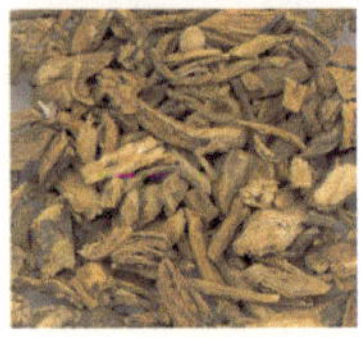	Dispels wind-damp, clears damp-heat, relieves pain	
	Peach Seed (Taoren)	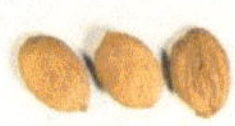	Promotes blood circulation, removes blood stasis, moistens intestines, relieves constipation	
	Gleditsia Seed (Zaojiaozhi)	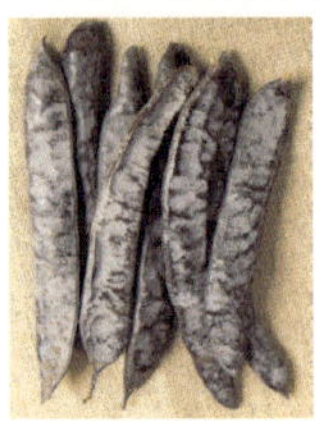	Resolves phlegm, opens orifices, reduces swelling, disperses nodules	
	Atractylodes Rhizome (Cangzhu)	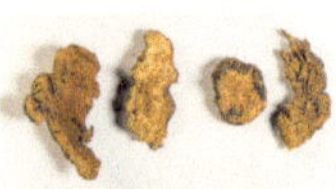	Dries dampness, strengthens the spleen, dispels wind, disperses cold	
	Saposhnikovia Root (Fangfeng)	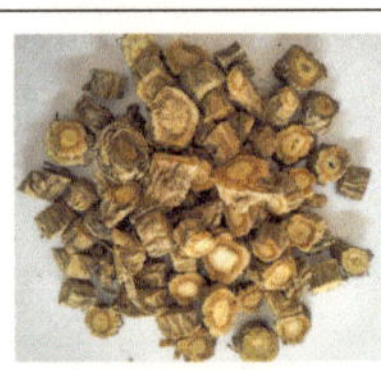	Dispels wind, releases the exterior, overcomes dampness, relieves pain	
	Phellodendron Bark (Huangbai)	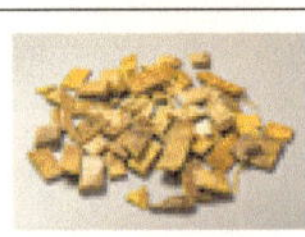	Clears heat, dries dampness, purges fire, detoxifies	
	Chinese Angelica Root Tail (Dangguiwei)	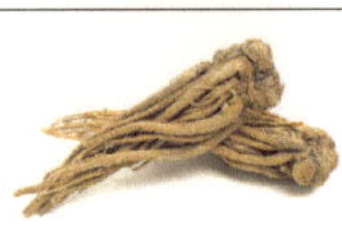	Promotes blood circulation, removes blood stasis, regulates menstruation, relieves pain	
	Alisma Rhizome (Zexie)	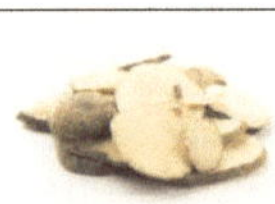	Promotes urination, drains dampness, clears heat	
	Areca Seed (Binglang)	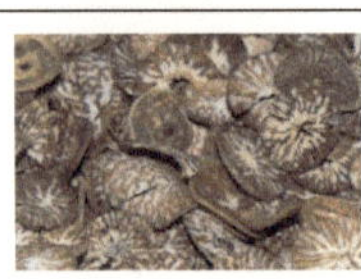	Kills parasites, relieves stagnation, moves qi, promotes urination	

Syndrome pattern	Chinese herbal medicine	Image	Efficacy	Notes
	Prepared Rhubarb Root (Shudahuang)	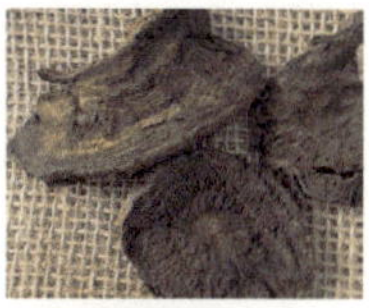	Purges accumulation, clears heat, purges fire	
	Garden Burnet Root (Diyu)	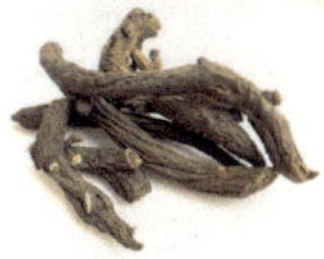	Cools blood, stops bleeding, detoxifies, heals sores	
	Pagoda Tree Flower (Huaihua)	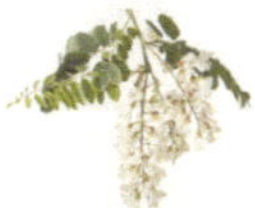	Cools blood, stops bleeding, clears liver fire	
	Schizonepeta Spike (Jingjiesui)	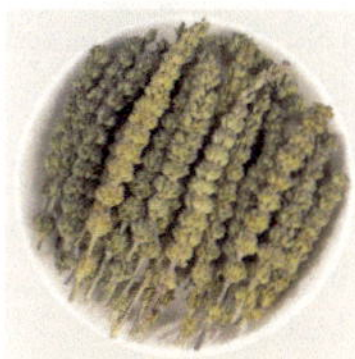	Releases the exterior, dispels wind, promotes rash eruption, relieves sores	
	Stephania Root (Fangji)	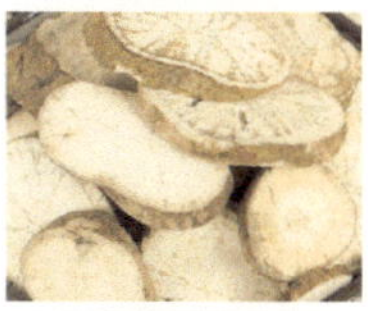	Dispels wind-damp, relieves pain, promotes urination, reduces swelling	
	Notopterygium Root (Qianghuo)	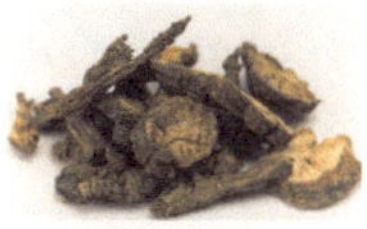	(Dispels wind, disperses cold, eliminates dampness, relieves pain	
	Green Tangerine Peel (Qingpi)	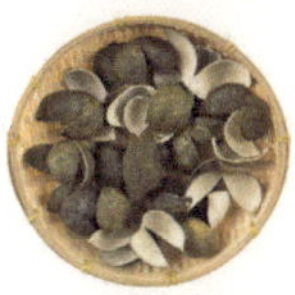	Soothes the liver, breaks qi stagnation, relieves accumulation	
	Corydalis Rhizome (Yanhusuo)	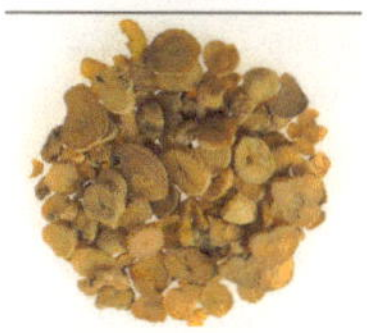	Promotes blood circulation, moves qi, relieves pain	
	Rehmannia Root (Shengdi)	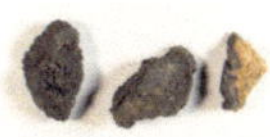	Clears heat, cools blood, nourishes yin, generates fluids	
	Moutan Bark (Danpi)	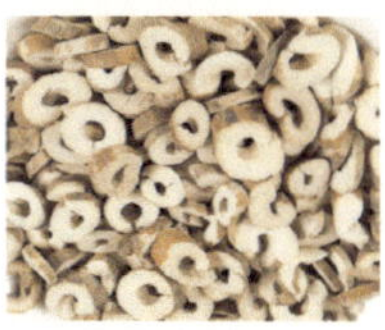	Clears heat, cools blood, promotes blood circulation, removes blood stasis	

Syndrome pattern	Chinese herbal medicine	Image	Efficacy	Notes
Spleen Deficiency and Qi Sinking	Astragalus Root (Huangqi)	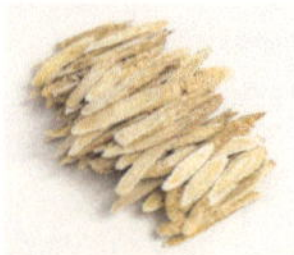	Tonifies qi, raises yang, secures the exterior, stops sweating, promotes urination, reduces swelling	
	Ginseng Root (Renshen)	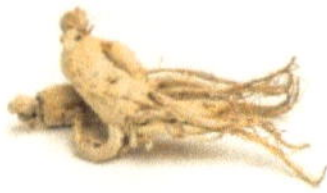	Greatly tonifies primordial qi, restores pulse, secures collapse, tonifies the spleen, benefits the lungs	
	Atractylodes Rhizome (Baizhu)	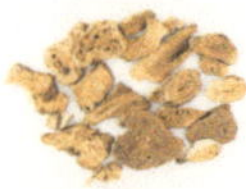	Strengthens the spleen, tonifies qi, dries dampness, promotes urination, stops sweating, calms the fetus	
	Chinese Angelica Root (Danggui)	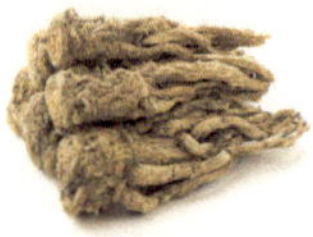	Tonifies blood, promotes blood circulation, regulates menstruation, relieves pain, moistens intestines, relieves constipation	
	Honey-fried Licorice root (Zhigancao)	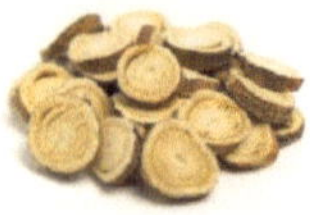	Tonifies the spleen, boosts qi, clears heat, detoxifies, harmonizes other herbs	
	Cimicifuga rhizome (Shengma)	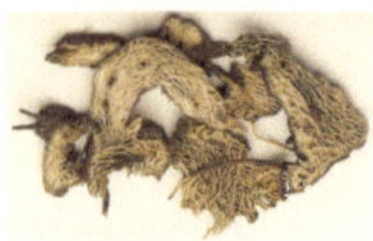	Releases the exterior, promotes rash eruption, clears heat, detoxifies, raises yang qi	
	Bupleurum root (Chaihu)	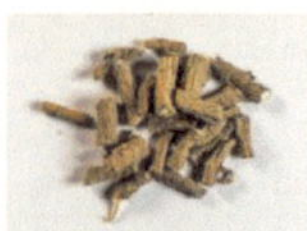	Soothes the liver, relieves stagnation, harmonizes the exterior and interior, raises yang qi	
	Tangerine peel (Chenpi)	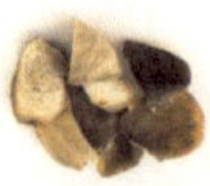	Regulates qi, strengthens the spleen, dries dampness, resolves phlegm	
	Cistanche herb (Roucongrong)	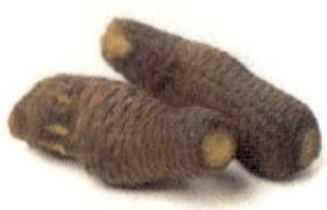	Tonifies kidney yang, benefits essence and blood, moistens intestines, relieves constipation	
	Hemp seed (Huomaren)	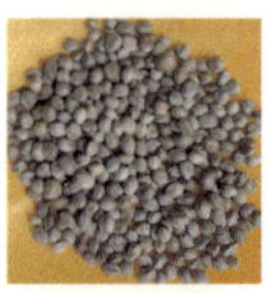	Moistens intestines, relieves constipation, nourishes deficiency	
	Codonopsis Root (Dangshen)	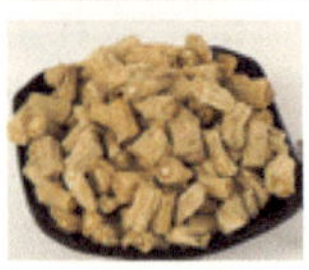	Tonifies middle qi, strengthens the spleen, benefits the lungs	

Syndrome pattern	Chinese herbal medicine	Image	Efficacy	Notes
	Charred Garden Burnet Root (Diyutan)	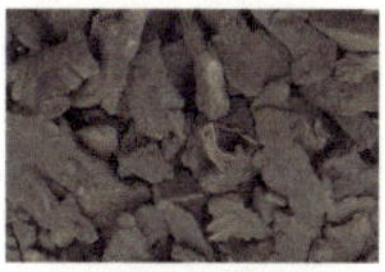	Astringes, stops bleeding, cools blood	
	Charred Pagoda Tree Flower (Huaihuatan)	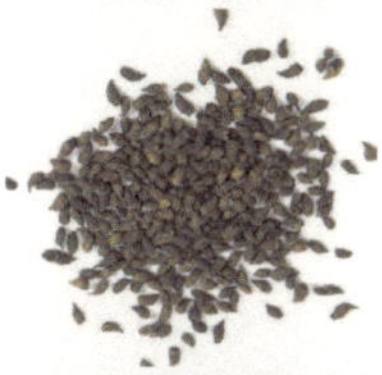	Astringes, stops bleeding, cools blood	
	Charred Biota Tops (Cebaitan)		Astringes, stops bleeding, cools blood	
	Honeysuckle flower (Jinyinhua)	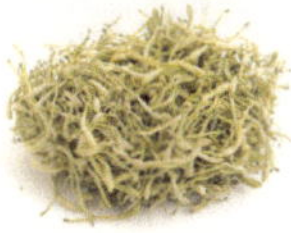	Clears heat, detoxifies, dispels wind-heat	
	Dandelion herb (Pugongying)	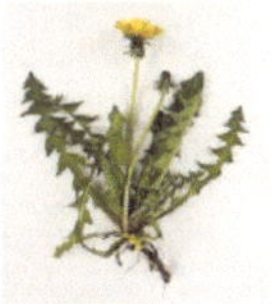	Clears heat, detoxifies, reduces swelling, disperses nodules	

Table A1.
Efficacy of various Chinese herbal medicines for the four major TCM syndrome patterns of hemorrhoids.

Author details

Yongfeng Liu[1*], Di Qiu[2], Tingyu Wang[2], Jinhuan Zhang[1], Xingxian Huang[1] and Haibo Yu[1]

1 Shenzhen Traditional Chinese Medicine Hospital, Shenzhen, China

2 The Fourth Clinical Medical College, Guangzhou University of Chinese Medicine, Shenzhen, China

*Address all correspondence to: 2934808419@qq.com

References

[1] Bo-kang G. Traditional Chinese Surgery. Beijing: People's Medical Publishing House; 2006. p. 165

[2] Changsen Y. Acupuncture and Moxibustion Therapy. Shanghai: Shanghai Scientific and Technical Publishers; 1985. p. 137

[3] Zhenguo T. Interpretation of Clinical Diagnosis and Treatment Guidelines in Traditional Chinese Medicine: Anorectal Diseases. Beijing: China Traditional Chinese Medicine Press; 2015. pp. 4-6

[4] Jiang S. Modified Liangxue Dihuang Decoction for the treatment of 43 cases of mixed hemorrhoids of the type with wind injuring the intestinal network. Journal of Gansu College of Traditional Chinese Medicine. 2011;**28**(03):31-32

[5] Jiali Y, Guiru W. Modified Liangxue Dihuang Decoction for the treatment of 31 cases of internal hemorrhoid strangulation with edema. Heilongjiang Traditional Chinese Medicine. 1995;**06**: 18-19

[6] Shi SY, Zhou Q, He ZQ, et al. Traditional Chinese medicine (Liang-Xue-Di-Huang Decoction) for hemorrhoid hemorrhage: Study Protocol Clinical Trial (SPIRIT Compliant). Medicine (Baltimore). 2020;**99**(16): e19720. DOI: 10.1097/ MD.0000000000019720

[7] Songshan C. Compound Zanglian Pill for the treatment of 47 cases of perinatal hemorrhoids. Jiangsu Journal of Traditional Chinese Medicine. 1986;**02**:35

[8] Yisen T. Zhitong Rushen Decoction for the treatment of bleeding from internal hemorrhoids. Shandong Journal of Traditional Chinese Medicine. 1995; **01**:35

[9] Weiquan W. Bu Zhong Yi Qi Tang in the clinical treatment of hemorrhoids. Shaanxi Journal of Traditional Chinese Medicine. 1999;**01**:25

[10] Zhou M, Jin W, Li P, Wang R, Guo X. Traditional Chinese medicine in the treatment of hemorrhoids—A review of preparations used and their mechanism of action. Frontiers in Pharmacology. 2023;**14**:1270339. DOI: 10.3389/fphar.2023.1270339

[11] Qianli T. Modified WuBei Zi Decoction in the preoperative treatment of strangulated hemorrhoids (with a comparative analysis of 50 cases). Guangxi. Journal of Traditional Chinese Medicine. 1993;**16**(06):1-2, 10

[12] Yong C, Xuan H, Xianming G, et al. Clinical efficacy of traditional Chinese medicine fumigation combined with biofeedback after stapled hemorrhoidopexy for rectal prolapse. Chinese Journal of Traditional Chinese Medicine. 2021;**36**(02):1192-1196

[13] Zhao JC, Zou BM. Application of Jiuhua Ointment in anorectal diseases. Liaoning Journal of Traditional Chinese Medicine. 1992;**10**:33. DOI: 10.13192/j. ljtcm.1992.10.35.zhaojch.022

[14] Ling H. Clinical Observation of Puji Hemorrhoids Suppository in the Treatment of Mixed Hemorrhoids after Surgery. Nanjing: Nanjing University of Traditional Chinese Medicine; 2011

[15] Yunxia L, Tianyu Y, Hongming X, et al. Meta-analysis of the efficacy and safety of traditional Chinese medicine enema in the treatment of internal hemorrhoids. Clinical Research of Traditional Chinese Medicine. 2024; **16**(18):126-130

[16] Zhong QM, Zeng EX, Li MD. Study on retention enema methods for patients with ulcerative colitis complicated by hemorrhoids. Basic Medical Forum. 2012;**16**(12):1524-1525

[17] Qian ZX, Li SL, Yin TB. Therapeutic effect of Zhiranxiao tablets on bleeding from internal hemorrhoids: A clinical observation in 569 cases. Journal of the First Military Medical University. 2003; **23**(5):508-509. Chinese

[18] Zhang H, Yao XY, Zhang DF, et al. Anti-hemorrhoidal activity of Lian-Zhi-San, a traditional Chinese medicine, in an experimental hemorrhoidal model in rats. Journal of Integrative Medicine. 2021;**19**(1):42-49. DOI: 10.1016/j.joim.2020.09.006

[19] Wenxuan X, Xinrong R, Tianpeng Z, et al. Effect of Jingwanhong combined with Dizhu Huajiao Pill on postoperative recovery of mixed hemorrhoids. Chinese Journal of Integrated Traditional and Western Medicine in Surgery. 2020; **26**(06):1111-1114

[20] Ning L, Hongbo H, Chengwei W, et al. Observation on the efficacy of electroacupuncture at Chengshan (BL57) and Changqiang (GV1) acupoints in the treatment of hemorrhoid pain. Chinese Acupuncture & Moxibustion. 2008; **28**(11):3. DOI: CNKI:SUN: ZGZE.0.2008-11-006

[21] Shaoling C, Jingbo H, Junhong C, et al. Observation on the efficacy of fumigation and hip bath with traditional Chinese medicine after anorectal surgery. Chinese Nursing Research: Mid-monthly Edition. 2006;**20**(7):2. DOI: 10.3969/j.issn.1009-6493.2006.20.024

[22] Xueyong S. Acupuncture and Moxibustion Meridians and Points. Beijing: China Press of Traditional Chinese Medicine; 2016

[23] Li S, Hairong X, Yamin Z. Treatment of 102 cases of hemorrhoids with needle-pricking therapy. Shanghai Journal of Traditional Chinese Medicine. 2001; **35**(12):1. DOI: 10.3969/j.issn.1007-1334.2001.12.021

[24] Yonghua W. Treatment of 120 cases of hemorrhoids with acupoint catgut embedding therapy. Chinese Acupuncture and Moxibustion. 1999;**05**: 42

[25] Yawei S. Treatment of hemorrhoids with fire needle therapy. Chinese Folk Therapy Journal. 2015;**23**(02):86. DOI: 10.19621/j.cnki.11-3555/r.2015.02.071

[26] Ligong L, Qinfeng H, Jie G, et al. Analysis of ancient moxibustion treatment characteristics for hemorrhoids. Shanghai Journal of Acupuncture and Moxibustion. 2010; **29**(05):273-274. DOI: 10.13460/j.issn.1005-0957.2010.05.027

[27] Weimin Y, Yiping L. Treatment of hemorrhoids with infection by cupping. Chinese Folk Therapy Journal. 2001;**12**: 21-22. DOI: 10.19621/j.cnki.11-3555/r.2001.12.026

[28] Jianhua X. Clinical report of auricular needle therapy for 50 cases of hemorrhoids. Journal of Clinical Acupuncture and Moxibustion. 1993;**Z1**: 32. DOI: 10.19917/j.cnki.1005-0779.1993.z1.025

[29] Jian C, Tie L, Xichen W. Application of acupuncture and moxibustion therapy in the treatment of hemorrhoids. Journal of Changchun University of Chinese Medicine. 2019;**35**(06):1230-1233. DOI: 10.13463/j.cnki.cczyy.2019.06.063

[30] Lei Z, Yamei C, Lihua X, et al. Effects of Qingre Xiaoyu formula fumigation and washing on pain, wound

healing, and anal function in patients with mixed hemorrhoids after surgery. Liaoning Journal of Traditional Chinese Medicine. 2024;**51**(11):116-119

[31] Jianie D, Shengjing R, Lianhui X, et al. Observation of the effect of transcutaneous electrical stimulation of the Baliao acupoints on postoperative pain in patients with mixed hemorrhoids. Liaoning Journal of Traditional Chinese Medicine. 2025. Available from: https://link.cnki.net/urlid/21.1128.R.20241106.0837.008 [Preprint online Nov. 6, 2024]

[32] Shu T, Li CH. Postoperative pain of hemorrhoids treated with thread embedding at Changqiang (GV 1). Chinese Acupuncture and Moxibustion. 2012;**32**(4):313-315. Chinese

[33] Hui L, Shan C. Observation of the analgesic effect of auricular seed therapy in hemorrhoid fistula surgery. Shandong Medical Journal. 2001;**16**:69

[34] Jing L, Min D, Chengzhan Z, et al. Therapeutic observation of Lei Huo moxibustion for postoperative urinary retention after hemorrhoid surgery. Liaoning Journal of Traditional Chinese Medicine. 2016;**43**(10):2179-2180

[35] Jing G, Li-Jiang J, Xin-Yuan Z, et al. Moxibustion in prevention of post-hemorrhoidectomy urinary retention of mixed hemorrhoids: A randomized clinical trial. World Journal of Acupuncture – Moxibustion. 2023;**33**(3):222-227

[36] Lihong Z, Wei H, Qiaomei L, et al. Therapeutic observation of retention enema with Kangfu Xin liquid for postoperative hemorrhoids. Chinese Journal of Anorectal Diseases. 2023;**43**(12):22

[37] Long Q, Li J, Wen Y. Clinical observation of auricular point sticking combined with Western medicine for preventing and treating postoperative complications of external excision and internal ligation in mixed hemorrhoids. Chinese Acupuncture and Moxibustion. 2015;**35**(3):237-240. Chinese

[38] Cai Erwei W, Yanyan. Clinical study of Zi Bai ointment for postoperative edema of mixed hemorrhoids. Chinese Journal of Traditional Chinese Medicine. 2013;**28**(09):2785-2787

[39] Qing J, Jianxin W, Juan H, et al. Clinical efficacy of Kuchan decoction combined with qi-regulating and blood-activating formula and Baliao Acupoint plaster in patients with severe perianal edema after mixed hemorrhoid surgery. Chinese Traditional Patent Medicine. 2024;**46**(08):2819-2822

Chapter 5

Cutting-Edge Strategies in Management of Hemorrhoids

Parshottambhai Patel

Abstract

This chapter introduces a transformative paradigm in hemorrhoid management by developing the 5PF method—Precise, Purposeful, Predictable, and Personalized fibrosis to Preserve Functions. This method advances care standards via a threefold strategy- rigorous analysis of prior research, identification of knowledge gaps, and targeted innovation. By shifting the focus from anatomical correction to functional preservation, 5PF sets a new benchmark in patient care and dramatically reduces healthcare costs. Traditional methods like Hemorrhoidectomy (EH), Laser Hemorrhoidoplasty (LHP), and Sclerotherapy (Sclero) use ablative techniques, resulting in excision or submucosal fibrosis. Stapler Hemorrhoidopexy (SH) and Stapled Transanal Rectal Resection (STARR) decreases rectal compliance, while Doppler-guided Hemorrhoidal Artery Ligation (DG-HAL), Infrared Coagulation (IRC), and emborrhoid reduce vascularity but do not address multifaceted pathophysiology. Except for EH, external hemorrhoids are not addressed. Secondary and circumferential hemorrhoids also remain unaddressed by all. The management of highly vascularized hemorrhoids presents a formidable challenge across methods. Existing approaches either control or cure with the trade-off of high recurrence rates or increased complications. Fibrosis induced by EH, LHP, sclerotherapy, SH, and STARR may impair functions. Diffuse fibrosis, submucous fibrosis, circular fibrosis, loss of anal cushion, and all hemorrhoids are not addressed are key problems.

Keywords: hemorrhoids management, 5PF technique, pathophysiology, sinusoidal congestion, precise fibrosis, functional preservation, transformative treatment, paradigm shift, lifetime costs, personalized care, value pyramid

1. Introduction

Hemorrhoid management is entering a transformative era where innovation meets simplicity to redefine patient outcomes. This chapter explores the forefront of hemorrhoid management, presenting next-generation treatment options that are highly efficient, minimally invasive, and eliminate the need for dressings or follow-up. These techniques not only deliver long-term value by minimizing lifetime costs but are also easy to learn, teach, and implement with minimal infrastructure.

Recent advances in pelvic floor anatomy [1], physiology [2], neurophysiology [3], pathophysiology [4], and fibrosis [5] have deepened our understanding of the anorectum and hemorrhoids. These insights underscore their pivotal role in maintaining continence and the delicate control of defecation [6].

Building on these breakthroughs, a more refined, precise, and minimally invasive treatment modality has emerged. This novel approach significantly improves patient outcomes by reducing complications and optimizing healthcare resource utilization [7].

Advancing high-quality patient care [8] requires synthesizing existing research, identifying knowledge deficits [9], and developing novel, evidence-based therapies. This progress is guided by six paradigms: disease pathophysiology, patient-centered outcomes, technological innovation, healthcare infrastructure, clinical expertise, and economic sustainability.

As science is cumulative, it demands continuous evaluation and innovation. This iterative process drives advancements in patient care, fostering a dynamic cycle of assessment, discovery, refinement, and transformation [10].

2. Building on the past: Paradigm shifts - Catalysts for transformation

Paradigm shifts redefine foundational frameworks, enabling innovative approaches to longstanding challenges. Despite advancements in pathophysiology [11] and technology, hemorrhoid management lacks a unified clinical and therapeutic strategy [12]. Decision-making remains influenced by training, experience, and cognitive biases, often leading to overgeneralizations [13]. Discernment—the ability to critically evaluate and refine perspectives—drives reassessment and transformative change [14].

2.1 Learning from history to advanced science

Historical insights provide essential context for addressing contemporary challenges [15, 16]. By analyzing patterns of progress, healthcare professionals can bridge past innovations with future strategies, *fostering continuous improvement* in care (**Figure 1**). The iterative cycle of assessment, discovery, and refinement remains central to developing evidence-based approaches [15].

2.2 Contributions of anatomical advancements

Anatomical understanding has been the *foundation of surgical innovation*. Galen (129–216 CE) pioneered empirical research through dissection. Andreas Vesalius (1514–1564) revolutionized anatomy by challenging assumptions through direct observation, laying the groundwork for evidence-based practice [17].

In anorectal surgery, St. Mark's Hospital has driven innovation for nearly two centuries [18]. The 1937 Milligan-Morgan procedure, rooted in anatomical precision, remains the *gold standard* for hemorrhoidectomy and exemplifies the integration of surgical strategy with anatomical dissection *by the surgeon himself* [19].

2.3 Advancements in hemorrhoid treatment

The management of hemorrhoids has evolved significantly over time (**Figure 1**), reflecting a dynamic interplay between *efficacy and safety*. Early approaches, such as Whitehead's ultra-radical excision [20], prioritized complete removal at the cost of high complication rates, including stricture and incontinence. Subsequently, radical

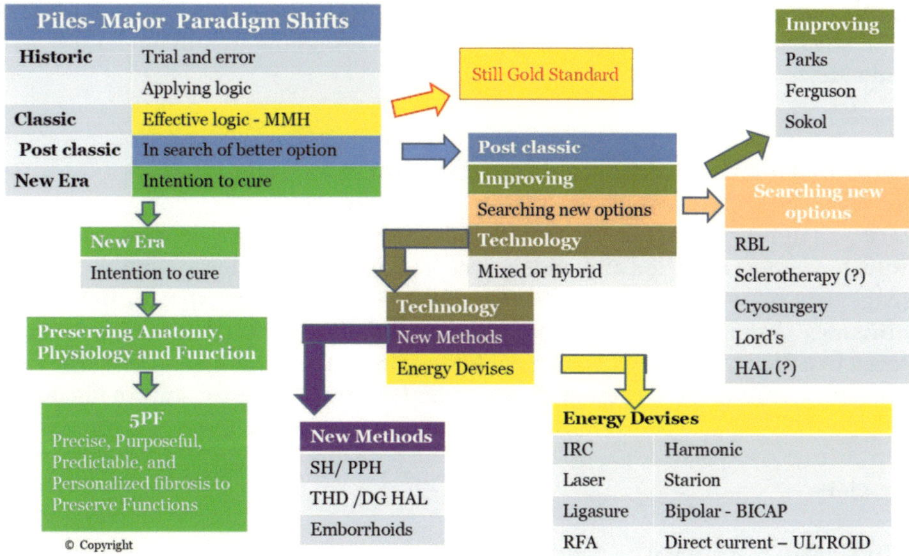

Figure 1.
Paradigm shifts in hemorrhoid treatment. A visual journey through the major advancements in hemorrhoid care.

techniques (EH) targeting the three main hemorrhoidal cushions [21] and destructive modalities like laser hemorrhoidoplasty (LHP) and sclerotherapy [22] became popular but often compromised long-term outcomes due to submucous fibrosis. Conversely, minimally invasive options like Doppler-guided hemorrhoidal artery ligation (DG-HAL) and infrared coagulation (IRC) [23], while safer, address only the pedicle. Stapled hemorrhoidopexy (SH) fails to address any part of the hemorrhoidal plexus and compromises rectal accommodation [24].

Cost-effective treatments like sclerotherapy and rubber band ligation continue to be widely utilized due to their affordability and proven effectiveness [25]. Meanwhile, advancements in vascular-targeted and energy-based technologies are enhancing both the safety and efficacy of hemorrhoid management. However, the success of surgical outcomes is *ultimately determined* not just by the available technology but by the surgeon's skillful approach and *strategic decision-making*.

This evolution highlights the *pressing need* for treatment paradigms that preserve anatomy and function without compromising effectiveness. The challenge lies in *bridging the gap* between over-aggressive and overly conservative strategies, paving the way for innovative approaches like the 5PF technique, which emphasizes precise, purposeful, and personalized intervention to achieve optimal outcomes with minimal complications.

2.4 The next transformation: Function-driven care

Anatomical advancements in hemorrhoid treatment have historically been transformative, yet the knowledge gained has often been cumulative, assimilative, or accommodative [26]. In contrast, the current approach marks a paradigm shift by prioritizing *functional preservation as the core principle* of care. This shift not only maintains critical functions but also reduces recurrence rates, minimizes postoperative complications, and optimizes long-term functionality. By integrating these principles, the approach offers a significant opportunity to improve patient outcomes and enhance quality of life on a global scale. This function-centered focus marks a critical advancement in hemorrhoid management, reshaping treatment paradigms worldwide.

3. Illuminating the unknown: Identification of knowledge gaps

Despite significant advancements in understanding pathophysiology and adopting new technologies, a unified and widely accepted approach to clinical and therapeutic management remains a challenge [9]. *Translating research into practice* is hindered by conflicting opinions on best practices and the need for individualized treatment plans tailored to patients' unique pathologies. Addressing knowledge gaps is key to advancing healthcare. Analyzing their origins enables targeted strategies, improving outcomes and driving progress. We will explore this in two parts: basics and examples.

3.1 Basics

Knowledge translation bridges research and practice, starting with identifying care gaps to turn evidence into action [11]. A *'knowledge-to-action gap'* occurs when evidence does not align with clinical practice, hindering care optimization [21]. Measuring these gaps aligns practices with evidence through targeted interventions. Knowledge gaps often stem from 'knowledge-to-action gap' (*'automatic pilot'*) and *unconscious adaptations*, perpetuating outdated methods [20]. Understanding these causes is crucial for effective solutions. Key assessment areas: Knowledge (align with evidence), Skills (identify gaps), Attitudes/Behaviors (assess barriers), and Outcomes (measure impact on patient outcomes) [14].

This chapter highlights key gaps in hemorrhoid management that the 5PF technique can address, providing a path to more effective, functional, and patient-centered care.

3.2 The role of anal cushions, mucosa, and submucosa

Anal cushions, mucosa, and submucosa are essential for fecal continence, supporting the anal region's function [4]. However, a knowledge-to-action gap exists, as current practices often focus on visible pathology, there is *no known techniques* that preserve these structures (**Figure 2**), leading to functional damage and poorer patient outcomes.

3.3 Addressing all types of hemorrhoids and effect of fibrosis

Figure 2 highlights persistent challenges—loss of mucosa and anal cushion, submucous, diffuse, and circular fibrosis, as well as unaddressed hemorrhoids—underscoring their significant impact on advanced hemorrhoid management. *Suboptimal* hemorrhoid treatment often leads to recurrence and/or long-term complications. Preserving epithelial barrier integrity is critical to preventing a *cascade* of chronic inflammation, fibrosis, and eventual stricture formation [27]. Strictures progress slowly, often remaining asymptomatic *until advanced* stages, making early pathological events challenging to study.

Loss of anal cushions: Leads to (**Figure 2**) compromised air and water-tight seals and anal lip functionality (e.g., EH, LHP, Sclero, and SH) [12]. *Loss of Mucosa*: Results in sensory deprivation and fibrosis (e.g., EH) [28]. *Diffuse Fibrosis*: Impairs ease of

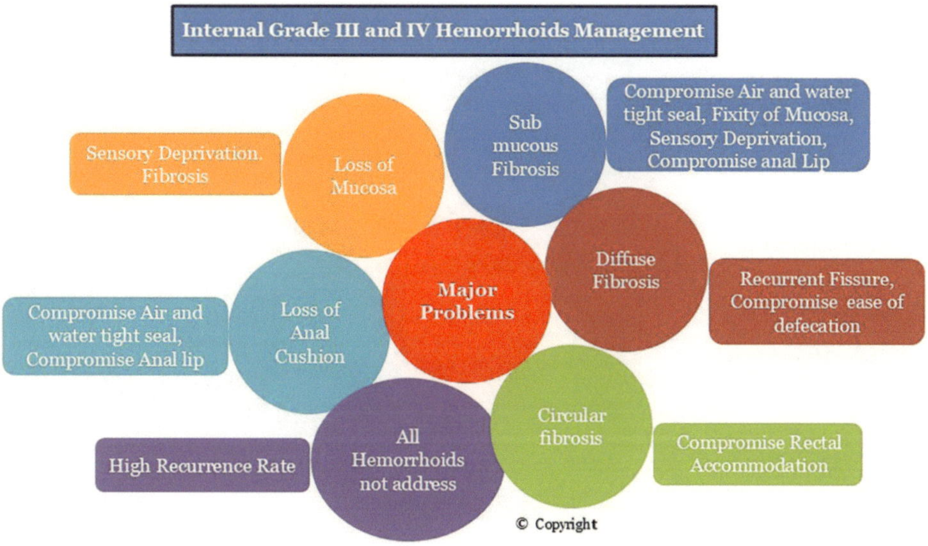

Figure 2.
Challenges in advanced hemorrhoid care.

defecation [5] – predisposes to recurrent fissures (e.g., EH) [22]. *Submucous Fibrosis*: Causes fixed mucosa, sensory loss, and recurrent fissures (e.g., LH and Scl) [24]. *Circular Fibrosis*: Often seen in SH, it compromises rectal accommodation [6].

3.4 Control or cure: A persistent dilemma in hemorrhoid management

Existing treatments often face a trade-off between control and potential cures (**Figure 3**), with high recurrence rates or/and complications. Excisional techniques may cure but cause significant pain and fibrosis, while less invasive methods provide relief yet often result in recurrence [29]. This *dilemma stems from prioritizing* immediate symptoms over long-term function and prevention of recurrence [30].

3.5 Too many methods: A double-edged sword in hemorrhoid management

Hemorrhoid management involves various treatments, such as EH, RBL, DH-HAL, IRC, HLP, Scl, LHP, SH, and STARR, each *offering distinct benefits*. However, the *dilemma of selecting the right approach* acts as a double-edged sword [30].

Innovative approaches like the 5PF technique, which prioritize functional preservation, offer a promising solution for achieving durable results with minimal complications. By emphasizing precision, personalization, and anatomical preservation, 5PF addresses the critical challenges in hemorrhoid management, providing a pathway to standardized and effective treatment.

4. Innovating for the future: The 5PF technique in hemorrhoid management

Ultimately, nothing surpasses the combined strength of reason and experience. Reality, however, is neither immediately evident nor straightforward—it is vast,

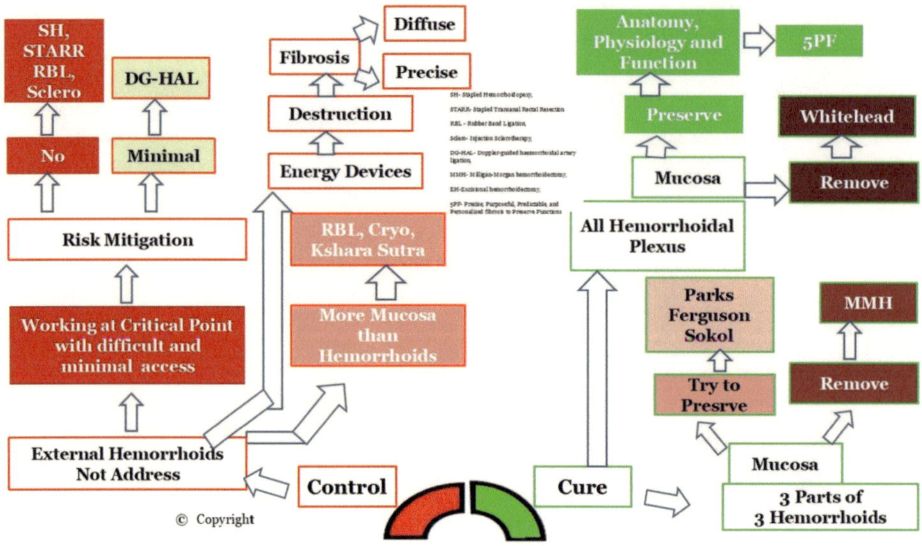

Figure 3.
Explores the dilemma of control vs. cure—at what cost, contrasting symptom-control methods with cure-oriented strategies.

intricate, and multifaceted [27]. Can we innovate and design strategies where function takes the lead? This is the central issue. The answer is a resounding yes, and it serves as the cornerstone of my approach (Video 1).

Objective: To target the pathophysiology of hemorrhoids by addressing sinusoidal congestion [28], while ensuring the preservation of anal structural and functional integrity.

Principles of Surgery (Video 2).

Conceptualizing hemorrhoids as a functional structure: Hemorrhoids are a dynamic, complex system of collapsible and distensible vascular channels within the mucosa and submucosa (**Figure 4**). Recognizing them as functional structures [6] *shifts the focus* from treating pathology to preserving function, enabling more refined, function-focused management strategies [3].

Addressing Sinusoidal Congestion through Targeted Precise Fibrosis: Sinusoidal congestion is a central hallmark of hemorrhoidal disease [28], characterized by engorgement and dilatation of vascular structures within the hemorrhoidal cushions (**Figure 5**). Effective treatment involves inducing *targeted, controlled fibrosis* in specific vascular regions, such as the submucosal plexus, while preserving the integrity of the mucosa and submucosa.

4.1 Precision and coordination in technique

The procedure requires delicate, precise, and coordinated movements, along with optimal lighting, to ensure both accuracy and effectiveness.

4.2 Goals of operation

Focus on the central issue—sinusoidal congestion—targeting it precisely to avoid morphological or structural damage to surrounding tissues.

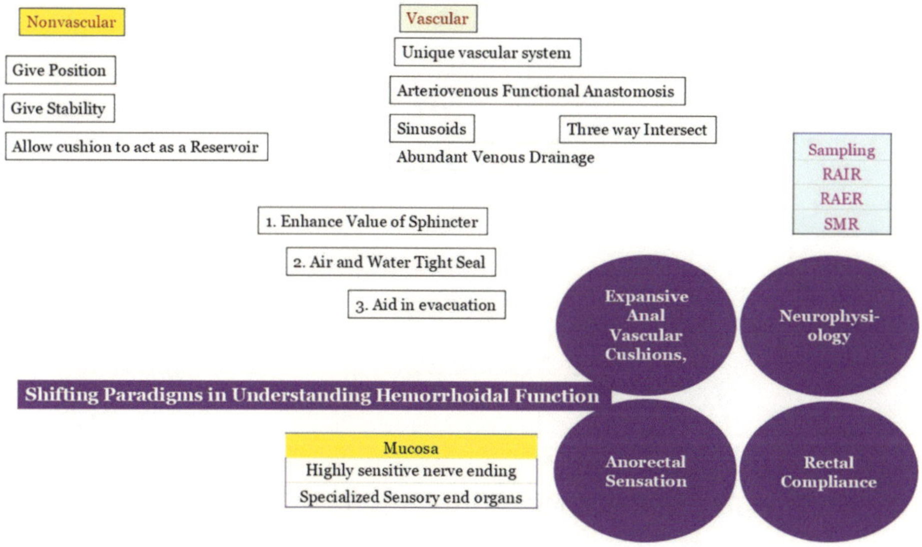

Figure 4.
Hemorrhoid function overview: explores the roles of vascular and nonvascular components in hemorrhoid function.

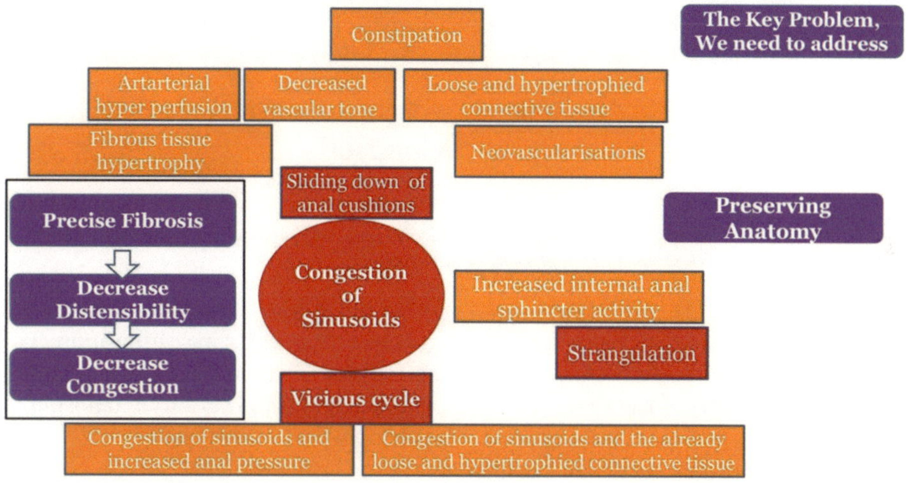

Figure 5.
Hemorrhoid Pathophysiology: This figure shows the vicious cycle of congestion, driven by constipation, decreased vascular tone, and fibrous hypertrophy, highlighting the need for precise fibrosis to reduce distensibility and congestion.

Targeted precise fibrosis should be applied across the entire hemorrhoidal plexus.

With precise execution, the paradigms presented in **Figure 6** can typically be achieved in nearly all cases.

Anorectal Surgery: Approach each part uniquely: Anorectal surgeries present a unique set of challenges due to the intricate anatomy [21] and physiology [4] of the region. Precision and specialized skills are paramount, as even minor procedures can disrupt critical functions, significantly affecting a patient's quality of life [5]. Both short-term success,

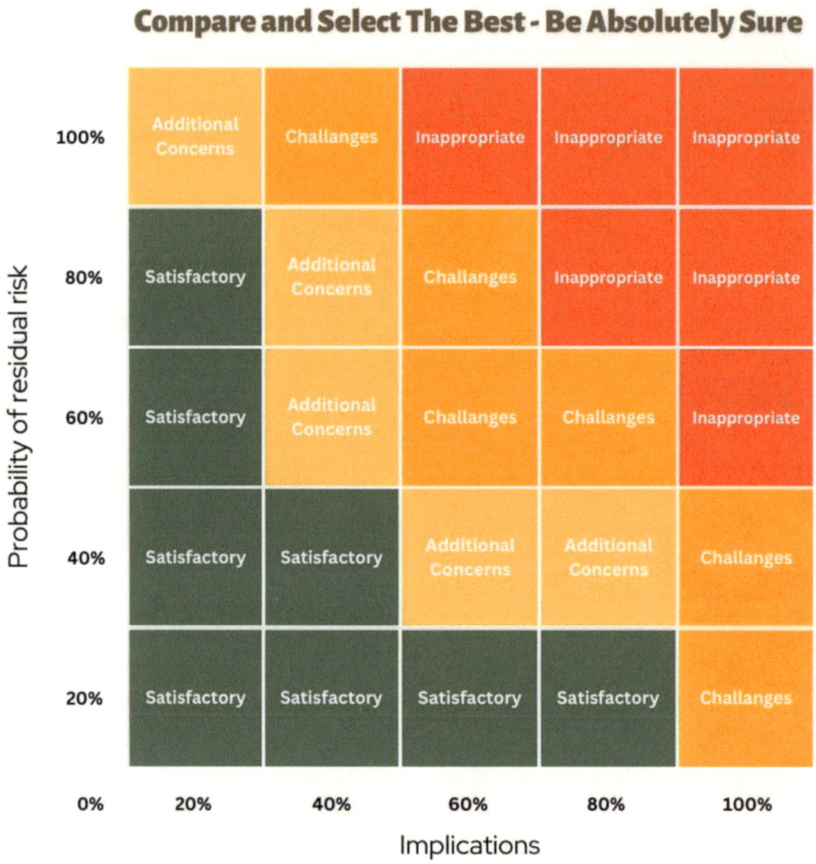

Figure 6.
The matrix visually compares all methods based on residual risks and implications, helping evaluate their effectiveness and guide the adoption of the most suitable approach.

and long-term functionality, hinge on a comprehensive understanding of the anorectal anatomy and its physiological interplay [31]. This chapter delves into the key anatomical and functional features of the anal canal, and discusses their implications in tailoring surgical techniques to enhance safety and optimize long-term outcomes.

Embryological development and regional anatomy: From a surgical perspective, the dentate (pectinate) line is the most critical landmark in the anal canal. This saw-toothed mucocutaneous junction divides the canal into two distinct regions with significant differences [32].

Upper two-thirds: Supplied by autonomic nerves and vascular structures derived from the hindgut, it is sensitive to stretch and distention but not pain. This makes internal hemorrhoids a focal point for surgical interventions (RBL, Scl, IRC, DGHAL, HLP, LHP, SH, and STARR).

Lower one-third: Innervated by somatic nerves and vascularized by ectoderm-derived structures, this region is highly sensitive to pain. Understanding these divisions is essential for tailoring surgical approaches [30].

Despite its compact 4 cm length, the anal canal is a remarkable anatomical structure shaped by its embryological origins. It is divided into three distinct zones [31], each with unique structural and functional characteristics: Upper Segment: Derived from the embryonic hindgut, this region features loosely attached epithelium. Middle Segment (Anal Transitional Zone, ATZ): region with firmly attached epithelium. Lower Segment: Derived from the ectoderm of the proctodeum, this segment has a loosely attached epithelium. These distinct zones illustrate the anal canal's intricate design, where embryological origins influence its structure, function, and susceptibility to specific pathological condition.

4.3 Structural components of the anal canal

Anal columns and crypts: The lumen of the anal canal is marked by longitudinal folds called columns of Morgagni, formed by the combined action of anal cushions and pleated tissue. These columns are interconnected by transverse anal valves, forming small recesses known as anal crypts (sinuses of Morgagni). These crypts house the excretory ducts of anal glands, which are prone to infection and inflammation, potentially leading to abscesses or fistulas [33].

Pectinate line and transition zones: The anal valves collectively form the pectinate line, where the intestinal mucosa transitions into squamous epithelium. This region marks a critical zone for understanding anorectal diseases and planning surgical interventions [29].

Vascular structures: Two arteriovenous plexuses are vital to the anal canal's anatomy: Internal Hemorrhoidal Plexus located above the dentate line; this structure is associated with the development of internal hemorrhoids. External Hemorrhoidal Plexus situated at the anal verge; this plexus plays a role in external hemorrhoid formation [33].

4.4 Epithelial lining and functional specialization

The anal canal features distinct epithelial layers, each reflecting specific structural and functional adaptations. The rectal mucosa (columnar epithelium) covers the hemorrhoidal pedicle, while the lower rectal mucosa (cuboidal and transitional epithelium) overlies the main hemorrhoidal mass [29]. The anoderm, located between the dentate line and the anal verge, consists of nonkeratinized squamous epithelium devoid of hair follicles or glands. This region is the least distensible of the three but is highly sensitive to pain due to dense sensory innervation. Injury to the anoderm [33], whether during surgery or due to chronic inflammation, can lead to severe complications such as anal stricture and debilitating pain [34].

4.5 Anorectal sampling and sensory mechanisms

Anorectal sampling is a physiological process enabling the periodic assessment of rectal contents. Transient relaxation of the internal anal sphincter (IAS) allows small amounts of rectal material to enter the upper anal canal, where specialized sensory receptors (e.g., Krause end-bulbs, Golgi–Mazzoni bodies, and Meissner's corpuscles) evaluate its composition. Occurring approximately every 8–10 minutes, this process maintains continence and aids in sensing rectal fullness. A thorough understanding of this mechanism is crucial for diagnosing and managing functional disorders [2].

4.6 The heart of the method: Execution - Precise fibrosis for function

Surgical innovation relies on precise execution. Precise fibrosis addresses pathology by reducing hemorrhoidal distensibility while integrating anatomical reconstruction and functional restoration. This adaptable technique ensures functional outcomes with minimal tissue disruption and delivers predictable, consistent results through reproducible fibrosis, confidently restoring function.

Technique: Absorbable sutures are placed at key points around hemorrhoidal tissues and tightened to reduce sinusoidal distensibility. Controlled trauma, ischemia, and infection induce fibrosis [5], influenced by suture type, location, applied force, and infection degree. The mucosa heals naturally, while fibrosis reinforces structure.

Intraoperative evaluation: The goals of intraoperative evaluation extend beyond reconfirming preoperative findings such as the type, grade, number, and vascularity of hemorrhoids. They also include assessing sphincter tone, volume, and movement; evaluating rectal contents; and performing deep palpation to examine surrounding structures. Additionally, a systematic and detailed study of the pelvic floor and pelvis is conducted to identify any unexpected findings. This process must be performed in a gentle and methodical manner to ensure accuracy and patient safety.

Indications: This method is specifically indicated for the management of internal hemorrhoids (Grades II, III, and IV), with or without associated with secondary, circumferential, or circumferentially prolapsing features, as well as external hemorrhoids unresponsive to conservative treatment. It is also recommended in cases of failed prior surgical interventions, concomitant surgical conditions, or individual patient preferences (Video 3).

Furthermore, this approach is invaluable in emergency settings. It is ideally suited for addressing highly vascular, complex hemorrhoidal cases and managing complications from earlier treatments. The versatility and efficacy of this method make it an indispensable tool in the surgical management of challenging anorectal conditions (Video 3).

Red flags in anorectal surgical management span diagnosis, planning, and management, with a critical focus on assessing contraindications. Persistent lower GI symptoms like pelvic or abdominal pain, first blood then stool, altered bowel habits, or abnormal stool color (e.g., black tarry stools or blood-stool mix) warrant detailed evaluation. Planning must address coexisting conditions such as urinary, respiratory issues, or coagulation concerns to prevent complications. Management focuses on sphincter integrity, pelvic abnormalities, and functional impairments. Contraindications, both absolute and relative (e.g., extreme obesity, joints immobility, nonresponding chronic constipation, or undiagnosed symptoms), require careful evaluation (Video 1).

Surgery in the anorectal region poses *unique challenges* due to its narrow, deep anatomy and the functional importance of the anal canal in continence and defecation. Factors like patient obesity, joint rigidity, and the pelvic floor's complexity further complicate the procedure, necessitating precision to avoid overstretching or tissue damage with significant postoperative consequences. Unlike straightforward pathologies, these require stepwise exploration, guided by logical planning, calm execution, and adaptive decision-making. Success hinges on cohesive teamwork, with the surgeon orchestrating every element—team coordination, positioning, instrumentation, and visibility—while staying within the site's constraints to minimize risks and optimize outcomes.

HemEvert Maneuver: The HemEvert maneuver is a *vital* technique in 5PF surgery, enhancing visibility and access by exposing internal hemorrhoids like an open book, ensuring effective treatment (Video 4).

Identify the most visible internal hemorrhoid, apply Allis forceps above the mucocutaneous junction, then *place a second* Allis forceps proximally and remove the first. Gently pull the hemorrhoid downward, apply *slight stretch, rotate clockwise*, and continue until fully exposed or reaching the gluteal region. The maneuver reveals additional hemorrhoids, typically at 3, 7, and 11 o'clock, with occasional presence of four or five hemorrhoids When the HemEvert maneuver fails due to access issues, positioning, or fibrosis, strategies include enhancing tissue mobility, repositioning the patient (e.g., table height, knee flexion, hip rotation, and head low), and gently adjusting tissues for improved visualization.

Proximal control: (Video: 5): A principle from vascular surgery is adapted in hemorrhoidal surgery to *prevent post-operative bleeding*, a known risk factor in procedures like EH, RBL, and SH. The pedicle is ligated with an early absorbable suture (e.g., chromic catgut), inducing controlled ischemia to promote fibrosis. It enhances hemostasis by targeting the vascular pedicle, minimizing bleeding. It ensures safety and simplicity requiring no additional intervention. This technique integrates with 5PF principles (Video 5).

4.7 Preserve the anal transitional zone (ATZ) and sensory structures for function

For internal hemorrhoids, place the first Allis forceps just above the dentate line to protect the ATZ and prevent trauma to the sensitive mucosa, followed by a second forceps above the first for *added safety*. For external hemorrhoids, address them externally.

4.8 Addressing pedicle and internal hemorrhoids: A scientific and harmonious approach

Harmonious hand technique: This technique thrives on the *seamless coordination* of three surgical team members and an assistant managing lighting. Every movement is synchronized, with all eight hands working in unison to achieve precision and efficiency.

4.9 Step-by-step procedure

4.9.1 Preparation and initial positioning

Begin the HemEvert maneuver to access the target hemorrhoid. Select the most suitable hemorrhoid for initial intervention. Use Allis forceps to gently pull the tissue downward with an inferior and clockwise motion, improving visualization and access. Gently grasp the hemorrhoid using Babcock forceps, applying downward tension without causing trauma. Incrementally reposition the forceps to fully expose the pedicle. *To Enhance Visualization*, the assistant uses the back of the forceps to retract adjacent hemorrhoids, providing a clear and unobstructed view of the target structure. Place 20 chromic catgut round body sutures below the pedicle with precision. To guide the needle, reverse the Allis forceps to create space, gently retract tissue to prevent obstruction, and ensure precise exit without contacting adjacent hemorrhoid. *To Securing the Knot*: Use the "*Pull-Down,*

Pull-Up, and Tie" method by passing the needle high on the pedicle, making an initial loose knot, pulling the hemorrhoid downward while lifting the knot into the rectum, and tightening the knot securely with the external thread (Video 5). Mock Verification: Conduct "demo" movements to confirm accurate needle placement and secure ligature positioning before finalizing. *Overcoming Challenges*: If access is restricted, gently reposition and reapply the stitch while preserving tissue integrity; adjust the assistant's retraction angle to enhance visualization without applying excessive force. *Management of Internal Hemorrhoids*: Place stitches 1 cm apart, adjusting for hemorrhoid size, vascularity, and redundancy; for large hemorrhoids, use two overlapping stitches if a single stitch is insufficient.

Achieving high placement on the pedicle: Place the stitch as high as possible on the pedicle, leaving it long to facilitate pulling and positioning subsequent stitches higher if necessary. *Avoiding Muscle Penetration*: Gently isolate the internal hemorrhoid from the rectal wall using Babcock forceps, and pass the needle close to the forceps, ensuring the muscle layer is not engaged. *Managing Complications*: Bleeding – Secure a knot immediately, apply pressure if needed, and place an additional stitch if bleeding persists. Hematoma – Apply sustained pressure and observe, placing a stitch if necessary. *Large Vascular Hemorrhoids*: Use the "*let it bleed*" technique by puncturing the hemorrhoid with an 18-gauge needle after proximal control to allow blood release, aiding in collapse and simplifying stitch placement (Video 7). *Mucosa-Sparing Technique*: Use submucosal stitches to minimize mucosal damage, particularly for larger hemorrhoids (Video 8). *Cutting Hemorrhoidal Tissue*: Generally unnecessary; if needed, limit tissue removal and use cautery sparingly.

Secondary and circumferential hemorrhoids: Manage with the same principles as primary internal hemorrhoids (Video 9).

Addressing external hemorrhoids: Treat after internal hemorrhoids, improve access with dressing and string retraction, evaluate number, size, vascularity (mostly clinical signs, occasionally puncture, or incisions), and identify diffuse involvement (Video 10).

4.10 Methods to induce precise fibrosis

Radial incisions: Limit blood supply, induce precise fibrosis, and reduce recurrence; indicated for highly vascular or localized enlargements; minimize excision to prevent complications. 2. *Needle and Low-Power Cautery*: Use a 26-gauge needle with low-power cautery (15 coagulation mode), spacing punctures ~15 mm apart based on vascularity. 3. *Edema Punctures*: Create multiple punctures for oedema fluid drainage; switch to cautery if bleeding occurs.

Scenario-based management: For normal external hemorrhoids, apply Method 3; for diffuse enlargement, use Method 2; for highly vascular or localized enlargements, combine Methods 1 and 2; excise skin tags directly.

Rationale for comprehensive treatment: Addressing all external hemorrhoids reduces postoperative complications, prevents recurrence and perianal hematomas, and lowers lifetime cost.

5. From principles to practice: A transformative approach to hemorrhoid management*

Study design and setting: This retrospective, single-center study conducted at a 15-bed facility investigated the management of grade III/IV internal (primary, secondary, circumferential, and circumferentially prolapsing) and external hemorrhoids focusing on the long-term outcomes of the 5PF technique in preserving functional integrity while minimizing recurrence and complications.

Study population: The cohort included 187 patients (123 males [66%] and 64 females [34%]) with a follow-up period of 1–13 years. Referral sources: 33% by relatives, 58% by patients/families (91% combined referral rate). Common symptoms: bleeding/prolapse (100%), constipation (146 cases), itching (57), and pain (38).

Methodology and surgical approach: Techniques focused on tissue preservation, minimizing damage, and ensuring optimal functional outcomes. Unique Challenges: Patients hesitated to seek treatment, fearing cancer due to the practitioner's oncology specialization, highlighting the need for education and trust-building.

Complication analysis: Complications were categorized as critical (impacting survival or long-term quality of life), important but not critical (affecting recovery, manageable without lasting effects), and minor (limited impact on patient outcome).

5.1 Critical complications

Immediate postoperative: All patients had moderate-to-severe pain managed with analgesics, local anesthetics (xylocaine jelly), fentanyl patches (110 cases), or injectable analgesics (7 cases post-discharge). Pain lasted 5–10 days (1 case: 22 days). No primary/secondary hemorrhage, reoperation, abscess, fistula, or dressing-related issues were observed.

Intermediate/long-term: No recurrence of bleeding/prolapse, stricture, or incontinence. Constipation (34 cases, including 6 with minor spotting) resolved with diet/ medical intervention.

Important but not critical complications: Procedures lasted 30–90 minutes under spinal anesthesia. Most patients (161) were discharged the next day, 17 stayed an extra day, and 9 required 2 days due to pain, urinary retention, or comorbidities.

Postoperative recovery: Urinary Retention: Associated with age, obesity, mobility, or large hemorrhoids. Preoperative catheterization (44%) mitigated risks; acute retention required intervention in 28 cases. Reddish Discharge: Lasted 10–40 days, managed with sanitary napkins, sitz baths, and patient education to differentiate from bleeding. Pruritus: Treated with antihistamines. Not That Important Complications: Minor complications included asymptomatic soft skin tags.

Recurrence as an 'unaddressed opportunity' rather than an 'unavoidable challenge': While it may be too early to draw definitive conclusions, data thus far supports the notion that recurrence is not inevitable but may be preventable with the right approach. Incorporating video observations has provided valuable insights for peer evaluation, showcasing key elements of the technique and outcomes. The next steps include extending follow-up (maximum follow-up 13 years) to capture long-term results, standardized metrics, and multicenter validation, and inviting further peer critique to refine and validate these promising findings (Video 11).

Comparing incomparable: Comparing diverse methods, each developed by experts and achieving significant success and patient satisfaction, is a challenging yet essential step toward understanding and improvement (**Figures 7–11**). This first-ever attempt seeks to highlight their strengths, identify opportunities for enhancement, and foster growth through fair and open evaluation. Acknowledging its imperfections and the need for iterative revisions, this effort aims to advance outcomes for practitioners and patients alike by providing a *transparent and comprehensive* framework for analysis.

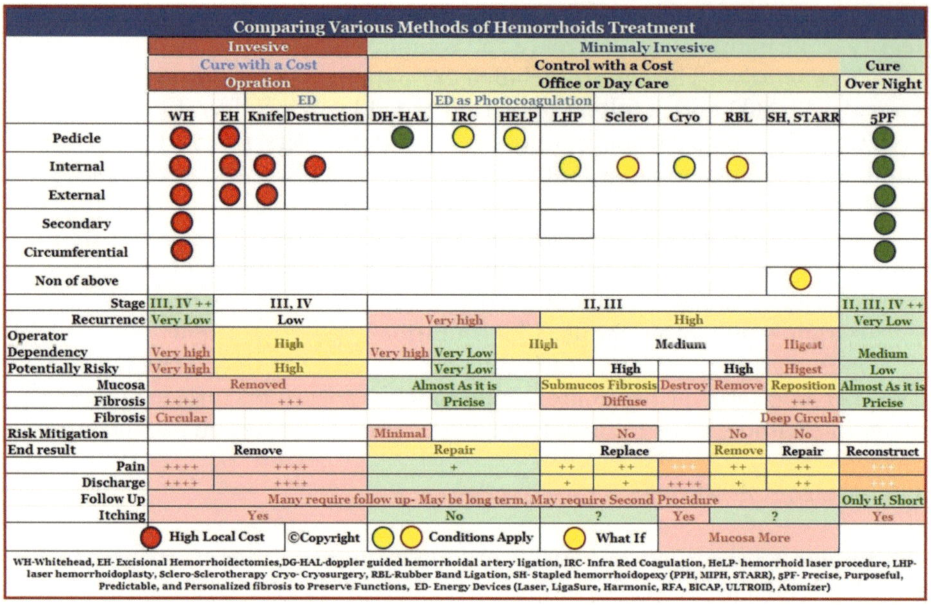

Figure 7.
Comparison aids in making informed decisions by identifying strengths, weaknesses, and the best options, leading to improved outcomes and well-defined priorities, while also enabling effective benchmarking.

Hemorrhoids - Ideological Classification of End Result of Treatment

Principle	Method	Sub methoc	MuEx	ExH	Examples
Remove	Excision	Complete	Full /Part	Yes	EH- Open, Closed, Semi, Sub
	Ligation	Incomplete	More than Hemorrhoid	No	RBL, Ayurvedic- KSHARA SUTRA
	Destruction	Energy devices	Diffuse Injury	No	Laser, Bipolar -BICAP, Direct current - ULTROID, LigaSure™, Harmonic, Starion™, RFA, Atomizer™
Repair	Fixation	Pull up	Above	No	Stapled hemorrhoidopexy
	Blood Supply	Arterial Ligation	No	No	DG-HAL, RAR maybe needed
	Blood Supply	Embolization	No	No	Emborrhoid
	Blood Supply	Coagulate	No	No	DG-Laser
	Tone	Reduction	No	No	Lord
Reconsruct	Fibrosis	5PF	Only if	Yes	5PF
Replace	Fibrosis	Precise	No	No	IRC
		Diffuse	Damage	No	Sclerotherapy, Cryosurgery, Laser
Mix		© copyright			

MuEX = Mucosal Excision, ExHe- External Hemorrhoids Addressed,

EH = Excisional Hemorrhoidectomy; 5PF- Precise, Purposeful, Predictable, and Personalized fibrosis to Preserve Functions

Figure 8.
It fosters objective benchmarking across methods, simplifies decision-making, identifies areas for improvement, enhances predictability, and facilitates advancements in evidence-based practice.

Implementation: The effectiveness of a treatment depends not only on its design but also on its execution. Proper implementation ensures the groundwork for achieving targeted clinical outcomes [35].

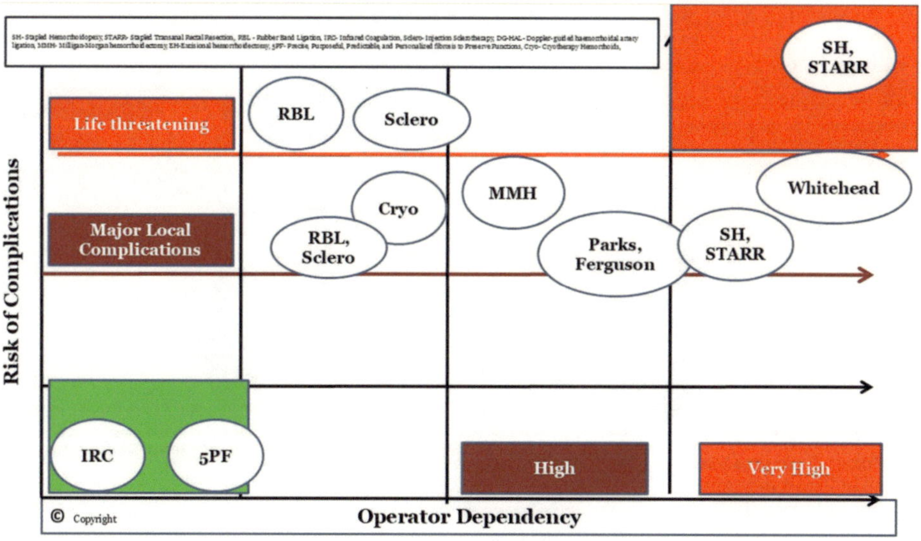

Figure 9.
Minimizing operator dependency and complication risks leads to safer, more predictable, and efficient procedures, enhancing procedural success and patient satisfaction, while reducing lifetime costs and supporting evidence-based practice.

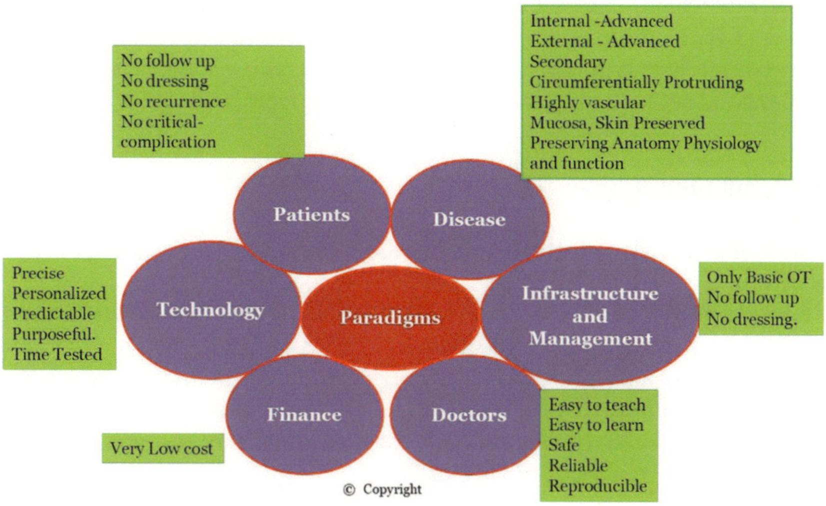

Figure 10.
This figure highlights the never-before paradigms selected and achieved for the 5PF approach.

6. Conclusion

The 5PF framework represents a scientifically grounded, patient-centered approach that prioritizes preserving function, setting a new standard in hemorrhoid management. By integrating patient needs, technological innovation, and sustainable practices, it addresses the *unmet global need* for treatments that improve quality of life and socialization. A major paradigm shift from anatomical correction to function preservation, the 5PF framework offers immediate benefits and long-term value.

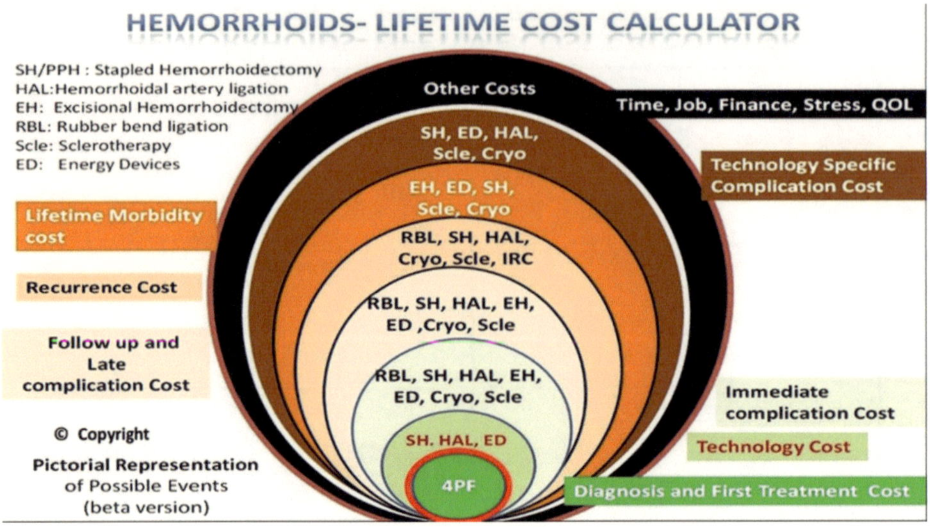

Figure 11.
By calculating lifetime costs, the tool empowers patients to make informed choices that balance immediate needs with long-term value, fostering smarter and more sustainable *health decisions.*

To *validate* its efficacy and support its broader adoption, a stepwise data-driven evaluation framework—encompassing comparative studies, longitudinal research, multicenter trials, randomized controlled trials, and systematic reviews—is essential. These comprehensive validations have the *potential to revolutionize* hemorrhoid management and set new care standards for millions worldwide.

Acknowledgements

The author acknowledges the use of ChatGPT for language polishing of the manuscript.

I extend my gratitude to all the participants of this study, whose time and effort were invaluable in completing this work.

Special thanks to Jaldip, Forum, Niyati, Ajay, Nimesh, and many more for their excellent technical support.

Finally, I would like to thank my family for their unwavering support and encouragement throughout the course of this research.

Video materials

Video materials referenced in this chapter are available online at: https://bit.ly/41kycwe

Conflict of interest

The authors declare no conflict of interest.

*Was presented at SAGES as an ePoster in 2024 - https://link.springer.com/article/10.1007/s00464-024-10893-w

DOI: http://dx.doi.org/10.5772/intechopen.1009663

Author details

Parshottambhai Patel[1,2]

1 Shiv Shraddha Nursing Home, Ahmedabad, India

2 Apollo Hospitals, Ahmedabad, India

*Address all correspondence to: cancervijay@gmail.com

References

[1] Rossetti SR. Functional anatomy of pelvic floor. Archivio Italiano di Urologia e Andrologia [Internet]. 2016;**88**(1):28-37. Available from: https://www.pagepressjournals.org/aiua/article/view/aiua.2016.1.28 [Accessed: December 9, 2024]

[2] Palit S, Lunniss PJ, Scott SM. The physiology of human defecation. Digestive Diseases and Sciences. 2012;**57**(6):1445-1464

[3] Santucci NR, Velez A. Physiology of lower gastrointestinal tract. Alimentary Pharmacology & Therapeutics [Internet]. 2024;**60**(S1):S1-S19. Available from: https://onlinelibrary.wiley.com/doi/abs/10.1111/apt.17900 [Accessed: December 9, 2024]

[4] Margetis N. Pathophysiology of internal hemorrhoids. Annals of Gastroenterology. 2019. Available from: http://www.annalsgastro.gr/files/journals/1/earlyview/2019/ev-01-2019-19-AG4360-0355.pdf;**32**:1-9 [Accessed: December 9, 2024]

[5] Henderson NC, Rieder F, Wynn TA. Fibrosis: From mechanisms to medicines. Nature [Internet]. 2020;**587**(7835):555-566. Available from: https://www.nature.com/articles/s41586-020-2938-9 [Accessed: December 9, 2024]

[6] Heitmann PT, Vollebregt PF, Knowles CH, Lunniss PJ, Dinning PG, Scott SM. Understanding the physiology of human defaecation and disorders of continence and evacuation. Nature Reviews Gastroenterology & Hepatology [Internet]. 2021;**18**(11):751-769. Available from: https://www.nature.com/articles/s41575-021-00487-5 [Accessed: June 5, 2023]

[7] Transformative Strategies for Hemorrhoid Management - A New Era of Preserving Anatomy, Physiology, and Function - Retrospective Longitudinal Consecutive Case Series [Internet]. Available from: https://scholar.google.com/citations?view_op=view_citation&hl=en&user=LstZZboAAAAJ&citation_for_view=LstZZboAAAAJ:ODE9OILHJdcC [Accessed: December 10, 2024]

[8] Hawkins AT, Davis BR, Bhama AR, Fang SH, Dawes AJ, Feingold DL, et al. The American Society of Colon and Rectal Surgeons clinical practice guidelines for the Management of Hemorrhoids. Diseases of the Colon & Rectum [Internet]. 2024. Available from: https://journals.lww.com/10.1097/DCR.0000000000003276;**67**:614-623 [Accessed: October 17, 2024]

[9] Kitson A, Straus SE. The knowledge-to-action cycle: Identifying the gaps. CMAJ [Internet]. 2010;**182**(2):E73-E77. Available from: https://www.cmaj.ca/content/182/2/E73 [Accessed: December 10, 2024]

[10] Holtrop JS, Scherer LD, Matlock DD, Glasgow RE, Green LA. The importance of mental models in implementation science. Frontiers in Public Health [Internet]. 2021;**9**:680316. Available from: https://www.frontiersin.org/journals/public-health/articles/10.3389/fpubh.2021.680316/full [Accessed: December 10, 2024]

[11] Knowles CH, Dinning P, Scott SM, Swash M, De Wachter S. New concepts in the pathophysiology of fecal incontinence. Annals of Laparoscopic and Endoscopic Surgery [Internet]. 2022;**7**:15-15. Available from: https://ales.amegroups.com/article/view/8307/html [Accessed: December 9, 2024]

[12] Wang L, Ni J, Hou C, Wu D, Sun L, Jiang Q, et al. Time to change? Present and prospects of hemorrhoidal classification. Frontiers in Medicine [Internet]. 2023;**10**:1252468. Available from: https://www.frontiersin.org/journals/medicine/articles/10.3389/fmed.2023.1252468/full [Accessed: December 10, 2024]

[13] Sibbel R, Huber A. How human decision-making biases influence health outcomes in patient care. European Journal of Management Issues [Internet]. 2021;**29**(2):64-72. Available from: https://www.ceeol.com/search/article-detail?id=978224 [Accessed: December 10, 2024]

[14] Affairs BC for R Peace and World. Discernment as a Tool for Decision-Making [Internet]. Available from: https://berkleycenter.georgetown.edu/responses/discernment-as-a-tool-for-decision-making [Accessed: December 10, 2024]

[15] Nutton V, editor. Principles of Anatomy According to the Opinion of Galen by Johann Guinter and Andreas Vesalius. London: Routledge; 2017. 202 p

[16] Hodson D. Teaching and Learning about Science: Language, Theories, Methods, History, Traditions and Values. Leiden: Brill; 2009. 440 p

[17] Pata F, Gallo G, Pellino G, Vigorita V, Podda M, Di Saverio S, et al. Evolution of surgical Management of Hemorrhoidal Disease: An historical overview. Frontiers in Surgery [Internet]. 2021;**8**:727059. Available from: https://www.frontiersin.org/journals/surgery/articles/10.3389/fsurg.2021.727059/full [Accessed: December 10, 2024]

[18] Dukes CE. Frederick salmon: Founder of St. Mark's hospital, London. Medical History [Internet]. 1959;**3**(4):312-316. Available from: https://www.cambridge.org/core/journals/medical-history/article/frederick-salmon-founder-of-st-marks-hospital-london/5709E3622FC80419E622C8A6A15E69A5 [Accessed: December 10, 2024]

[19] Milligan ETC, Naunton Morgan C, Jones Lionel E, Officer R. Surgical anatomy of the anal canal, and the operative treatment of hæmorrhoids. The Lancet [Internet]. 1937;**230**(5959):1119-1124. Available from: https://linkinghub.elsevier.com/retrieve/pii/S0140673600884652 [Accessed: December 10, 2024]

[20] Graham ID, Logan J, Harrison MB, Straus SE, Tetroe J, Caswell W, et al. Lost in knowledge translation: Time for a map? Journal of Continuing Education in the Health Professions [Internet]. 2006;**26**(1):13. Available from: https://journals.lww.com/jcehp/abstract/2006/26010/lost_in_knowledge_translation__time_for_a_map_.3.aspx [Accessed: December 14, 2024]

[21] Kahneman D. Thinking, Fast and Slow. New York, NY, US: Farrar, Straus and Giroux; 2011. 499 p. (Thinking, fast and slow)

[22] Alfredsson J, Wick MJ. Mechanism of fibrosis and stricture formation in Crohn's disease. Scandinavian Journal of Immunology [Internet]. 2020;**92**(6):e12990. Available from: https://onlinelibrary.wiley.com/doi/abs/10.1111/sji.12990 [Accessed: December 9, 2024]

[23] Chimenti I, Sattler S, del Monte-Nieto G, Forte E. Editorial: Fibrosis and inflammation in tissue pathophysiology. Frontiers in Physiology [Internet]. 2022;**12**:830683. Available from: https://www.frontiersin.org/journals/physiology/articles/10.3389/

fphys.2021.830683/full [Accessed: December 9, 2024]

[24] Iwata K, Mikami Y, Kato M, Yahagi N, Kanai T. Pathogenesis and management of gastrointestinal inflammation and fibrosis: From inflammatory bowel diseases to endoscopic surgery. Inflammation and Regeneration [Internet]. 2021;**41**(1):21. DOI: 10.1186/s41232-021-00174-7

[25] Ng KS, Holzgang M, Young C. Still a case of "No pain, No gain"? An updated and critical review of the pathogenesis, diagnosis, and management options for hemorrhoids in 2020. Annals of Coloproctology [Internet]. Jun 2020;**36**(3):133-147. Available from: https://www.ncbi.nlm.nih.gov/pmc/articles/PMC7392573/ [Accessed: December 11, 2024]

[26] Mott T, Latimer K, Edwards C. Hemorrhoids: Diagnosis and treatment options. American Family Physician [Internet]. 2018;**97**(3):172-179. Available from: https://www.aafp.org/pubs/afp/issues/2018/0201/p172.html [Accessed: December 11, 2024]

[27] Larson JL. Reason and Experience [Internet]. Berkeley, CA: University of California Press; 1971. Available from: https://www.degruyter.com/document/doi/10.1525/9780520411777/html [Accessed: December 14, 2024]

[28] Lohsiriwat V. Hemorrhoids: From basic pathophysiology to clinical management. World Journal of Gastroenterology [Internet]. 2012;**18**(17):2009-2017. Available from: http://www.wjgnet.com/1007-9327/full/v18/i17/2009.htm [Accessed: December 10, 2024]

[29] Jorge JMN, Habr-Gama A. Anatomy and Embryology of the Colon, Rectum, and Anus. In: Wolff BG, Fleshman JW, Beck DE, Pemberton JH, Wexner SD, editors. The ASCRS Textbook of Colon and Rectal Surgery. New York, NY: Springer; 2007. pp. 1-22

[30] Lee JM, Kim NK. Essential anatomy of the Anorectum for colorectal surgeons focused on the gross anatomy and histologic findings. Annals of Coloproctology [Internet]. 2018;**34**(2):59-71. Available from: https://www.ncbi.nlm.nih.gov/pmc/articles/PMC5951097/ [Accessed: December 11, 2024]

[31] The Anal Canal - Structure - Arterial Supply - TeachMeAnatomy [Internet]. Available from: https://teachmeanatomy.info/abdomen/gi-tract/anal-canal/ [Accessed: December 11, 2024]

[32] Thompson-Fawcett MW, Warren BF, Mortensen NJM. A new look at the anal transitional zone with reference to restorative proctocolectomy and the columnar cuff. British Journal of Surgery [Internet]. 1998;**85**(11):1517-1521. DOI: 10.1046/j.1365-2168.1998.00875.x

[33] Ahmed A, Arbor TC, Qureshi WA. Anatomy, Abdomen and Pelvis: Anal Canal. In: StatPearls [Internet]. Treasure Island (FL): StatPearls Publishing; 2024. Available from: http://www.ncbi.nlm.nih.gov/books/NBK554531/ [Accessed: December 11, 2024]

[34] Grizzi F, Chiriva-Internati M. The complexity of anatomical systems. Theoretical Biology & Medical Modelling. Dec 2005;**2**(1):26

[35] Wensing M, Wilson P. Making implementation science more efficient: Capitalizing on opportunities beyond the field. Implementation Science [Internet]. 2023;**18**(1):40. DOI: 10.1186/s13012-023-01298-9

Chapter 6

Hemorrhoids in Pregnancy and Breastfeeding

Arum Linangkung

Abstract

Hemorrhoid is the fourth leading outpatient gastrointestinal disease. In pregnancy, hemorrhoids are a challenging yet most common disease in the second and third trimesters. The hormonal changes, weight gain, pressure from the growing uterus, changes in blood flow, and constipation contribute to the causes. Bleeding and painful bowel movements can affect the growing baby and the quality of breastfeeding if not well treated during and after pregnancy. Worsening conditions, such as prolapsed, strangulated, and thrombosed hemorrhoids, contribute to serious management and surgical intervention. Hemorrhoids are also responsible for considerable socioeconomic cost and personal suffering, which results in loss of productivity and quality of life.

Keywords: hemorrhoids, pregnancy, breastfeeding, prolapsed hemorrhoids, piles

1. Introduction

Hemorrhoids are a common condition affecting the anorectal area, marked by the enlargement and displacement of the normal anal cushions. This condition impacts millions globally and constitutes a significant medical and socioeconomic concern. Hemorrhoids are common during pregnancy. The rate of hemorrhoids during pregnancy is considerably higher in women with a history of hemorrhoids and those experiencing multifetal pregnancies [1]. The most reported symptoms include burning, itching, perianal pain, and rectal bleeding. In the third trimester and postpartum period, the symptoms usually worsen; constipation or chronic diarrhea sometimes occurs, and patients seek medical help. The incidence of hemorrhoids varies widely, with studies estimating a prevalence between 15% and 41%, and in certain populations, it may reach as high as 85%. The likelihood of hemorrhoids development increases with maternal age and the number of pregnancies [2]. Due to the significant impact of hemorrhoids on maternal health, a comprehensive understanding of their pathophysiology, prevention, and management is essential for achieving long-term optimal care during pregnancy and breastfeeding.

2. Epidemiology

The exact incidence of hemorrhoidal disease remains underreported, as many affected individuals do not seek medical evaluation. Hemorrhoids are one of the most frequently diagnosed gastrointestinal conditions in outpatient settings in the United States, accounting for an estimated 4 million healthcare visits each year. Approximately 75% of the population is expected to experience hemorrhoid symptoms at some stage in life. Reported prevalence rates vary widely, ranging between 4 and 40%. The condition appears most common in Caucasians aged 45–65 and individuals from higher socioeconomic groups. However, these patterns may be influenced by differences in healthcare access and reporting bias [3].

The risk of developing hemorrhoids is closely linked to the number of pregnancies and deliveries, with a significant percentage of patients having experienced at least one previous pregnancy. After the first pregnancy, hemorrhoids occur in a notable percentage of women, and this number increases with subsequent pregnancies. Childbirth increases the risk of developing hemorrhoids almost eight times [4]. Pregnancy and spontaneous vaginal delivery are well-known risk factors for developing hemorrhoids in women, primarily due to increased intra-abdominal pressure from uterine expansion, hormonal changes, and constipation, which affects 38% of pregnant women. Clinical studies show that hemorrhoids are most common during the third trimester of pregnancy and within the first month after delivery, with approximately 25–35% of pregnant women experiencing this condition. Specifically, thrombosed hemorrhoids are more prevalent during the last trimester (7.8%) and immediately after childbirth (20%). The likelihood of symptomatic hemorrhoids in pregnant women rises with age and parity [3, 5].

3. Anatomy and physiological changes during pregnancy

Several anatomical and physiological changes during pregnancy are involved in the development of hemorrhoids. The primary major change is the increased abdominal pressure from the growing uterus. The mechanical effect of the expanding uterus and fetal growth put pressure on the rectum, the inferior vena cava, and the portal vein. The pressure causes impairment of the venous return, leading to venous stasis and blood pooling in the rectal veins. Additionally, the pressure on pelvic veins from the enlarging uterus creates vascular dilation in the pelvic area and contributes to hemorrhoid development. The secondary factor is the change in circulating blood volume, which rises by 25–40% during pregnancy. The increasing blood flow causes further engorgement of blood vessels, including those in the rectum, leading to hemorrhoids. The third factor is the hormonal changes, particularly the rising progesterone level has a significant role in the development of hemorrhoids. Progesterone relaxes the walls of veins and makes them more susceptible to swelling and dilation. It creates blood pooling in the veins, which exacerbates hemorrhoid symptoms. Estrogen also plays a role in altering vascular tone, contributing to venous dilation and increased susceptibility to hemorrhoids. The pregnancy-related gastrointestinal changes due to the increase in progesterone level slow gastrointestinal motility, leading to constipation, which is a common problem during pregnancy. Due to constipation, straining is required during bowel movements, which elevates the intra-abdominal pressure and develops hemorrhoids.

Fluid retention and edema are common during pregnancy due to hormonal changes and increased blood volume. The swelling effect affects the rectal area, increasing the likelihood of hemorrhoids. The change in circulatory dynamics, particularly from the compression of the inferior vena cava by the enlarged uterus, reduces venous return from the lower body and pelvic organs, contributing to venous stasis in the hemorrhoidal veins [6, 7].

Pelvic floor dysfunction happened due to weakened pelvic floor muscle from the growing uterus and vaginal delivery. Prolonged labor, forceful pushing, and instrumentation can stretch the pelvic floor muscles and hinder venous drainage from the rectal area, contributing to the development of hemorrhoids.

4. Pathophysiology of hemorrhoids in pregnancy and breastfeeding

There are several proposed theories in the pathophysiology of hemorrhoids. The varicose vein theory has been disproven. The vascular hyperplasia that hemorrhoids are erectile tissue and hypertonia of the internal anal sphincter have some validity, yet are not entirely conclusive. The cushion theory is widely accepted. It suggests the sliding anal canal process that hemorrhoids result from the abnormal displacement of anal cushions during defecation.

Four main pathophysiological events in the development of hemorrhoids are sliding of the anal cushions, degeneration of the connective tissue, impairment of the venous return during defecation, and blood stagnation within the dilated plexus. These key events occur due to chronic intra-abdominal pressure and the absence of valves in rectal veins, restricting venous drainage during defecation. Various factors such as upright posture, pregnancy, obesity, and straining during defecation can all increase abdominal pressure, contributing to hemorrhoid formation. Squatting position during defecation is better for toilet habits than sitting posture, which fails to straighten the anorectal and requires greater intra-abdominal pressure [6, 8].

Anal cushions move in opposing directions during defecation, resulting in repetitive stretching of Treitz's muscle. These structures are attached to the internal sphincter and the conjoined longitudinal muscle after returning to their normal position spontaneously. When the muscle fibers disintegrate, the sliding anal cushions persist in dan prolapse.

The weakening of supportive connective tissue also accelerates the prolapse of anal cushions. Mechanisms of impairment are muscle damage, collagen abnormalities (aging or Ehlers-Danlos syndrome), and increased activity of matrix metalloproteinases. The stretched mucosa contributes to fibrous tissue hypertrophy, elasticity loss, and retraction failure. Recently, chronic diarrhea, which can increase pressure on the venous system, is now considered a stronger risk factor than constipation for hemorrhoid development [9]. In contrast to constipation, persistent diarrhea often manifests as a prolonged inflammation from Crohn's disease or ulcerative colitis. However, some studies proved chronic diarrhea as a result of maternal hormonal fluctuation. Both constipation and chronic diarrhea prolong the defecation time, however, they should be treated from their etiologies individually.

Blood congestion is usually exacerbated by increased abdominal pressure and impaired venous return. Arterial hyper-perfusion and decreased vascular tone also contribute to this event. Passive congestion occurs when the ability of hypertrophied connective tissue fails to support the vascular network. The condition becomes more severe as the internal anal sphincter activity impedes venous return.

The progression of hemorrhoids transforms enlarged and engorged anal cushions into abnormal cushions or hemorrhoids or piles that prolapse through the anal canal. A series of vicious cycles progresses from congestion, increased anal pressure, and venous obstruction continuously. In acute prolapse, hemorrhoid tissue may become strangulated as the piles are trapped by the sphincter and the venous return is in a complete obstruction. Prolapsed hemorrhoids are inflamed and fragile.

Chronic inflammation affects both the vascular and supportive tissues, making the vessels in the lamina propria vulnerable to erosion, causing bleeding during defecation. Thrombosed hemorrhoids are a result of an ischemic, ulcerated, and necrotic condition of the piles. Without any intervention this condition leads to further tissue damage and complications [8].

Many investigations have been conducted by gathering anatomical, functional, and histopathological data to study, yet the underlying causes of hemorrhoids are not completely understood. Whether hemorrhoids are primary or secondary conditions, we still need future research to clarify the etiology. Researchers agreed that hemorrhoid has multifactorial and numerous potential causes. In every patient, there is a unique individual combination of triggers and pathophysiological events that result in a personalized sequence of disease.

Understanding the modifiable factors in the pathophysiology of hemorrhoids during pregnancy and breastfeeding can be beneficial in preventing hemorrhoids from becoming symptomatic and complicated. In **Figure 1**, we can evaluate two important factors in maternal health status. The protector sign is the green light to protect the anal cushion from hemorrhoid formation or to prevent complications. The initiator sign is the opposite or the red light, which can trigger symptomatic hemorrhoids and increase their severity. Good stress management, adequate spiritual strength, an educative healthy lifestyle, and a supportive socioeconomic life are also important in pregnancy and breastfeeding well-being. An educative healthy lifestyle is contagious in this era of social media, including eating well, taking probiotics, being physically active, having enough sleep, and managing mental health.

Maternal health literacy will also improve the mechanical and hormonal factors consecutively. An excessive weight gain and massive increase in body mass index as a risk factor of hemorrhoids during gestation and lactation can be controlled. Controlled fetal growth is also helpful in the process of delivery in preventing prolonged labor, forceful pushing, instrumentation, perianal trauma, and pelvic floor dysfunction. Awareness and attention should be prioritized in older pregnant mothers as they are also facing degenerative issues, particularly during the third trimester and after childbirth, to improve their quality of life.

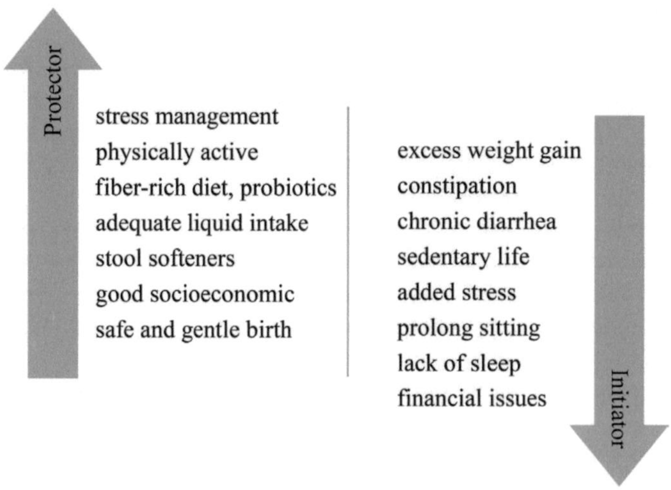

Figure 1.
Hemorrhoids' protector and initiator during pregnancy and breastfeeding.

Mental health in maternal well-being plays a key role in the development of hemorrhoids. The increase in progesterone can contribute to hemorrhoid formation by the fluctuation of the progesterone level [8]. Impaired mental health status also causes psychosomatic issues, lowering immunity status, which leads to ulcerative colitis or chronic diarrhea. Future research in the gut-brain connection during pregnancy is needed to be further investigated.

Constipation and chronic diarrhea increase intra-abdominal pressure and impede venous return, especially with prolonged defecation and straining, which exerts pressure on anal cushions. The risk factors for constipation and chronic diarrhea during pregnancy can be divided into four categories: (a) dietary changes due to iron supplementation, and inadequate fluid intake due to nausea and vomiting during pregnancy; (b) behavioral changes as a result of decreased physical activity, physical and social stress; (c) hormonal changes that impaired bowel movement as the effect of fluctuation of progesterone and estrogen levels, also from motilin concentration change; (d) other causes from the fetal and uterus growth in pregnancy and the painful hemorrhoids. Almost every pregnancy experiences nutritional alterations and gastrointestinal issues.

Constipation, chronic diarrhea, and hemorrhoid disease have a strong negative impact on both the physical and emotional well-being of maternal health, further worsening their quality of life after childbirth [4].

5. Diagnosis

Diagnosis of hemorrhoids should begin with a comprehensive medical history to identify relevant symptoms and risk factors, supported by physical examination findings. A thorough medical history should focus on symptoms associated with hemorrhoids and the risk factors such as constipation, low fiber intake, a sedentary lifestyle, and pregnancy status. A history of chronic or uncontrolled portal hypertension should be considered to distinguish hemorrhoid disease from anorectal varices. It is also important to investigate any history of inflammatory bowel disease and symptoms related to impaired anal continence to determine the most appropriate treatment [10].

6. Symptoms

The primary symptoms of hemorrhoids include rectal bleeding and prolapse of tissue, which are often the main reasons patients seek medical attention. The secondary symptoms, such as irritation and discomfort, may occur but are frequently attributed to other underlying conditions. Contrary to popular belief, pain is not a characteristic symptom of hemorrhoids and is usually indicative of complications such as thrombosis or strangulation [6]. Rectal bleeding is the most reported symptom of hemorrhoidal disease, often characterized by bright red blood that is typically painless. However, if the bleeding is accompanied by pain, other diagnoses, such as an anal fissure, should be considered. This bleeding generally occurs during or immediately after defecation. Prolapse occurs when internal hemorrhoids protrude through the anal canal, which can lead to discomfort and hygiene issues. Mucus discharge may occur due to irritation from prolapsed hemorrhoids. This should be distinguished from other conditions, such as rectal adenoma or carcinoma, to avoid misdiagnosis.

Pain is typically associated with prolapsed hemorrhoids that become strangulated or thrombosed. In the absence of prolapse, pain may suggest other conditions, including anal fissures or abscesses. Anemia, although rarely caused directly by hemorrhoids, can result from chronic hemorrhoid bleeding. If anemia persists, it should prompt screening for other potential causes, including colorectal carcinoma. Altered bowel habits, such as changes in stool caliber or narrowed stool, are not typically caused by hemorrhoids. These symptoms should be further evaluated for other conditions, such as colon cancer. Fecal incontinence can occur with large, prolapsed hemorrhoids, leading to mild incontinence. However, any instance of incontinence should be assessed carefully to rule out other conditions like rectal prolapse. Irritation and discomfort are common when persistent inflammation from hemorrhoids leads to itching and general discomfort in the perianal area. Swelling may occur with external hemorrhoids, causing perianal swelling. This can worsen with prolonged sitting or straining. Pruritus, or itching, is often caused by skin irritation from mucus discharge but may also result from infections or underlying dermatological conditions [11].

7. Physical examination

Physical examination should confirm the presence of hemorrhoid disease and rule out other anorectal conditions. This includes inspecting the perianal area, conducting a digital anorectal exam, and evaluating the degree of hemorrhoid prolapse during straining. Examination using an anoscope should also be part of the examination, with the Sims position being preferred as it is less uncomfortable for the patient compared to the prone position. For patients with hemorrhoid disease and rectal bleeding, a screening colonoscopy is recommended to exclude other potential colorectal conditions. In Western countries, hemorrhoid disease is one of the most common causes of severe acute lower gastrointestinal bleeding. However, rectal bleeding is also an early sign of colorectal cancer and other colorectal conditions, such as inflammatory bowel disease, diverticular disease, and angiodysplasia. Therefore, screening colonoscopy is essential to rule out these other conditions. Colonoscopy should be a mandatory indication for older patients or those with a personal or family history of colorectal cancers, advanced adenomas, inflammatory bowel disease, altered bowel habits, significant weight loss, or abnormal laboratory findings such as iron deficiency anemia or positive fecal occult blood tests (FOBT). When colonoscopy is contraindicated, flexible sigmoidoscopy may be used as an alternative screening method, often in conjunction with FOBT. Sigmoidoscopy and colonoscopy should be integrated with anoscopy, which has shown a higher detection rate for perianal pathology. Although an increased maximum resting anal pressure is commonly seen in non-prolapsing hemorrhoids, manometry is not routinely performed for diagnosis. Moreover, anorectal endosonography is generally not indicated for diagnosing hemorrhoid disease but may reveal thickening of the submucosal tissue or internal/external anal sphincter involvement [3, 6].

8. Preventive care medical treatment

Prevention care can be achieved with a healthy lifestyle and the understanding of maintaining the physiological changes not to become pathological and less symptomatic (**Figure 1**). A collaborative approach among multidisciplinary teams: family physician, proctologist, nutritionist, occupational therapist, obstetrician and gynecologist, leads to improved maternal health outcomes. Conservative pharmacologic management is often used for patients with mild prolapsed hemorrhoids. Medications such as topical and suppository treatments are commonly prescribed to reduce inflammation, itching, and pain in the affected area. Oral medications such as fiber supplementation or stool softeners can reduce straining during bowel movements and improve the symptoms. Analgesics including acetaminophen and ibuprofen are often used to manage mild pain. These medications are typically recommended for mild to moderate cases to provide temporary relief but not address the underlying issue, which may require surgical intervention. In acute cases. Oral and topical flavonoids are considered safe, acceptable, and effective in pregnancy, however, breastfeeding is not yet confirmed [3, 10]. Recent innovation in the biological agent for reducing inflammation in chronic hemorrhoids and refractory cases is still under research.

9. Surgical treatment

Surgical intervention is considered when conservative methods fail and the hemorrhoid piles are large and cause significant discomfort or complications. Open hemorrhoidectomy, the excision of the hemorrhoidal tissue, is considered the gold standard for advanced cases of hemorrhoid prolapse. This procedure has a high success rate and lowest recurrence rate but can be associated with significant postoperative pain and longer recovery time. This conventional hemorrhoidectomy is considered safe during pregnancy without risk to the fetus. Excision under local anesthesia can be performed safely in selective cases without special monitoring or increased risk of preterm labor or miscarriage [3, 9]. Stapled hemorrhoidopexy using a specialized stapling device to produce a circular ring of mucosal resection proximal to the piles and to suspend them. This procedure offers less operating time, an earlier return of bowel function, shorter hospital stays, less pain, faster functional recovery with shorter time off work, an earlier return to normal activities, and better wound healing. However, the incidence of recurrence and the need for future re-operations are also significantly higher when compared to the conventional method [3, 8].

10. Minimal invasive procedures

Minimally invasive procedures are typically used for patients with moderate symptoms, unfit for surgery, multi-comorbidities, or when there is a need for a faster recovery. Rubber band ligation (RBL) is one of the most common minimally invasive treatments, in which a rubber band is placed around the base of the hemorrhoid, leading to ischemia and the eventual detachment of the hemorrhoid. RBL is a safe and effective procedure in pregnancy and lactation [12]. Infrared photocoagulation can also be used for other treatment options that fail conservative treatment. However, its effectiveness is still debatable. Injection sclerotherapy, first described by Morgan in 1869, involves the injection of sclerosing agents into the apex of the internal hemorrhoidal complex above the dentate line. This causes tissue destruction, scarring, fibrosis, and fixation of the hemorrhoid tissue. Sclerosing agents like 5% phenol in almond oil, aluminum potassium sulfate and tannic acid (ALTA), and 50% dextrose water are commonly used, with ALTA being the most effective. In low-resource countries, 50% dextrose water may be a safe and effective alternative treatment option. Other minimally invasive options are Transanal Hemorrhoidal Dearterialization (THD), Doppler-guided Hemorrhoidal Artery Ligation (DGHAL) with rectoanal repair, and Anal Cushion Lifting (ACL). Those methods identify and ligate the feeding vessels of the hemorrhoids, reducing blood flow to the piles and restoring the anatomical position of the prolapsed mucosa.

The newest method of minimally invasive surgery is laser hemorroidoplasty. It appears to be more effective than the suture hemorrhoidopexy but less effective than hemorrhoidectomy and offers a less painful recovery process. The procedure using CO_2, argon, diode or Nd-YAG laser to create non-excisional convolution. It is feasible and safe, which seems to cause no significant changes in the anorectal physiology.

11. Rehabilitation and follow-up

Rehabilitation following hemorrhoid treatment focuses on preventing recurrence, managing postoperative symptoms, and facilitating recovery. Dietary modifications are essential, with an emphasis on increasing fiber intake and adequate hydration to avoid constipation and straining during bowel movements, which can exacerbate hemorrhoidal issues. Regular physical activity is also recommended to help promote bowel regularity, reduce weight gain, and prevent constipation. Anal hygiene is crucial in avoiding infection and recurrence, and patients are advised on proper cleaning methods and the use of sitz baths to alleviate discomfort. For pain management, patients are encouraged to use ice packs, sitz baths, and prescribed pain medications in the early stages of recovery. Sitz baths have been shown to significantly promote complete healing in pregnant women compared to conservative treatments such as anorectal creams.

Follow-up is vital for assessing healing, preventing complications, and detecting any recurrence of symptoms. The first follow-up visit typically occurs within 2–4 weeks after treatment to ensure proper healing and to address any issues such as pain or bleeding. For surgical procedures, such as hemorrhoidectomy or stapled hemorrhoidopexy, follow-up visits are essential to monitor for complications, including infection or bleeding. Long-term follow-up is recommended for all patients, particularly those who underwent minimally invasive treatments like rubber band ligation, as there is a higher risk of recurrence [13, 14].

12. Conclusion

Hemorrhoids in pregnancy and breastfeeding are common diseases and the first-line therapy should be conservative. Increasing fiber-rich diet and liquid intake, being physically active, having good stress management, reducing excessive weight gain, avoiding constipation, using stool softeners, and maintaining no-straining toilet habits can minimize the risk factors of hemorrhoids. Topical remedies, sitz baths, and suppositories can be used to help the symptomatic hemorrhoids spontaneously heal. When the symptoms worsen, surgical intervention should be individualized and tailored based on patients' severity and personal preference. Maintaining a healthy lifestyle after intervention is crucial to prevent future recurrence and achieve a better quality of life.

Conflict of interest

The authors declare no conflict of interest.

Author details

Arum Linangkung
Division of Digestive Surgery, Department of Surgery, Dr. Suhardi Hardjolukito Central Air Force National Hospital – Academic Hospital of Faculty of Medicine, Public Health and Nursing, Universitas Gadjah Mada, Yogyakarta, Indonesia

*Address all correspondence to: arum.linangkung@gmail.com

References

[1] Chen YY, Chang CY, Lin CH, Cheng LY, Shih WT, Chen KJ, et al. Prevalence, characteristics, and treatment of hemorrhoids during pregnancy: A nationwide population-based cohort study in Taiwan. Journal of Women's Health. 2023;**32**(12):1394-1401. DOI: 10.1089/jwh.2023.0124

[2] Boughton RS, Brophy C, Corbett G, Murphy S, Clifford J, Hanly A, et al. Haemorrhoids and anal fissures in pregnancy: Predictive factors and effective treatments. Cureus. 2024;**16**(2):e53773

[3] Gallo G, Martellucci J, Sturiale A, Clerico G, Milito G, Marino F, et al. Consensus statement of the Italian Society of Colorectal Surgery (SICCR): Management and treatment of hemorrhoidal disease. Techniques in Coloproctology. 2020;**24**(2): 145-164

[4] Bužinskienė D, Sabonytė-Balšaitienė Ž, Poškus T. Perianal diseases in pregnancy and after childbirth: Frequency, risk factors, impact on women's quality of life and treatment methods. Frontiers in Surgery. 2022;**9**:788823

[5] Poskus T, Sabonyte-Balsaitiene Z, Jakubauskiene L, Jakubauskas M, Stundiene I, Barkauskaite G, et al. Preventing hemorrhoids during pregnancy: A multicenter, randomized clinical trial. BMC Pregnancy and Childbirth. 2022;**22**(1):374. DOI: 10.1186/s12884-022-04688-x

[6] Ryu HS. Treatment of hemorrhoid in unusual condition-pregnancy. The Ewha Medical Journal. 2022;**45**(4):e11. DOI: 10.12771/emj.2022.e11

[7] Kazma JM, van den Anker J, Allegaert K, Dallmann A, Ahmadzia HK. Anatomical and physiological alterations of pregnancy. Journal of Pharmacokinetics and Pharmacodynamics. 2020;**47**(4):271-285

[8] Margetis N. Pathophysiology of internal hemorrhoids. Annals of Gastroenterology. 2019;**32**(3):264-272

[9] Hong YS, Jung KU, Rampal S, et al. Risk factors for hemorrhoidal disease among healthy young and middle-aged Korean adults. Scientific Reports. 2022;**12**:129. DOI: 10.1038/s41598-021-03838-z

[10] Hawkins AT et al. The American Society of Colon and Rectal Surgeons clinical practice guidelines for the management of hemorrhoids. Diseases of the Colon and Rectum. 2024;**67**(5):614-623. DOI: 10.1097/DCR.0000000000003276

[11] Kothari S et al. AGA clinical practice update on pregnancy-related gastrointestinal and liver disease: Expert review. Gastroenterology. 2024;**167**(5):1033-1045

[12] Stavrou G, Tzikos G, Malliou P, Panidis S, Kotzampassi K. Rubber band ligation of hemorrhoids: Is the procedure effective for the immunocompromised, hemophiliacs and pregnant women? Annals of Gastroenterology. 2022;**35**(5):509-513. DOI: 10.20524/aog.2022.0737

[13] Miyamoto H. Minimally invasive treatment for advanced hemorrhoids. Journal of the Anus, Rectum, and Colon. 2023;**7**(1):8-16. DOI: 10.23922/jarc.2022-068

[14] Rao SSC. Constipation, hemorrhoids, and anorectal disorders in pregnancy. The American Journal of Gastroenterology. 2022;**117**(10S):16-25. DOI: 10.14309/ajg.0000000000001962

Section 3

Rectal and Anal Tumors

Chapter 7

HPV, Anal and Rectal Cancer: Gender Norms, Health Behaviors, and Screening Disparities in Women

Ashley Parks and Adriana Jovanov

Abstract

Human papillomavirus (HPV) is a significant etiological factor in the development of anal and rectal cancers. Despite preventive measures such as vaccination and screening, disparities in incidence and outcomes persist between genders. This chapter explores the intersection of HPV-related health behaviors, gender norms, and systemic resource and screening disparities for women. It examines the epidemiology of HPV, biological mechanisms of carcinogenesis, and health behaviors that mitigate cancer risk. A critical analysis of gender norms reveals how societal expectations influence health behaviors and access to care. The chapter concludes with strategies to improve screening rates and resource allocation, aiming to create a more equitable healthcare landscape.

Keywords: HPV, human papillomavirus, anal cancer, anal cancer screening, rectal cancer, gender norms, health behaviors, screening, Women's health

1. Introduction

Human papillomavirus (HPV) is a pervasive virus with a well-established role in the development of various cancers, including those of the anal and rectal regions. Despite advancements in preventive measures such as vaccination and screening, significant disparities remain in the incidence and outcomes of these cancers between genders. This chapter aims to explore the complex interplay of HPV-related health behaviors, gender norms, and systemic disparities in resources and screening for women.

Advancements in preventive measures have significantly impacted the management of HPV and related cancers. The introduction of HPV vaccines, such as Gardasil and Cervarix, has been a major breakthrough in reducing the incidence of HPV infections and subsequent cancers. These vaccines are effective against the most oncogenic HPV strains, including HPV-16 and HPV-18, which are responsible for the majority of HPV-related cancers [1]. Additionally, recent studies have shown that a single dose of the HPV vaccine can provide long-term protection, potentially simplifying vaccination schedules and increasing coverage [2, 3].

Screening for anal and rectal cancers has also seen improvements. High-resolution anoscopy (HRA) and anal cytology are now recommended for high-risk populations, such as individuals with HIV, to detect precancerous lesions early [4]. The ANCHOR study demonstrated that treating these precancerous lesions can significantly reduce the risk of developing anal cancer [5]. These advancements underscore the importance of early detection and intervention in preventing the progression of HPV-related diseases.

Despite these advancements, women continue to face unique challenges in accessing preventive measures. Societal norms and gender-specific barriers often hinder women's participation in vaccination and screening programs. For instance, cultural taboos and misconceptions about anal cancer can lead to delays in seeking medical advice and lower screening rates [6, 7]. This chapter will delve into these issues, presenting evidence from recent studies and expert opinions to underscore the urgent need for targeted interventions.

2. Gender differences in the epidemiology of HPV and anal/rectal cancer

Human papillomavirus (HPV) is the most common sexually transmitted infection globally, with certain strains being highly oncogenic. HPV is responsible for nearly all cervical cancers and many cancers of the vagina, vulva, penis, anus, rectum, and oropharynx [8]. According to the Centers for Disease Control and Prevention (CDC), an estimated 47,984 new cases of HPV-associated cancers are reported annually in the United States, with 26,280 among females and 21,704 among males [8].

Anal and rectal cancers, though less common than cervical cancer, have shown increasing incidence rates, particularly among women. Anal cancer is slightly more common in women than men, with an incidence rate of 1.9 per 100,000 people per year [9]. The five-year relative survival rate for anal cancer is approximately 70.6% [9]. The incidence of anal cancer has been rising over the past few decades. From 1975 to 2020, the rate of new cases of anal cancer increased from 0.82 per 100,000 persons to 2.01 per 100,000 persons [9]. This increase is partly attributed to the higher prevalence of HPV infection and the aging population. HPV types 16 and 18 are the most common high-risk strains associated with anal cancer, accounting for approximately 90% of cases [10].

Gender differences in the epidemiology of anal and rectal cancers are notable. Men generally have higher rates of rectal cancer compared to women, while women have a slightly higher incidence of anal cancer [11]. For instance, the incidence rate of rectal cancer in men is approximately 4.3 per 100,000 compared to 3.2 per 100,000 in women [12]. These differences may be influenced by various factors, including hormonal differences, lifestyle factors, and differences in the uptake of screening [13].

HPV vaccination has been shown to significantly reduce the incidence of HPV-associated cancers. The CDC recommends HPV vaccination for all preteens at ages 11 to 12 years old, with catch-up vaccination for all adults through age 26 years [7]. Despite these recommendations, vaccination coverage remains suboptimal. As of 2021, only 58.6% of adolescents aged 13–15 years had received the recommended doses of the HPV vaccine [7].

The burden of HPV-associated cancers varies by demographic factors such as race and ethnicity. Non-Hispanic American Indian/Alaska Native females have the highest incidence rates of HPV-associated cancers compared to other racial and ethnic groups, while non-Hispanic Asian/Pacific Islander females have the lowest rates [8]. These disparities underscore the urgent need for targeted public health interventions aimed at increasing vaccination and screening rates among high-risk populations, ensuring equitable access to preventive care.

3. Biological mechanisms of HPV-induced carcinogenesis

Before delving into health behaviors and differences across groups, it is essential to understand the biology of human papillomavirus (HPV) and its role in carcinogenesis. HPV is a small, double-stranded DNA virus from the Papillomaviridae family, with a genome of approximately 8 kilobase pairs. The virus infects epithelial cells and has more than 200 identified types, over 40 of which can be transmitted through sexual contact and infect the genital and anal regions [8].

HPV types are categorized into low-risk and high-risk groups based on their oncogenic potential. Low-risk types, such as HPV-6 and HPV-11, typically cause benign lesions like genital warts. In contrast, high-risk types, such as HPV-16 and HPV-18, are associated with various cancers, including cervical, anal, and oropharyngeal cancers [14]. Nearly all cervical cancers and a significant proportion of other anogenital cancers are attributed to high-risk HPV infections [14].

The progression from HPV infection to cancer follows a series of critical steps. Initially, HPV enters the basal cells of the epithelium through micro-abrasions. Once inside, the viral DNA may remain episomal (non-integrated) or integrate into the host genome, setting the stage for potential cellular changes that can lead to cancer development. Integration of high-risk HPV types, such as HPV-16 and HPV-18, is a critical event in carcinogenesis. This integration disrupts the E2 gene, leading to the overexpression of the E6 and E7 oncoproteins [4]. These oncoproteins interfere with tumor suppressor proteins p53 and retinoblastoma (pRb), respectively, leading to uncontrolled cell proliferation and genomic instability [4].

E6 oncoprotein promotes the degradation of p53, a key regulator of the cell cycle and apoptosis. By inactivating p53, E6 prevents the cell from undergoing apoptosis in response to DNA damage, allowing the accumulation of genetic mutations [13]. E7 oncoprotein binds to pRb, releasing E2F transcription factors that drive the cell cycle forward, leading to uncontrolled cell division [13]. The combined action of E6 and E7 oncoproteins disrupts normal cell cycle control, promoting the development of cancer.

Persistent HPV infection can result in the accumulation of additional genetic and epigenetic changes that propel the process of carcinogenesis. Furthermore, inflammation and oxidative stress serve as critical cofactors in HPV-mediated cancer development, creating an environment that fosters tumor progression. Chronic inflammation can result in the production of reactive oxygen species (ROS), which cause DNA damage and promote genetic instability [15]. Additionally, HPV infection can induce epigenetic modifications, such as DNA methylation and histone modification, which can alter gene expression and contribute to cancer progression [15].

HPV-driven carcinogenesis is a multistep process influenced by both viral and host factors. The initial outcome of carcinogenesis is modulated by the type of HPV (high-risk versus low-risk), the integration of HPV DNA into the host genome, and the host's immune response [16]. High-risk HPV types, such as HPV-16 and HPV-18, are more likely to integrate into the host genome and cause cancer compared to low-risk types, which are typically associated with benign lesions like genital warts [16].

Understanding the molecular mechanisms of HPV-induced carcinogenesis is crucial for developing targeted therapies and preventive strategies. Current research is focused on identifying therapeutic targets to prevent and reverse HPV integration, such as DNA damage response inhibitors, siRNA approaches, and epigenetic modifiers [8]. These strategies hold promise for improving the management and treatment of HPV-related cancers.

4. Strategies for risk mitigation: Vaccination and screening

4.1 HPV vaccination

Vaccination against HPV is a critical preventive measure, significantly reducing the risk of infection with high-risk strains. The HPV vaccine is highly effective in preventing infections with HPV types 16 and 18, which are responsible for approximately 70% of cervical cancers and a significant proportion of other anogenital cancers [8]. Despite its effectiveness, HPV vaccination coverage remains suboptimal. In 2022, only 58.6% of adolescents aged 13–15 years in the United States had received the recommended 2 or 3 doses of the HPV vaccine [17]. This low coverage is influenced by various factors, including lack of awareness, vaccine hesitancy, and access to healthcare services [18].

Barriers to HPV vaccination are multifaceted. A study identified several key barriers, including scheduling conflicts, lack of strong recommendations from healthcare providers, and concerns about vaccine safety and efficacy [19]. Additionally, socioeconomic factors such as lower income and education levels are associated with lower vaccination rates [20]. Addressing these barriers requires targeted public health interventions, including educational campaigns, policy changes to improve access to healthcare, and training for healthcare providers to effectively communicate the importance of HPV vaccination [19].

4.2 Safe sexual practices

Safe sexual practices are another important aspect of HPV risk mitigation. Using condoms and dental dams during vaginal, anal, and oral sex can reduce the risk of HPV transmission, although they do not provide complete protection as HPV can infect areas not covered by these barriers [21]. Limiting the number of sexual partners and avoiding sexual activity with individuals who have had many other partners can also lower the risk of HPV exposure [22]. Education on safe sexual practices is crucial, especially for young people who are at the highest risk of acquiring HPV.

4.3 Regular screening

Regular screening for HPV and related cancers is essential for early detection and treatment. The Pap test and HPV test are effective tools for detecting precancerous changes and HPV infections in the cervix. The CDC recommends that women start getting Pap tests at age 21 and continue with regular screenings as advised by their healthcare provider [23]. For women aged 30 to 65, co-testing with both the Pap test and HPV test every 5 years is recommended [24]. Despite these recommendations, many women face barriers to accessing screening services, including lack of insurance, limited access to healthcare providers, and cultural stigmas associated with sexual health [19].

Screening plays a crucial role in detecting cervical precancers, allowing for early treatment and preventing them from progressing into cancer. The HPV test looks for the virus that can cause cell changes on the cervix, while the Pap test looks for precancers, cell changes on the cervix that might become cervical cancer if not treated appropriately [23]. Regular screening and follow-up treatment are crucial in preventing cervical cancer and other HPV-related cancers [25].

5. Gender norms and health behaviors

Societal expectations and stereotypes heavily influence health behaviors, particularly when it comes to screening for anal and rectal cancers. Women often encounter unique barriers to accessing care, including the stigma tied to these cancers. Gender norms can further discourage women from seeking screening and treatment, deepening disparities in health outcomes. This section delves into the factors contributing to lower screening rates for anal and rectal cancers among women and highlights the risks associated with these disparities.

5.1 Stigma and cultural taboos

A major barrier to screening for anal and rectal cancers in women is the stigma and cultural taboos surrounding these diseases. Anal cancer, in particular, is often linked to sexual behavior, which can evoke feelings of shame or embarrassment, deterring women from seeking essential screenings and care. Women may be reluctant to discuss symptoms or seek screening due to fear of judgment or misunderstanding from healthcare providers and their communities [8]. This stigma is compounded by the lack of public awareness and education about anal cancer, leading to misconceptions and delays in seeking medical advice [26].

5.2 Lack of awareness and education

Many women remain unaware of the risks associated with anal and rectal cancers or the importance of regular screenings. While public health campaigns have heavily emphasized awareness for breast and cervical cancers, this focus has created a significant gap in understanding and education about less common but equally critical cancers like anal and rectal cancers. This lack of awareness means that women may not recognize the symptoms of these cancers or understand the need for regular screening [18]. Educational initiatives are crucial to inform women about the risks and encourage proactive health behaviors. It is vital to ensure that healthcare providers are equipped with adequate education, training, and materials for patients throughout the community they serve. The lack of awareness and education surrounding HPV, anal cancer, and rectal cancer significantly contributes to the stigma and misinformation associated with these health issues. Many individuals remain uninformed about the risks associated with HPV and the importance of early detection and prevention strategies. By enhancing the education and training of healthcare providers, we can empower them to effectively communicate the risks, prevention methods, and screening options to their patients. This, in turn, fosters a more informed community, reduces stigma, and promotes proactive health behaviors, ultimately leading to improved outcomes in the fight against these preventable cancers.

5.3 Healthcare provider barriers

Healthcare providers play a critical role in recommending and conducting cancer screenings. However, there is often a lack of training and comfort among providers in discussing and performing anal and rectal cancer screenings. This can result in missed opportunities for early detection and intervention. Additionally, some providers may not be aware of the latest guidelines for screening high-risk populations, further contributing to the low screening rates [19]. Training programs and resources for healthcare providers are essential to improve screening practices and patient communication.

5.4 Socioeconomic factors

Socioeconomic challenges play a significant role in shaping disparities in screening rates. Women from lower-income backgrounds often face barriers that limit their access to essential healthcare services, including lifesaving cancer screenings. Financial barriers, such as lack of insurance or high out-of-pocket costs, can prevent women from seeking preventive care. Additionally, women in rural or underserved areas may face logistical challenges, such as long travel distances to healthcare facilities, which can deter them from getting screened [20]. Addressing these socioeconomic barriers is vital to improving access to screening and reducing disparities.

5.5 Risks of not screening

The risks associated with not screening for anal and rectal cancers are considerable. Early detection plays a crucial role in enabling more effective treatment and improving patient outcomes. In the absence of regular screening, these cancers may be identified at a more advanced stage, making them more challenging to treat and resulting in lower survival rates. Without regular screening, cancers may be diagnosed at a more advanced stage, when they are harder to treat and survival rates are lower. For example, the five-year relative survival rate for localized anal cancer is approximately 82%, but this drops to 30% for distant-stage disease [27]. Regular screening can detect precancerous lesions and early-stage cancers, allowing for timely intervention and improved prognosis [28].

5.6 Strategies to improve screening rates

To address these challenges, several strategies can be implemented to improve screening rates for anal and rectal cancers in women:

- *Educational campaigns*: Public health campaigns should focus on raising awareness about the risks of anal and rectal cancers and the importance of screening. These campaigns can help reduce stigma and encourage women to seek preventive care. For example, campaigns that include testimonials from survivors can personalize the message and make it more relatable [29].

- *Training for healthcare providers*: Providing training and resources for healthcare providers can improve their ability to discuss and perform screenings. This includes education on the latest screening guidelines and techniques for high-risk populations. Workshops and continuing education courses can be effective in updating providers' knowledge and skills [26].

- *Policy changes*: Implementing policies that reduce financial barriers to screening, such as expanding insurance coverage for preventive services, can increase access to care for underserved populations. Policies that mandate coverage for HPV vaccination and screening can also play a crucial role [7].

- *Community-based initiatives*: Local health organizations can play a crucial role in providing resources and support to women, helping them navigate the healthcare system and access necessary services. Community health workers can provide education and support to encourage screening. For instance, mobile clinics can bring screening services to rural and underserved areas, reducing logistical barriers [25].

These strategies will be more fully explored in Section 7, where we will discuss specific interventions and programs that have been successful in increasing screening rates and improving health outcomes for women.

6. Implications for education and healthcare

The implications of HPV and anal/rectal cancer extend beyond individual health, affecting both education and healthcare systems. Understanding these implications is crucial for developing effective strategies to prevent and manage these cancers, particularly among women who face unique challenges due to gender norms and health behaviors.

6.1 Implications for health education

Educational initiatives play a vital role in raising awareness about HPV and its associated risks. Comprehensive sex education programs that include information about HPV, its transmission, and the importance of vaccination can significantly reduce the incidence of HPV-related cancers. These programs should target not only adolescents but also parents and educators to ensure a broad understanding of the benefits of HPV vaccination and regular screening [8]. For example, integrating HPV education into school curricula can help normalize discussions about sexual health and reduce stigma.

Public health campaigns are a vital element of education in this area. By addressing misconceptions and reducing the stigma surrounding anal and rectal cancers, these campaigns can encourage open discussions and increase awareness, ultimately promoting early detection and treatment. For instance, campaigns that feature testimonials from cancer survivors can personalize the message and make it more relatable, encouraging more women to seek preventive care [26]. Additionally, integrating HPV education into routine healthcare visits can provide ongoing opportunities for patients to learn about their risks and the steps they can take to protect themselves [18].

6.2 Implications for healthcare

Healthcare providers are on the front lines of HPV prevention and cancer screening. Ensuring that providers are well-informed about the latest guidelines for HPV vaccination and cancer screening is crucial. Training programs and continuing education courses can help providers stay updated on best practices and improve their ability to communicate effectively with patients about the importance of vaccination and screening [19]. For example, workshops on cultural competency can help providers address the specific needs and concerns of diverse patient populations.

Healthcare systems must also address the barriers that prevent women from accessing preventive care. This includes expanding insurance coverage for HPV vaccination and cancer screening, particularly for underserved populations. Policies that reduce out-of-pocket costs and provide financial assistance can make these services more accessible [20]. Additionally, healthcare facilities should strive to create a welcoming and non-judgmental environment where women feel comfortable discussing their health concerns and seeking care [27]. Implementing patient navigation programs can help guide women through the healthcare system, ensuring they receive timely and appropriate care.

6.3 Public health implications

From a public health perspective, increasing HPV vaccination rates and improving screening for anal and rectal cancers can significantly reduce the burden of these diseases. Public health initiatives should focus on high-risk populations, including women with a history of HPV-related cancers, individuals with HIV, and those engaging in high-risk sexual behaviors [28]. Community-based programs that provide education, vaccination, and screening services can help reach these populations and reduce disparities in cancer outcomes [29]. For example, mobile health clinics can bring services directly to underserved communities, overcoming barriers related to transportation and access.

Research and data collection are also critical components of public health efforts. Monitoring vaccination rates, screening uptake, and cancer incidence can help identify gaps in care and inform targeted interventions. Collaboration between public health agencies, healthcare providers, and community organizations is essential to develop and implement effective strategies for HPV prevention and cancer control [26]. For instance, partnerships with local schools and community centers can facilitate outreach and education efforts.

7. Strategies for addressing gender disparities in access and outcomes

To improve screening rates and resource allocation for women, several strategies can be implemented. This section will explore policy changes, educational campaigns, community-based initiatives, and programs that empower women, providing real-life examples and evidence-based sources to illustrate their effectiveness.

7.1 Policy changes

Implementing policies that require coverage for HPV vaccination and screening can greatly enhance access to essential preventive services. A notable example is the HPV Cancer Prevention Program at St. Jude Children's Research Hospital, which has played a pivotal role in advocating for policy changes aimed at increasing HPV vaccination coverage and ensuring more individuals benefit from these crucial health services. Their analysis identified several factors that influence vaccination rates, such as Medicaid income eligibility, insurance coverage, and access to primary care physicians. Based on these findings, they developed policy recommendations, including leveraging meningococcal conjugate vaccination as a model for HPV vaccination education and recommendations, and opposing non-medical vaccination exemptions [30].

Another successful policy initiative is the Healthy People 2030 objective set by the U.S. Department of Health and Human Services, which aims to increase HPV vaccination rates to 80% among adolescents aged 13 through 15. This objective has driven legislative efforts to introduce and enforce vaccination requirements, particularly in states with low vaccination rates [31]. For instance, Rhode Island implemented a policy requiring HPV vaccination for all students entering seventh grade, resulting in a significant increase in vaccination coverage [32].

In Australia, the National HPV Vaccination Program provides free HPV vaccines to school-aged children, which has led to one of the highest vaccination rates globally. This program has significantly reduced the incidence of HPV-related cancers and serves as a model for other countries [33]. Similarly, Scotland's national HPV vaccination program has achieved high coverage rates and a substantial reduction in cervical precancerous lesions among vaccinated cohorts [34].

7.2 Educational campaigns

Public health campaigns play a crucial role in educating women about the risks of HPV and the importance of regular screening. The European Cancer Organization's HPV Action Network launched the "HPV Testimonies" campaign, which features personal stories from individuals affected by HPV-related cancers. These testimonials highlight the importance of vaccination and screening, making the message more relatable and impactful [35].

In the United States, the CDC's "Inside Knowledge" campaign aims to raise awareness about gynecologic cancers, including cervical cancer caused by HPV. The campaign provides educational materials, public service announcements, and survivor stories to educate women about the symptoms, risk factors, and the importance of regular screening [36]. Additionally, the "Protect Them" campaign by the American Cancer Society focuses on educating parents about the benefits of HPV vaccination for their children, emphasizing the vaccine's role in cancer prevention [37].

The "Be Clear on Cancer" campaign in the UK has also been effective in raising awareness about various cancers, including cervical cancer. This campaign uses mass media, including TV and radio ads, to reach a broad audience and encourage early detection and screening [38]. Another example is the "Get Checked" campaign in New Zealand, which promotes regular health checks and cancer screenings through community events and social media outreach [39].

7.3 Community-based initiatives

Local health organizations can provide resources and support to women, helping them navigate the healthcare system and access necessary services. The Clinton Health Access Initiative (CHAI) has implemented community-based HPV self-testing programs in several African countries, including Zimbabwe, Kenya, and Malawi. These programs deliver self-sampling kits directly to women in their homes and community health posts, making screening more accessible and increasing uptake. Preliminary findings show that community-based HPV testing achieves comparable rates of follow-up care to facility-based models, with women reporting that the self-collection process is easy and convenient [40].

In the United States, the Take CARE (Clinical Avenues to Reach Health Equity) initiative focuses on reducing cervical cancer incidence and mortality in Appalachian communities. This program includes three evidence-based initiatives: "I Vaccinate" for HPV vaccination, "Break Free" for smoking cessation, and "HOME" for cervical cancer screening. By engaging community members and healthcare providers, the program addresses barriers to vaccination and screening, such as transportation and healthcare access, and promotes health equity [41].

The "Pink Ribbon Red Ribbon" initiative, launched by the George W. Bush Institute, focuses on reducing cervical and breast cancer in sub-Saharan Africa and Latin America. This program partners with local governments and organizations to provide education, vaccination, and screening services, significantly improving cancer prevention and treatment in these regions [42]. Another example is the "Screen Our Circle" initiative by the American Indian Cancer Foundation, which aims to increase cancer screening rates among Native American women through culturally tailored education and outreach [43].

7.4 Empowering women

Programs that empower women to take charge of their health can significantly boost participation in preventive measures and screenings. For instance, the Rural Health Network's women's health initiative highlights the importance of regular check-ups and screenings, offering comprehensive guides and support tailored to women at various life stages. This approach not only fosters awareness but also encourages proactive health management among women. By offering in-person and telehealth services, the program ensures that women have convenient access to care, regardless of their location [44].

Another exemplary initiative is the Women's Health and Wellness Clinic, which offers a range of services including gynecological health care, mental health check-ups, and heart health evaluations. The clinic focuses on educating women about the significance of preventive care, empowering them to make informed decisions regarding their health and well-being. This holistic approach not only enhances awareness but also fosters a proactive attitude toward health management. This holistic approach addresses both physical and mental health, recognizing the interconnectedness of overall well-being [45].

The "Every Woman Every Child" initiative, launched by the United Nations, aims to improve the health and well-being of women and children worldwide. This program focuses on empowering women through education, healthcare access, and economic opportunities, leading to better health outcomes and increased participation in preventive care [46]. Additionally, the "Strong Women, Strong World" initiative by World Vision focuses on empowering women in developing countries through health education, vocational training, and community support [47].

8. Conclusion

Addressing the disparities in HPV-related anal and rectal cancers requires a multifaceted approach that includes policy changes, educational efforts, and community support. By understanding and addressing the unique challenges faced by women, we can create a more equitable healthcare landscape where all individuals have access to the necessary tools for cancer prevention and early detection.

Throughout this chapter, we have explored various strategies to improve screening rates and resource allocation for women. These strategies encompass policy changes, educational campaigns, community-based initiatives, and programs that empower women.

8.1 Policy changes

Implementing policies that mandate coverage for HPV vaccination and screening can significantly increase access to preventive services. Successful policy initiatives, such as the Healthy People 2030 objective set by the U.S. Department of Health and Human Services, aim to increase HPV vaccination rates among adolescents [31]. Similarly, the National HPV Vaccination Program in Australia provides free HPV vaccines to school-aged children, resulting in one of the highest vaccination rates globally [33]. These policy changes have proven effective in increasing vaccination coverage and reducing the incidence of HPV-related cancers.

8.2 Educational campaigns

Public health campaigns play a crucial role in educating women about the risks of HPV and the importance of regular screening. Campaigns like the CDC's "Inside Knowledge" and the American Cancer Society's "Protect Them" focus on raising awareness about gynecologic cancers and the benefits of HPV vaccination [36, 37]. These campaigns use various media channels to reach a broad audience, making the message more relatable and impactful. By providing educational materials, public service announcements, and survivor stories, these campaigns help women understand the importance of preventive care.

8.3 Community-based initiatives

Local health organizations can provide resources and support to women, helping them navigate the healthcare system and access necessary services. Programs like the Clinton Health Access Initiative's community-based HPV self-testing in African countries have made screening more accessible and increased uptake [40]. In the United States, the Take CARE initiative focuses on reducing cervical cancer incidence and mortality in Appalachian communities by addressing barriers to vaccination and screening [41]. These community-based initiatives are essential in reaching underserved populations and promoting health equity.

8.4 Empowering women

Programs that empower women to take charge of their health can lead to increased participation in preventive measures and screenings. The Rural Health Network's women's health initiative and the Women's Health and Wellness Clinic provide comprehensive guides and support for women at different life stages [44, 45]. These programs emphasize the importance of regular check-ups and screenings, ensuring that women have convenient access to care. Additionally, global initiatives like the United Nations' "Every Woman Every Child" and World Vision's "Strong Women, Strong World" focus on empowering women through education, healthcare access, and economic opportunities [46, 47]. By empowering women, these programs contribute to better health outcomes and increased participation in preventive care.

8.5 Addressing gender norms and health behaviors

Societal expectations and stereotypes significantly influence health behaviors, especially when it comes to screening for anal and rectal cancers. Women encounter distinct challenges in accessing healthcare, including the stigma associated with these cancers. These entrenched gender norms can deter women from seeking necessary screenings and treatments, ultimately worsening disparities in health outcomes. Addressing these challenges requires targeted educational campaigns to raise awareness and reduce stigma, as well as training for healthcare providers to improve their ability to discuss and perform screenings [8, 19, 26].

8.6 Addressing biological mechanisms of HPV-induced carcinogenesis

Understanding the molecular mechanisms of HPV-induced carcinogenesis is crucial for developing targeted therapies and preventive strategies. HPV-driven carcinogenesis involves the integration of viral DNA into the host genome, leading to the overexpression of oncoproteins that disrupt normal cell cycle control and promote cancer development [4, 13]. Research focused on identifying therapeutic targets to prevent and reverse HPV integration holds promise for improving the management and treatment of HPV-related cancers [8].

8.7 Considering the implications for education and healthcare

Educational initiatives play a vital role in raising awareness about HPV and its associated risks. Comprehensive sex education programs and public health campaigns can significantly reduce the incidence of HPV-related cancers by informing individuals about the importance of vaccination and regular screening [8, 26]. Healthcare providers must be well-informed about the latest guidelines for HPV vaccination and cancer screening, and healthcare systems must address barriers that prevent women from accessing preventive care [19, 20].

In conclusion, addressing the disparities in HPV-related anal and rectal cancers requires a comprehensive approach that includes policy changes, educational efforts, and community support. By implementing effective policies, launching impactful educational campaigns, supporting community-based initiatives, and empowering women, we can create a more equitable healthcare landscape. These strategies not only improve screening rates and resource allocation but also ensure that all individuals have access to the necessary tools for cancer prevention and early detection. By continuing to build on these efforts, we can make significant strides in reducing the burden of HPV-related cancers and improving health outcomes for women worldwide.

Acknowledgements

The authors would like to acknowledge the support of their respective institutions in providing them with the time and resources to complete this chapter. The author acknowledges the use of CoPilot, a ChatGPT 4 tool, for language polishing of the manuscript and Zotero for the polishing of all reference formatting.

Conflict of interest

The authors declare no conflict of interest.

Notes/thanks/other declarations

The authors with to thank their families for their consistent support as they pursue meaningful careers as women in public health.

Author details

Ashley Parks[1*] and Adriana Jovanov[2]

1 Appalachian State University, Boone, NC, USA

2 OneLegacy, Murrieta, CA, USA

*Address all correspondence to: parksav@appstate.edu

References

[1] Kreimer AR, Struyf F, Del Rosario-Raymundo MR, et al. Efficacy of fewer than three doses of an HPV-16/18 AS04-adjuvanted vaccine: Combined analysis of data from the Costa Rica vaccine and PATRICIA trials. The Lancet Oncology. 2015;**16**(7):775-786. DOI: 10.1016/S1470-2045(15)00047-9

[2] Palefsky JM, Giuliano AR, Goldstone S, et al. HPV vaccine against anal HPV infection and anal intraepithelial neoplasia. The New England Journal of Medicine. 2011;**365**(17):1576-1585. DOI: 10.1056/NEJMoa1010971

[3] National Cancer Institute. Single Dose of HPV Vaccine. Available from: https://www.cancer.gov/news-events/cancer-currents-blog/2020/hpv-vaccine-single-dose-long-term-protection

[4] D'Souza G, Wiley DJ, Li X, et al. Incidence and epidemiology of anal cancer in the Multicenter AIDS cohort study. Journal of Acquired Immune Deficiency Syndromes. 2008;**48**(4):491-499. DOI: 10.1097/QAI.0b013e31817aebfe

[5] National Cancer Institute. ANCHOR Study. Available from: https://anchorstudy.org/sites/default/files/newsletters/anchor_press_release_07oct2021.pdf

[6] Darragh TM, Colgan TJ, Cox JT, et al. The lower Anogenital squamous terminology standardization project for HPV-associated lesions: Background and consensus recommendations from the College of American Pathologists and the American Society for Colposcopy and Cervical Pathology. Archives of Pathology & Laboratory Medicine. 2012;**136**(10):1266-1297. DOI: 10.5858/arpa.LGT200570

[7] Centers for Disease Control and Prevention. HPV Vaccination. Available from: https://www.cdc.gov/hpv/parents/vaccine.html

[8] Senapati R, Senapati NN, Dwibedi B. Molecular mechanisms of HPV mediated neoplastic progression. Infect Agents Cancer. 2016;**11**:59. DOI: 10.1186/s13027-016-0107-4

[9] National Cancer Institute. Cancer Stat Facts: Anal Cancer. 2024. Available from: https://seer.cancer.gov/statfacts/html/anus.html

[10] Centers for Disease Control and Prevention. Cancers Linked with HPV each Year. 2024. Available from: https://www.cdc.gov/cancer/hpv/cases.html

[11] Gao RN, Neutel CI, Wai E. Gender differences in colorectal cancer incidence, mortality, hospitalizations and surgical procedures in Canada. Journal of Public Health (Oxford, England). 2008;**30**(2):194-201. DOI: 10.1093/pubmed/fdn019

[12] Park IJ, Lee C. Sex disparities in colorectal cancer. In: Sex/Gender-Specific Medicine in Clinical Areas. Springer; 2024. pp. 345-353. DOI: 10.1007/978-981-97-0130-8_19

[13] Cubie HA. Diseases associated with human papillomavirus infection. Virology. 2013;**445**(1-2):21-34. DOI: 10.1016/j.virol.2013.06.007

[14] Wang X, Huang X, Zhang Y. Involvement of human papillomaviruses in cervical cancer. Frontiers in Microbiology. 2018;**9**:2896. DOI: 10.3389/fmicb.2018.02896

[15] National Cancer Institute. HPV and Cancer. 2024. Available from:

https://www.cancer.gov/about-cancer/causes-prevention/risk/infectious-agents/hpv-and-cancer

[16] Doorbar J, Quint W, Banks L, et al. The biology and life-cycle of human papillomaviruses. Vaccine. 2012;**30S**:F55-F70. DOI: 10.1016/j.vaccine.2012.06.083

[17] National Cancer Institute. HPV Vaccination. 2024. Available from: https://progressreport.cancer.gov/prevention/hpv_immunization

[18] Escoffery C, Riehman K, Watson L, Priess AS, Borne MF, Halpin SN, et al. Facilitators and barriers to the implementation of the HPV VACs (vaccinate adolescents against cancers) program: A consolidated framework for implementation research analysis. Preventing Chronic Disease. 2019;**16**:180406. DOI: 10.5888/pcd16.180406

[19] Batur P. The HPV Vaccine: Understanding and addressing barriers to vaccination. Cleveland Clinic Journal of Medicine. 2020;**87**(9):545-552. DOI: 10.3949/ccjm.87a.ccc051

[20] Villarroel MA, Galinsky AM, Lu PJ, Pingali C. Human papillomavirus vaccination coverage in children ages 9-17 years: United States, 2022. NCHS Data Brief. 2024;**495**:1-8. DOI: 10.15620/cdc:123456

[21] Planned Parenthood. How Do you Prevent HPV? 2024. Available from: https://www.plannedparenthood.org/learn/stds-hiv-safer-sex/hpv/how-can-i-make-sure-i-dont-get-or-spread-hpv

[22] American Cancer Society. How to Protect against HPV. 2024. Available from: https://www.cancer.org/cancer/risk-prevention/hpv/hpv-prevention.html

[23] Centers for Disease Control and Prevention. Screening for Cervical Cancer. 2024. Available from: https://www.cdc.gov/cervical-cancer/screening/index.html

[24] Centers for Disease Control and Prevention. Preventing HPV-Associated Cancers. 2024. Available from: https://www.cdc.gov/cancer/hpv/preventing-hpv-associated-cancers.html

[25] World Health Organization. Human Papillomavirus (HPV) and Cervical Cancer. 2024. Available from: https://www.who.int/news-room/fact-sheets/detail/human-papillomavirus-(hpv)-and-cervical-cancer

[26] National Cancer Institute. Anal Cancer Advances Open Door to Screening and Prevention. Available from: https://www.cancer.gov/news-events/cancer-currents-blog/2024/anal-cancer-screening-self-collected

[27] American Cancer Society. Risk Factors for Anal Cancer. 2024. Available from: https://www.cancer.org/cancer/types/anal-cancer/causes-risks-prevention/risk-factors.html

[28] OncoLink. Anal Cancer Screening for People at High Risk. 2024. Available from: https://www.oncolink.org/cancers/gastrointestinal/anal-cancer/risk-and-prevention/anal-cancer-screening

[29] American Cancer Society. Why we Screen for some Cancers and Not Others. 2024. Available from: https://www.cancer.org/cancer/latest-news/why-we-screen-for-some-cancers-and-not-others.html

[30] St. Jude Children's Research Hospital. Updated Analysis of Public Policy Decisions and Factors Driving HPV Vaccination Coverage in the

United States. 2024. Available from: https://www.stjude.org/research/comprehensive-cancer-center/hpv-cancer-prevention-program/analysis-hpv-vaccination-coverage-us.html

[31] U.S. Department of Health and Human Services. Healthy People 2030. 2024. Available from: https://health.gov/healthypeople

[32] Rhode Island Department of Health. HPV Vaccination Requirement for School Entry. 2025. Available from: https://health.ri.gov/immunization/for/schools

[33] Australian Government Department of Health. National HPV Vaccination Program. 2024. Available from: https://www.health.gov.au/initiatives-and-programs/national-hpv-vaccination-program

[34] Public Health Scotland. HPV Vaccination Programme. 2024. Available from: https://www.publichealthscotland.scot/our-areas-of-work/immunisation/hpv-vaccination-programme/

[35] European Cancer Organisation. Real-Life Stories of HPV-Related Cancers Underline Urgent Need for Access to Vaccination and Screening. 2024. Available from: https://www.europeancancer.org/resources/news/real-life-stories-of-hpv-related-cancers-underline-urgent-need-for-access-to-vaccination-and-screening.html

[36] Centers for Disease Control and Prevention. Inside Knowledge: Get the Facts about Gynecologic Cancer. 2024. Available from: https://www.cdc.gov/cancer/gynecologic/knowledge/index.htm

[37] American Cancer Society. Protect Them: HPV Vaccine Campaign. 2024. Available from: https://www.cancer.org/healthy/hpv-vaccine.html

[38] Public Health England. Be Clear on Cancer. 2024. Available from: https://www.nhs.uk/be-clear-on-cancer/

[39] Ministry of Health New Zealand. Get Checked Campaign. 2024. Available from: https://www.health.govt.nz/your-health/healthy-living/get-checked

[40] Clinton Health Access Initiative. Advancing Cervical Cancer Prevention: Empowering Women, Saving Lives, and Driving Elimination Efforts. 2024. Available from: https://www.clintonfoundation.org/press-and-news/clinton-health-access-initiative/advancing-cervical-cancer-prevention-empowering-women-saving-lives-and-driving-elimination-efforts/

[41] St. Jude Research. Community-Engaged Approaches to Cervical Cancer Prevention in Appalachia. 2024. Available from: https://www.stjude.org/research/comprehensive-cancer-center/hpv-cancer-prevention-program/resources/news-hpv-program/wos-electra-paskett.html

[42] George W. Bush Institute. Pink Ribbon Red Ribbon. 2024. Available from: https://www.bushcenter.org/explore-our-work/pink-ribbon-red-ribbon.html

[43] American Indian Cancer Foundation. Screen our Circle. 2024. Available from: https://www.americanindiancancer.org/screen-our-circle/

[44] Rural Health Network. Empowering Women's Health: Key Screening and Diagnostic Tests. 2024. Available from: https://www.ruralhealthnetworkinc.com/blog/empowering-women-s-health-key-screening-and-diagnostic-tests

[45] Women's Health and Wellness Clinic. Empowering Women: A Guide to Women's Health Screenings and Check-Ups. 2024. Available from: https://www.womenshealthandwellnessclinic.com/post/empowering-women-a-guide-to-women-s-health-screenings-and-check-ups

[46] United Nations. Every Woman every Child. 2024. Available from: https://www.everywomaneverychild.org/

[47] World Vision. Strong Women, Strong World. 2025. Available from: https://www.worldvision.org/strong-women-strong-world

Chapter 8

Predictive Factors in Tumor Response for Neoadjuvant Chemoradiotherapy in Rectal Cancer Patients

Yusif Aliyarov

Abstract

Reaching complete pathological response is one of the main goals in the treatment of patients with locally advanced rectal cancer. Factors that predict the response to neoadjuvant chemoradiotherapy are the issue of many scientific researches. In our study of 270 patients with locally advanced rectal cancer, we studied patient-associated and tumor-related factors. Among these factors, patient-related factors such as age and body mass index, and tumor-related factors such as tumor location and tumor size, and relatively oncomarker carcinoembryonic antigen (CEA) levels were defined as predictive factors of tumor response. Using these predictive factors, we can predict the prognosis of patients and develop personalized treatment strategies.

Keywords: rectal cancer, neoadjuvant chemoradiotherapy, oncomarker CEA, body mass index, tumor regression grade

1. Introduction

Neoadjuvant chemoradiotherapy and total mesorectal excision have become the gold standard of care for patients with clinical stages II and III rectal cancer [1]. Approximately 10–30% of patients with rectal cancer get a complete pathological response after neoadjuvant treatment [2]. However, some patients did not respond to neoadjuvant chemoradiotherapy. Patients with complete pathological response have a favorable oncological prognosis, with high 5-year disease-free and overall survival [3].

The ability to predict the efficacy of neoadjuvant chemoradiotherapy for rectal cancer has important clinical significance.

T-tumor, N-node, M-Metastasis (TNM) staging alone is insufficient for predicting tumor response after chemoradiotherapy (CRT) for locally advanced rectal cancer. Several studies aimed to develop a nomogram to better predict tumor regression grade after CRT. Factors such as sex, age, carcinoembryonic antigen (CEA) level, tumor location, induction chemotherapy, consolidation chemotherapy, perineural invasion, and lymphovascular invasion were analyzed. The variables significantly associated with tumor response are used to build a nomogram that was validated in

IntechOpen

both the training and validation cohorts. Given the importance of risk stratification and prognosis prediction, a stable and easily computable prediction model is needed for clinical applications to help clinicians accurately predict the probability of tumor response after CRT for patients with LARC [4].

Neoadjuvant therapy is increasingly used in rectal cancer treatment. To assess the residual cancer pathologically, we have two main kinds of methods: TNM and tumor regression grade. In 1994, Mandard suggested the first semi-quantitative tumor regression grade, which was used in squamous cell carcinoma (SCC) esophageal cancer. It consisted of 5 grades and has become the source of many other systems. In 1997, Dworak, by collapsing the 5-grade tumor regression grade (TRG) into a 4-tier TRG, suggested that TRG obtained a new system that had better consistency and used it in the assessment of rectal cancer. In 2002, Wheeler reviewed 42 patients with advanced rectal adenocarcinoma who underwent neoadjuvant chemoradiation and built a 3-tier TRG, also named RCRG (Rectal Cancer Regression Grade) [5]. In 2005, Ryan investigated specimens from 247 locally advanced rectal cancer patients who underwent neoadjuvant treatment, and by collapsing Mandard TRG 1–5 into TRG 1–2 vs. 3 vs. 4–5, he suggested a new system that could improve the kappa value from 0.64 to 0.84. So they reclassified the latter as Ryan TRG 1–3. In 2005, Rodel, referring to Dworak TRG, on the basis of comparing the amount of residual tumor with fibrosis, quantified the proportion of tumor regression in the previous tumorous area, or tumor bed, by using the cutoff values of 25 and 50% and suggested a 5-grade system. But nowadays, among multiple tumor regression grading classifications, Mandard's and Dworak's TRG systems remain the most utilized systems in assessing the response of rectal cancer to neoadjuvant treatment [6].

Radiomics interrogates quantitative features on imaging that cannot be seen with the naked eye. Radiomics in rectal cancer is one of the most promising emerging methods for advancing imaging assessment, whether based on CT, MRI, or PET/CT. Radiomics has been investigated as a novel approach to predict treatment outcomes following neoadjuvant chemotherapy. Almost 26 studies are dedicated to using radiomics to predict tumor response in patients with locally advanced rectal cancer undergoing neoadjuvant chemoradiation. 24 studies involved the extraction of radiomic features from MRI T2-weighted images, and two studies have extracted radiomic features specifically from CT images. Petresc et al. used MRI T2-weighted radiomic features to build a radiomic score, which showed an AUC (areas under the curve) of 0.94 in the training set and an AUC of 0.80 in the validation set. Zhou et al. extracted radiomic features from MRI diffusion-weighted images and apparent diffusion coefficient maps to predict non-responders, and the resulting model achieved an AUC of 0.82 in the training set and an AUC of 0.77 in the validation set. Results from these studies suggest that radiomics, particularly MRI-based radiomics, are promising for predicting treatment outcomes after neoadjuvant chemotherapy [7].

Approximately 10–15% of sporadic stage II-III colorectal cancer has microsatellite instability (MSI). In rectal cancer, the incidence of MSI is low, 7% of cases. Several studies investigated the impact of MSI on tumor response after neoadjuvant chemotherapy treatment. Cercek et al. found MSI to be an indicator of poor response to neoadjuvant chemotherapy. Contrary to this, Ye et al. found that MSI was associated with improved disease-free survival (DFS) in patients who received neoadjuvant chemotherapy but was associated with worse DFS in those who received neoadjuvant chemoradiotherapy. De Rosa et al. stated that, in their cohort, MSI patients treated with neoadjuvant chemoradiation had the best pathological complete rates (pCR)—27%. While it remains clear that MMR status should be reported in rectal cancer diagnosis, further research with bigger cohorts is warranted to understand the prognostic implications [8].

Despite this, it is still very difficult to predict the response of rectal cancer after neoadjuvant treatment, and relevant research is needed. In our study, we tried to evaluate the clinical factors that can predict tumor response to neoadjuvant chemoradiotherapy in rectal cancer patients.

2. Material and methods

Our study included 270 patients with locally advanced rectal cancer, histologically verified as adenocarcinoma with a disease stage of cmr T2-T4 N0-N+ M0 (CRM+), who were treated at the National Center of Oncology of the Ministry of Health of the Azerbaijan Republic from 2016 to 2023. Among these patients, 123 (45.6%) were women, and 147 (54.4%) were men. The patients' ages ranged from 24 to 82 years (mean age: 58.1 ± 9.75 years). To classify patients by age, we used the WHO classification. According to this classification, the study cohort included 25 (9.3%) young patients aged 18–44 years, 117 (43.3%) middle-aged patients aged 45–59 years, 123 (45.6%) elderly patients aged 60–74 years, and 5 (1.8%) senile patients aged 75–90 years.

Before treatment, all patients underwent a standardized diagnostic protocol, which included rectosigmoidoscopy, colonoscopy, MRI of the pelvic organs, contrast-enhanced CT of the chest, contrast-enhanced CT of the abdominal cavity, esophagogastroduodenoscopy (EGD), and electrocardiography (ECG). Based on MRI data, stage T2 was diagnosed in 15 (5.6%) patients, T3 in 221 (81.8%) patients, and T4 in 34 (12.6%) patients. Regional lymph node metastases were detected in 221 (81.9%) patients.

All patients underwent prolonged neoadjuvant chemoradiotherapy according to the standard protocol. After CT simulation on a CLINAC linear accelerator with 6 MeV photon beams, external beam radiotherapy was performed using the radical RapidArc program. The single focal dose for the rectal tumor bed and regional lymph nodes was 1.8 Gy, with a total dose of 46 Gy, plus a "boost" single focal dose of 1.8 Gy, with a total boost dose of 7.2 Gy. Concomitant chemotherapy was administered during the first and fifth weeks of radiotherapy, following the 5-fluorouracil regimen: 750 mg intravenously on days I–IV, combined with calcium folinate at 35 mg intravenously on days I–IV. The tumor response to neoadjuvant chemoradiotherapy was evaluated in all patients at week 8 using MRI of the pelvic organs.

All patients underwent surgical treatment. The pathological tumor regression grade (TRG) was determined according to the Dworak classification. Based on the degree of tumor regression, patients were divided into four clinical groups:

- The first group included patients with no response or a weak response to preoperative chemoradiotherapy (TRG1 by Dworak)—58 patients (21.5%).
- The second group included patients with partial tumor regression in response to treatment (TRG2 by Dworak)—95 patients (35.2%).
- The third group included patients with an almost complete clinical response (TRG3 by Dworak)—81 patients (30.0%).
- The fourth group included patients with a complete pathological response, in whom no tumor cells were detected in the postoperative pathological examination (TRG4 by Dworak)—36 patients (13.3%).

Gender	
female	123(45,6%)
male	147(54,4%)
Age	
18–44	25(9,3%)
45–59	95(35,2%)
60–74	123(45,6%)
75–90	5(1,8%)
T-stage	
T2	15(5,6%)
T3	221(81,8%)
T4	34(12,6%)
N-stage	
N-	49(18,1%)
N+	221(81,9%)

Table 1.
Patient charachteristics.

Patient characteristics are presented in **Table 1**. Predictive factors for tumor response to neoadjuvant chemoradiotherapy were divided into two groups. The first group included patient-related factors such as sex, age, and body mass index. The second group included tumor biology-related factors such as CEA tumor marker levels, tumor localization in the rectum, tumor differentiation grade, and tumor size.

For statistical analysis, Pearson's χ^2 test was used with IBM SPSS Statistics 20, and cross-tabulations were performed.

3. Results

3.1 Patient-related factors

At first, we studied patient-associated factors.

Recent studies have shown gender disparities in colorectal cancer patients' survival [9–13]. One of the aims of our study was also to check if there exists any gender-related difference in tumor response after neoadjuvant treatment in rectal cancer patients.

Among female patients:

- Partial tumor regression (TRG II) was observed in 35%, and grade III regression was observed in 27.6%.
- No treatment effect was observed in 22.8%, while a complete response to treatment was recorded in 14.6%.

Among male patients:

- Partial regression (TRG II) was observed in 35.4%, and near-complete regression (TRG III) was seen in 32%.
- Grade I regression occurred in 20.4%, with a complete response in 12.2%.

Table 2 shows the crosstabulation of tumor regression grades and gender.

Comparing the distribution of tumor regression grades between male and female patients reveals nearly identical patterns. Pearson's chi-square test results ($\chi^2(3) = 0.882$, $p = 0.830$) indicate no statistically significant association between gender and tumor regression grade (based on the Dworak scale). This suggests that the differences in TRG categories between males and females are minimal and do not indicate a gender-related influence on tumor response in this study [14–19].

Colorectal cancer is generally thought to be a malignancy affecting elderly patients [20]. But over the last decades, the incidence of colorectal cancer, and especially rectal cancer, has increased in young individuals [21]. Young patients present with a more aggressive pathological subtype and poor prognosis. While most studies were focused on old patients, few studies have focused on the young [22]. Zhang et al., in their study, showed that young patients with locally advanced rectal cancer were associated with lower complete pathological response after neoadjuvant radiochemotherapy [20].

In our patients' cohort, according to age stratification, most patients fell into the middle-aged (43.3%) and elderly (45.6%) groups. Young patients constituted 9.3%, while very elderly patients (75 and older) made up just 1.8%.

Analysis of these age groups revealed:

- Among young patients (18–44 years), the majority exhibited weak regression (40%), with partial and near-complete regression observed in 32% and 20%, respectively. Only 8% achieved complete regression.
- Middle-aged patients (45–59 years) predominantly showed partial (36.8%) and near-complete regression (33.3%), with 17.1% showing no response and 12.8% achieving complete pathological response.
- Elderly patients (60–74 years) were the largest group (45.6%). Partial regression (TRG II) was observed in 35%, near-complete regression in 28.5%, no response in 21.1%, and complete regression in 15.4%.

Tumor regression grade	Women	Men	Total
TRG I	28 (22.8%)	30 (20.4%)	58(21,5%)
TRG II	43 (35.0%)	52 (35.4%)	95(35,2%)
TRG III	34 (27.6%)	47 (32.0%)	81(30.0%)
TRG IV	18 (14.6%)	18 (12.2%)	36(13,3%)
Total	123(100%)	147(100%)	270(100%)

Table 2.
Crosstabulation of tumor regression grades by gender.

- The very elderly (75 and older) represented the smallest group (1.8%), with no complete responses observed. Two patients showed no response, two had near-complete regression, and one had partial regression. The primary goal of treatment for rectal cancer is achieving complete clinical or pathological response. Our analysis revealed an intriguing trend: the proportion of patients achieving complete pathological response increased with age, with the highest rates observed in patients aged 45–74. Literature highlighting the aggressive tumor biology in younger patients aligns with our findings [23–25].

Obesity is a worldwide health concern associated with numerous chronic morbidities [26, 27]. Obesity has been shown to be a risk factor for the occurrence and progression of colorectal cancer [28–30]. Patient characteristics such as obese body habitus and internal distribution of adipose tissue have the potential to affect radiation dosing and delivery, and therefore may lead to significant response differences and survival outcomes [31–35]. Sun et al. [31], in their study, which was conducted in Asian patients, showed that obesity was associated with poorer T downstaging and tumor regression grade.

In our study, the body mass index (BMI) at the time of diagnosis ranged from a minimum of 15.00 to a maximum of 56.00. The average BMI was 26.36, indicating that the average patient fell into the "overweight" category according to the WHO classification (25–29.9). The standard deviation was 4.78, reflecting some variability in BMI among the patients; however, the majority of values were concentrated around the average. In this study, patients were divided into five groups based on their BMI at the time of diagnosis. The division criteria were as follows: Group 1 (BMI < 18.5)—underweight, Group 2 (BMI 18.5–24.9)—normal weight, Group 3 (BMI 25.0–29.9)—overweight, Group 4 (BMI 30.0–34.9)—obesity class I, and Group 5 (BMI ≥ 35.0)—obesity class II and III. **Table 3** shows the distribution of patients by BMI.

The distribution of patients across the groups showed that the largest category was overweight, comprising 117 patients (43.3%). The normal weight group included 79 patients (29.3%), while the obesity class I group consisted of 57 patients (21.1%). Together, these three groups represented the majority of the sample. Fewer patients were observed in the underweight group, with only 11 individuals (4.1%), and the obesity class II and III group, with six individuals (2.2%). These data suggest that overweight and obese individuals predominated among the patients, potentially influencing the development of diseases associated with elevated BMI. In **Table 4**, we can see the crosstabulation between tumor regression grade (TRG) and BMI.

Obesity level	Number of patients	%
Underweight	11	4,1
Normal weight	79	29,3
Overweight	117	43,3
Obesity Class I	57	21,1
Obesity Class II and III	6	2,2
Total	270	100

Table 3.
Distribution of patients by obesity level after neoadjuvant chemoradiotherapy.

TRG	Underweight	Normal weight	Overweight	Obesity Class I	Obesity Class II-III	
TRG1	2(18,2%)	14(17,7%)	24(20,5%)	17(29,8%)	1(16,7%)	58
TRG2	5(45,5%)	29(36,7%)	34(29,1%)	24(42,1%)	3(50%)	95
TRG3	3(27,3%)	24(30,4%)	40(34,2%)	13(22,8%)	1(16,7%)	81
TRG4	1(9,1%)	12(15,2%)	19(16,2%)	3(5,3%)	1(16,7%)	36

Table 4.
Crosstabulation between tumor regression grade(TRG)G and BMI.

In the underweight group (BMI < 18.5), 45.4% of patients exhibited partial tumor regression (TRG by Dworak 2), 27.3% showed near-complete regression (TRG by Dworak 3), 18.2% had no response to treatment (TRG by Dworak 1), and only 9.1% achieved complete tumor regression (TRG by Dworak 4).

Among patients with normal weight (BMI 18.5–24.9), who represented 29.3% of all patients undergoing neoadjuvant chemoradiotherapy, partial tumor regression (TRG2) was most prevalent, observed in 29 patients (36.7%). Near-complete regression (TRG3) was noted in 24 patients (30.4%). Patients with weak regression or no response (TRG1) comprised 14 individuals (17.75%), while complete pathological response (TRG4) was identified in 12 patients (15.2%). Overweight patients (BMI 25–29.9), who accounted for 43.3% of the total (117 patients), showed the following distribution based on pathological regression: The third degree of tumor regression by Dworak (TRG3) was most common, observed in 40 patients (34.2%). This was followed by the second degree of regression (TRG2) in 34 patients (29.1%), no response in 24 patients (20.5%), and complete pathological response in 19 patients (16.2%). Patients with class I obesity (BMI 30.0–34.9) represented 21.1% of those undergoing neoadjuvant chemoradiotherapy (57 patients). Among these, second-degree tumor regression (TRG2) predominated, observed in 24 patients (42%). Thirteen patients (22.8%) had third-degree regression (TRG3), while only three patients (5.3%) achieved complete tumor regression. Weak or no regression (TRG1) was noted in 17 patients (29.8%). In the group with class II and III obesity (BMI ≥ 35.0), there were only six patients, representing 2.2% of the total. Half of these patients (50.0%) demonstrated partial regression, with one patient each (16.7%) in the remaining regression categories. Analyzing the data, the highest percentage of patients with a complete clinical response was observed in the normal weight and overweight groups (15.2 and 16.2%, respectively). In contrast, the class I obesity group had a lower rate of complete responses (5.3%). The small number of patients in the underweight and class II and III obesity groups limits the ability to fully characterize these groups and determine associations between them and the degree of tumor regression. The results of Pearson's chi-square test ($\chi^2(12) = 11.300$, $p < 0.05$) indicate a statistically significant association between BMI groups and the degree of tumor regression according to the Dworak scale. Our study findings support the evidence that obesity is associated with a poor response to neoadjuvant treatment in rectal cancer patients [36–40].

4. Predictive factors associated with the tumor biology

Carcinoembryonic antigen (CEA) is a tumor-associated antigen with significant clinical value for monitoring and evaluating treatment efficacy in colorectal cancer. In colon cancer, the CEA level is a crucial prognostic factor in stages I and II, where elevated pre-treatment CEA levels are associated with a higher risk of both local recurrence and distant metastases.

Few studies have examined the impact of CEA levels on treatment outcomes in rectal cancer patients. Tierman et al. [41] demonstrated the predictive role of CEA in achieving complete pathological response in a study of 609 rectal cancer patients who underwent neoadjuvant chemoradiotherapy. Riesterer et al. [42] found that tumor cells with high CEA density exhibited radioresistance. Beddy et al. [43] showed that pre-treatment CEA levels and their reduction post-treatment are independent predictors of complete tumor regression. Wallin et al. [44] also demonstrated the predictive role of pre-treatment CEA levels on complete pathological response [45], but this correlation was only observed in non-smoking patients. In our study, patients were divided into three groups based on CEA levels: Group 1 – CEA ≤ 5 ng/ml, Group 2 – CEA 5.1–20 ng/ml, and Group 3 – CEA ≥ 20 ng/ml. Analysis showed that pre-treatment CEA levels ≥20 ng/ml significantly reduced the percentage of patients achieving a complete pathological response.

The impact of tumor localization in the rectum on treatment outcomes has been the subject of many scientific studies. For a long time, there was a dogma that tumors in the lower rectum were more radiosensitive. Das et al. [46] demonstrated in their work that tumors located more than 5 cm from the anal verge had a higher percentage of complete pathological response. Huang et al. [47] compared the treatment outcomes of patients with tumors in the upper rectum and those with tumors in the middle and lower rectum. According to their study, patients with upper rectal tumors had better overall survival compared to those with middle and lower rectal tumors. However, there were no significant differences in recurrence-free survival or complete pathological response after neoadjuvant chemoradiotherapy. De la Pinta et al. [48] also noted that tumors in the upper rectum showed a higher rate of complete regression compared to other localizations.

In our study, patients were divided into three groups based on the tumor's localization in the rectum: 0–5 cm (lower rectum), 5–10 cm (middle rectum), and > 10 cm (upper rectum) from the anal verge. **Table 5** shows the crosstabulation of TRG and tumor localization in the rectum.

The majority of patients had lower rectal tumors (155 patients, 57.4% of the total cohort). Middle rectal cancer was diagnosed in 112 patients, accounting for 41.5%. Only three patients (1.1%) with tumors located more than 10 cm from the anal verge underwent neoadjuvant chemoradiotherapy.

Among patients with upper rectal tumors, pathological examination revealed grade 1 tumor regression (TRG1) in two patients and grade 3 regression (TRG3) in one patient.

Tumor Regression Grade	Upper Rectum	Middle Rectum	Lower Rectum	Total
TRG I	2 (4.0%)	17 (34%)	31(62.0%)	50 (100.0%)
TRG II	0	39 (40,2%)	58 (59.8%)	97 (100.0%)
TRG III	1 (1.1%)	36 (40.9%)	51 (58%)	88 (100.0%)
TRG IV	**0 (0.0%)**	**20 (57.1%)**	**15 (42.9%)**	**35 (100.0%)**
Total	3(1,1%)	112(41,5%)	155(57,4%)	270(100%)

Table 5.
Shows the cross-tabulation of tumor regression grades and tumor localization in the rectum.

The majority of patients with middle rectal tumors had grade 2 regression (34.8%) and grade 3 regression (32.2%). Grade 1 tumor regression was observed in 17 patients (15.2% of this group). Complete pathological response was achieved in 17.9% of patients in this group.

In the group of patients with lower rectal cancer, most also had grade 2 regression by Dworak (37.3%) and grade 3 regression (33%). There were more patients with radioresistant tumors in this localization (20%) compared to the middle rectum (15.2%). Complete pathological response was diagnosed in only 8.7% of patients in this group, which was significantly lower than the rate observed in middle rectal tumors (17.9%). To study the relationship between tumor localization in the rectum and tumor regression grade (TRG) using the Dworak scale, a χ^2 test of independence was conducted. The results of the crosstabulation show that patients with TRG1 (minimal regression) accounted for 18.5% of the total cohort, with the majority in this group having lower rectal tumors (62%). In the groups with TRG2 and TRG3, most tumors were also located in the lower rectum (59.8 and 58%, respectively). Tumors in all three sections of the rectum were predominantly found in segments with TRG2 and TRG3. The highest percentage of complete regression (TRG4) was observed in the middle third of the rectum, 57.1%. The χ^2 test results showed that the relationship between tumor localization and regression grade was not statistically significant, $\chi^2(9) = 13.649$, $p = 0.135$, indicating no strong association between these variables.

A one-way analysis of variance (ANOVA) was conducted to assess the relationship between the tumor's distance from the anal verge and the tumor regression grade (TRG) in patients with rectal cancer. **Table 6** shows the crosstabulation between tumor regression grade and tumor distance from the anal verge. The ANOVA results showed that the mean distance of tumors from the anal verge significantly differed among TRG groups, $F(3, 266) = 2.811$, $p = 0.040$. Multiple comparisons using the least significant difference (LSD) criterion revealed statistically significant differences between certain group pairs. Specifically, the TRG4 group had a significantly greater mean tumor distance from the anal verge compared to the TRG1 and TRG2 groups. The difference between TRG4 and TRG1 was 1.44 cm ($p = 0.008$), and between TRG4 and TRG2 was 1.05 cm ($p = 0.029$). Although the difference between TRG4 and TRG3 was not statistically significant ($p = 0.175$), there was a trend toward greater distance in the TRG4 group.

Figure 1 shows the mean tumor distance from the anal verge with 95% confidence intervals for each TRG group (from 1 to 4). It is evident that as the regression grade increases (TRG4), the mean tumor distance from the anal verge also increases, reflecting a relationship between tumor regression grade and localization.

TRG	Tumor distance from anal verge			
	0–3 sm	3-5sm	5-8sm	>8sm
TRG1	21(24,4%)	11(14,1%)	11(11,7%)	1(8,3%)
TRG2	33(38,4%)	27(34,6%)	33(35,1%)	4(33,3%)
TRG3	20(23,3%)	29(32,2%)	34(36,2%)	5(41,7%)
TRG4	12(14%)	11(14,1%)	16(17%)	2(16,7%)
	86	78	94	12

Table 6.
Crosstabulation between tumor regression grade (TRG) and tumor distance from anal verge.

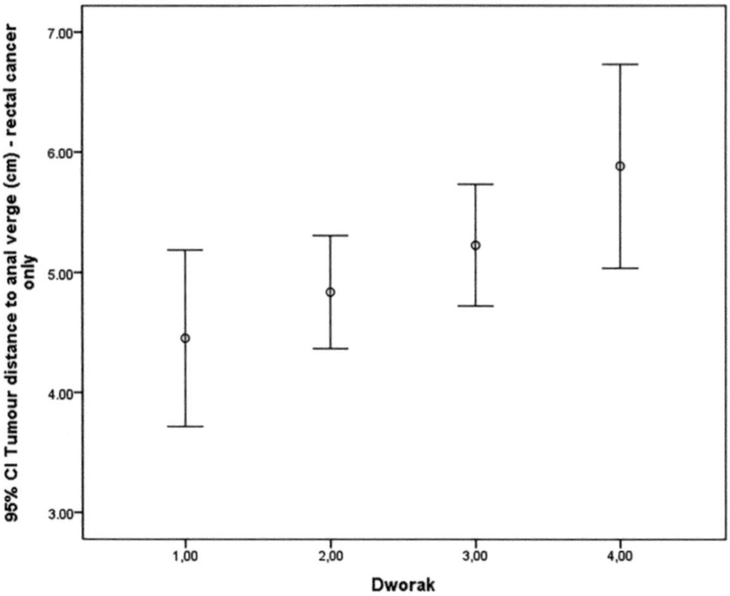

Figure 1.
Comparison of mean tumor distance from the anal verge between clinical groups.

Thus, it can be concluded that the tumor's distance from the anal verge is associated with the regression grade in rectal cancer patients, with the greatest distances observed in the TRG4 group.

We also studied the impact of tumor differentiation on the response to neoadjuvant chemoradiotherapy. The primary group consisted of patients with moderate differentiation, making up 72.2% of the cohort. Patients with low differentiation totaled 40, comprising 14.9% of the group, while 35 patients were diagnosed with highly differentiated adenocarcinoma based on tumor biopsy, accounting for 12.9% of the total.

The relationship between clinical groups based on tumor regression and tumor differentiation levels was analyzed using Pearson's chi-square test. **Table 7** presents data on the distribution of patients by clinical groups and tumor differentiation levels. The highest number of patients with highly differentiated adenocarcinoma was observed in the TRG 3 tumor regression group, with 16 patients (45.7% of those with high differentiation). Only four patients (11.4%) in this group had a low differentiation grade. Complete tumor regression was detected in 12 patients (34.4%) with highly differentiated tumors.

Tumor Regression Degree	G1 - Highly Differentiated.	G2 - Moderately Differentiated.	G3 - Poorly Differentiated	
TRG 1	4 (11,4%)	32 (16,4%)	14 (35%)	50 (100.0%)
TRG2	3 (8.5%)	83 (42,6%)	11 (27,5%)	97 (100.0%)
TRG 3	16 (45,7%)	65 (33,3%)	7 (17,5%)	88 (100.0%)
TRG 4	**12 (34.4%)**	**15 (7,7%)**	**8 (20%)**	**35 (100.0%)**
Total	35(12,9%)	195(72,2%)	40(14,9%)	270

Table 7.
Crosstabulation of tumor regression degree and tumor differentiation degree.

Among patients with moderately differentiated tumors, the largest number was found in the TRG 2 tumor regression group, with 83 patients (42.6%). Complete tumor regression was observed in 15 patients (7.7% of those with moderately differentiated adenocarcinoma). Finally, the largest number of patients with poorly differentiated tumors showed a weak response to neoadjuvant chemoradiotherapy, with 14 patients (35%).

The results of Pearson's chi-square test indicate statistically significant differences in the distribution of patients across clinical groups depending on tumor differentiation levels: $\chi^2(6, N = 181) = 24.12$, $p < 0.001$. These findings confirm a significant association between clinical groups and tumor differentiation levels, which may have important clinical implications for prognosis assessment and treatment strategy selection for patients [49].

The influence of tumor size and volume on treatment outcomes after neoadjuvant therapy in rectal cancer has been the subject of several studies. For example, a study by Fan Yang et al. explored the relationship between tumor volume and regression degree after neoadjuvant therapy in rectal cancer. A tumor volume of 37.3 cm^3 was identified as the threshold above which the likelihood of achieving complete tumor regression sharply declined. In our study, we measured the vertical tumor size based on MRI data. The vertical tumor size in our cohort ranged from 3.5 to 11.5 cm. **Figure 2** shows the comparison of tumor sizes on MRI before treatment among groups based on TRG. Analysis of variance (ANOVA) revealed statistically significant differences in tumor sizes on MRI before treatment among the groups based on tumor regression by Dworak: $F(3, 187) = 3.362$, $p = 0.020$. This indicates that at least one group, classified by tumor regression according to Dworak, differed in average tumor size prior to treatment.

Multiple comparison tests using the LSD method showed that the average tumor size in the TRG 1 by Dworak group was significantly larger compared to the TRG 4 by Dworak group (mean difference = 1.597 cm, $p = 0.003$). A significant difference was

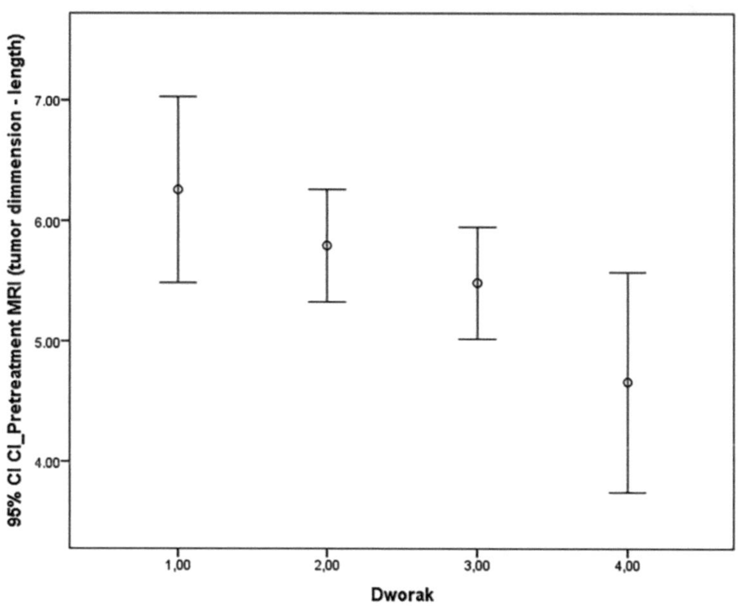

Figure 2.
Comparison of tumor sizes on MRI before treatment among groups based on tumor regression.

also observed between the TRG 2 by Dworak and TRG 4 by Dworak groups (mean difference = 1.131 cm, $p = 0.014$). Other comparisons did not reveal statistically significant differences at the 0.05 level.

Thus, groups with higher tumor regression levels according to the Dworak scale (especially TRG 3 and TRG 4) had smaller tumor sizes on MRI before treatment. This may indicate a correlation between the degree of tumor response and the initial tumor size.

5. Conclusion

After analyzing the obtained data, we concluded that factors such as young patient age and excessive weight negatively impact treatment outcomes in patients with rectal cancer. Among younger patients, a higher percentage present with locally advanced disease at the time of diagnosis. Additionally, mucinous and signet-ring cell carcinomas, which are known for their resistance to neoadjuvant therapy, are more prevalent in this group.

Obese patients also exhibit a predominance of radioresistant tumors, most likely due to a reduced dose of ionizing radiation reaching the tumor area as a result of significant mesorectal and pararectal fat.

Regarding tumor-related factors, the longstanding belief that lower-ampullary rectal cancer is highly radiosensitive was not confirmed in our study. On the contrary, tumors located more than 5 cm from the anal verge showed a higher rate of complete tumor regression.

A CEA tumor marker level of ≥20 ng/ml appears to be a critical threshold, above which the rate of complete tumor regression significantly decreases. Finally, patients with highly differentiated tumors demonstrated the highest percentage of complete pathological response.

These findings may help clinicians predict patient prognosis and develop individualized treatment strategies. Personalizing treatment is the future of rectal cancer management, and exploration of new predictive factors of tumor response will guide us to determine a group of patients with favorable prognoses, and intensification of treatment in these patients will lead to a clinically complete response.

Ethics approval.

The present study protocol was approved by the local Ethics Committee of the National Centre of Oncology (reference number: 0102160).

Author details

Yusif Aliyarov
National Centre of Oncology, Baku, Azerbaijan

*Address all correspondence to: yusifaliyarov@yahoo.com

References

[1] Sauer R, Becker H, Hohenberger W, et al. Preoperative versus postoperative chemoradiotherapy for rectal cancer. The New England Journal of Medicine. 2004;**351**:1731-1740

[2] Martin ST, Heneghan HM, Winter DC. Systematic review and meta-analysis of outcomes following pathological complete response to neoadyuvant chemoradiotherapy for rectal cancer. British Journal of Surgery. 2012;**99**:918-928

[3] Alwers E, Jansen L, Kather J, Amitay E, Bläker H, Kloor M, et al. Response to neoadjuvant treatment among rectal cancer patients in a population-based cohort. International Journal of Colorectal Disease. 2021;**36**(1):177-185. DOI: 10.1007/s00384-020-03744-2

[4] Zhang JW, Cai Y, Xie XY, Bin HH, Ling JY, Wu ZH, et al. Nomogram for predicting pathological complete response and tumor downstaging in patients with locally advanced rectal cancer on the basis of a randomized clinical trial. Gastroenterology Report. 2020;**8**(3):234-241. DOI: 10.1093/gastro/goz073

[5] Berkovich L, Lahav L, Kidron D, Mishaeli M, Yahya NH, Avital S. Lack of pathological response of rectal cancer to neoadjuvant chemoradiotherapy is associated with poorer long-term oncological outcomes. Clinical Oncology Research and Reports. 2019;**2**(5):2-6. DOI: 10.31487/j.COR.2019.5.18

[6] Mancini R, Pattaro G, Diodoro MG, Sperduti I, Garufi C, Stigliano V, et al. Tumor regression grade after neoadjuvant chemoradiation and surgery for low rectal cancer evaluated by multiple correspondence analysis: Ten years as minimum follow-up. Clinical Colorectal Cancer. Mar 2018;**17**:13-19. DOI: 10.1016/j.clcc.2017.06.004 C

[7] Bulens P, Couwenberg A, Intven M, Debucquoy A, Vandecaveye V, Van Cutsem E, et al. Predicting the tumor response to chemoradiotherapy for rectal cancer: Model development and external validation using MRI radiomics. Radiotherapy and Oncology. 2020;**142**:246-252. DOI: 10.1016/j.radonc.2019.07.033

[8] Ye S-B, Cheng Y-K, Zhang L, Zou Y-F, Chen P, Deng Y-H, et al. Association of mismatch repair status with survival and response to neoadjuvant chemo(radio) therapy in cancer. npj Precision Oncology. 2020;**4**(1):1-9. DOI: 10.1038/s41698-020-00132-5

[9] Sarasqueta C, Zunzunegui MV, Enríquez Navascues JM, Querejeta A, Placer C, Perales A, et al. Gender differences in stage at diagnosis and preoperative radiotherapy in patients with rectal cancer. BMC Cancer. 2020;**20**:759. DOI: 10.1186/s12885-020-07195-4

[10] Hendifar A, Yang D, Lenz F, Lurje G, Pohl A, Lenz C, et al. Gender disparities in metastatic colorectal cancer survival. Clinical Cancer Research. 2009;**15**(20):6391-6397. DOI: 10.1158/1078-0432

[11] Yang Y, Wang G, He J, Ren S, Wu F, Zhang J, et al. Gender differences in colorectal cancer survival: A meta-analysis. International Journal of Cancer. 2017;**141**(10):1942-1949. DOI: 10.1002/ijc.30827

[12] Abancens M, Bustos V, Harvey H, McBryan J, Harvey BJ. Sexual

dimorphism in colon cancer. Frontiers in Oncology. 2020;**10**:607909. DOI: 10.3389/fonc.2020.607909

[13] Wagner AD, Oertelt-Prigione S, Adjei A, Buclin T, Cristina V, Csajka C, et al. Gender medicine and oncology: Report and consensus of an ESMO workshop. Annals of Oncology. 2019;**30**(12):1914-1924. DOI: 10.1093/annonc/mdz414

[14] On J, Shim J, Mackay C, Murray G, Samuel L, Parnaby C, et al. Pathological response post neoadjuvant therapy for locally advanced rectal cancer is an independent predictor of survival. Colorectal Disease. 2021;**23**(6):1326-1333

[15] Fischer J, Eglinton TW, Richards SJ, Frizelle FA. Predicting pathological response to chemoradiotherapy for rectal cancer: A systematic review. Expert Review of Anticancer Therapy. 2021;**128**:1-12. Available from: https://www.tandfonline.com/doi/full/10.1080/14737140.2021.1868992

[16] Clarke TL, White DA, Osborne ME, Shaw AM, Smart NJ, Daniels IR. Predicting response to neoadjuvant chemoradiotherapy in locally advanced rectal cancer with serum biomarkers. Annals of the Royal College of Surgeons of England. May 2017;**99**(5):373-377. DOI: 10.1308/rcsann.2017.0030

[17] Conde-Muíño R, Cuadros M, Zambudio N, Segura-Jiménez I, Cano C, Palma P. Predictive biomarkers to chemoradiation in locally advanced rectal cancer. BioMed Research International. 2015;**2015**:921435. DOI: 10.1155/2015/921435. Epub 2015 Oct 4

[18] Jia H, Shen X, Guan Y, Xu M, Tu J, Mo M, et al. Predicting the pathological response to neoadjuvant chemoradiation using untargeted metabolomics in locally advanced rectal cancer. Radiotherapy and Oncology. 2018;**128**(3):548-556. DOI: 10.1016/j.radonc.2018.06.022

[19] Lai S, Huang L, Luo S, Liu Z, Dong J, Wang L, et al. Systemic inflammatory indices predict tumor response to neoadjuvant chemoradiotherapy for locally advanced rectal cancer. Oncology Letters. 2020;**20**(3):2763-2770. DOI: 10.3892/ol.2020.11812

[20] Zhang Y, Yan L, Yong W, Meifang X, Liu X, Guan G. Worse treatment response to neoadjuvant chemoradiotherapy in young patients with locally advanced rectal cancer. BMC Cancer. 2020;**20**(854):1-10. DOI: 10.1186/s12885-020-07359-2

[21] Cai X, Wu H, Peng J, Zhu J, Cai S, Cai G, et al. Tolerability and outcomes of radiotherapy or chemoradiotherapy for rectal cancer in elderly patients aged 70 years and older. Radiation Oncology. 2013;**8**:86

[22] Patel SG, Ahnen DJ. Colorectal cancer in the young. Current Gastroenterology Reports. 2018;**20**:15

[23] Dossa F, Chesney TR, Acuna SA, Baxter NN. A watch-and-wait approach for locally advanced rectal cancer after a clinical complete response following neoadjuvant chemoradiation: A systematic review and meta-analysis. The Lancet Gastroenterology and Hepatology. 2017;**2**(7):501-513. Available from: https://pubmed.ncbi.nlm.nih.gov/28479372/

[24] O'Connell JB, Maggard MA, Liu JH, Etzioni DA, Ko CY. Are survival rates different for young and older patients with rectal cancer. Diseases of the Colon and Rectum. 2004;**47**:2064-2069

[25] Li Q, Cai G, Li D, Wang Y, Zhuo C, Cai S. Better long-term survival in young patients with non-metastatic colorectal

cancer after surgery, an analysis of 69,835 patients in SEER database. PLoS One. 2014;**9**:e93756

[26] Liu H, Wei R, Li C, Zhao Z, Guan X, Yang M, et al. BMI may be a prognostic factor for local advanced rectal cancer patients treated with long-term neoadjuvant chemoradiotherapy. Cancer Management and Research. 2020;**12**:10321-10332

[27] Aldaqal SM, Maqbul AA, Alhammad AA, Alghamdi AS, Alharbi BA, Alharbi MT, et al. The impact of body mass index on the clinicopathological and prognostic factors of colorectal cancer in Saudi Arabia. Cureus. 2020;**12**(11):e11789. DOI: 10.7759/cureus.11789

[28] Carr PR, Amitay EL, Jansen L, Alwers E, Roth W, Herpel E, et al. Association of BMI and major molecular pathological markers of colorectal cancer in men and women. The American Journal of Clinical Nutrition. 2020;**111**(3):562-569. DOI: 10.1093/ajcn/nqz315

[29] Shahjehan F, Merchea A, Cochuyt JJ, Li Z, Colibaseanu DT, Kasi PM. Body mass index and long-term outcomes in patients with colorectal cancer. Frontiers in Oncology. 2018;**8**:620. DOI: 10.3389/fonc.2018.00620

[30] Bull CJ, Bell JA, Murphy N, Sanderson E, Davey Smith G, Timpson NJ, et al. Adiposity, metabolites, and colorectal cancer risk: Mendelian randomization study. BMC Medicine. 2020;**18**(1):396. DOI: 10.1186/s12916-020 01855-9

[31] Sun Y, Xu Z, Lin H, Lu X, Huang Y, Huang S, et al. Impact of body mass index on treatment outcome of neoadjuvant chemoradiotherapy in locally advanced rectal cancer. EJSO. 2017;**43**:1828e1834

[32] Moghaddam AA, Woodward M, Huxley R. Obesity and risk of Colo rectal cancer: A meta-analysis of 31 studies with 70,000 events. Cancer Epidemiology, Biomarkers & Prevention. 2007;**16**:2533e47

[33] Renehan AG, Tyson M, Egger M, Heller RF, Zwahlen M. Body-mass index and incidence of cancer: A systematic review and meta-analysis of prospective observational studies. Lancet. 2008;**371**:569e78

[34] Ma Y, Yang Y, Wang F. Obesity and risk of colorectal cancer: A sys tematic review of prospective studies. PLoS One. 2013;**8**:e53916

[35] Meyerhardt JA, Tepper JE, Niedzwiecki D, Hollis DR, McCollum AD, Brady D, et al. Impact of body mass index on out comes and treatment-related toxicity in patients with stage II and III rectal cancer: Findings from intergroup trial 0114. Journal of Clinical Oncology. 2004;**22**:648-657

[36] Park IJ, You YN, Skibber JM, Rodriguezbigas MA, Das P, Eng C, et al. Oncologic and functional hazards of obesity among patients with locally advanced rectal cancer following neoadjuvant chemora diation therapy. American Journal of Clinical Oncology. 2017;**40**:277e82. DOI: 10.1097/. COC.0000000000000150

[37] Aytac E, Lavery IC, Kalady MF, Kiran PR. Impact of obesity on operation performed, complications and long term outcomes in terms of restoration of intestinal continuity for patients with mid and low rectal cancer. Diseases of the Colon and Rectum. 2013;**56**:689e97

[38] You JF, Tang R, Changchien CR, Chen JS, You YT, Chiang JM, et al. Effect of body mass index on the outcome of

patients with rectal cancer receiving curative anterior resection: Disparity between the upper and lower rectum. Annals of Surgery. 2009;**249**:783e7

[39] Clark W, Siegel EM, Chen YA, Zhao X, Parsons CM, Hernandez JM, et al. Quantitative measures of visceral adiposity and body mass in dex in predicting rectal cancer outcomes after neoadjuvant chemora diation. Journal of the American College of Surgeons. 2013;**216**:1070e81

[40] Chern H, Chou J, Donkor C, Shia J, Guillem JG, Nash GM, et al. Effects of obesity in rectal cancer surgery. Journal of the American College of Surgeons. 2010;**211**:55e60

[41] Tierman JP, Perry SL, Vergbese ET, West NP, Yeluri S, Jayne DG, et al. Carcinoembryonic antigen is the preferred biomarker for in vivo colorectal cancer targeting. British Journal of Cancer. Feb 2013;**108**(3):662-667. DOI: 10.1038/bjc.2012.605

[42] Riesterer O, Milas L, Ang KK. Use of molecular biomarkers for predicting the response to radiotherapy with or without chemotherapy. Journal of Clinical Oncology. 2007;**25**(26). DOI: 10.1200/JCO.2007.11.8497

[43] Beddy D, Hyland JMP, Winter DC, Lim C, White A, Moriarty M, et al. A simplified tumor regression grade correlates with survival in locally advanced rectal carcinoma treated with neoadjuvant. Chemoradiotherapy. 2008;**15**(12):3471-3477. DOI: 10.1245/s10434-008-0149-y. Epub 2008 Oct 10

[44] Wallin U, Rothenberger D, Lowry A, Luepker R, Mellgren A. CEA - A predictor for pathologic complete response after neoadjuvant therapy for rectal cancer. Diseases of the Colon & Rectum. 2013;**56**(7):859-868. DOI: 10.1097/DCR.0b013e31828e5a72

[45] Barbaro B, Leccisotti L, Vecchio FM, Di MM, Serra T, Salsano M, et al. The potential predictive value of MRI and PET-CT in mucinous and nonmucinous rectal cancer to identify patients at high risk of metastatic disease. The British Journal of Radiology. 2017;**90**:20150836

[46] Das P, Skibber JM, Rodriguez-Bigas MA, Feig BW, Chang GJ, Wolff RA, et al. Predictors of tumour response and downstaging in patients who receive preoperative chemoradiation for rectal cancer. Cancer. 2007;**109**(9):1750-1755

[47] Huang M-Y, Lee H-H, Tsai H-L, Huang C-W, Yeh Y-S, Ma C-J, et al. Comparison of efficacy and safety of preoperative chemoradiotherapy in locally advanced upper and middle/lower rectal cancer. Radiation Oncology. 2018;**13**:53. DOI: 10.1186/s13014-018-0987-0

[48] De La Pinta C, Martín M, Sempere C, Hervás A, Fernández-Iizarbe E, López F, et al. Magnetic resonance imaging value to predict pathologic staging in Locally Advanced Rectal Cancer after neoadjuvant chemoradiation. Turkish Journal of Colorectal Disease. 2019;**29**:39-45

[49] Reggiani BL, Lionti S, Domati F, Pagliani G, Mattioli E, Barresi V. Histological grading based on poorly differentiated clusters is predictive of tumour response and clinical outcome in rectal carcinoma treated with neoadjuvant chemoradiotherapy. Histopathology. 2017;**71**:393-405

Chapter 9

Presacral Tumors

Jin K. Kim, Kaylee Smith and Jorge Marcet

Abstract

Presacral tumors are rare and are of a broad tissue origin which are most often benign than malignant. This chapter seeks to review the current medical literature to provide readers an updated approach to the modern diagnosis and management of presacral tumors. Emphasis will be given to selection of the most appropriate modern imaging modalities and laboratory analysis to arrive at a differential diagnosis. Surgical approaches will be reviewed, including minimally (invasive laparoscopic, robotic) techniques. Multidisciplinary management of complex malignant presacral tumors will be covered. The chapter seeks to be a comprehensive review on this subject. The discussion of the various tumors will be presented within the context of congenital and acquired, and further categorized into benign and malignant tumors.

Keywords: Presacral tumors, retrorectal tumors, presacral cysts, dermoid tumors, malignant presacral tumor, chordoma, acquired, congenital, duplication cyst, sarcoma, tailgut cyst

1. Introduction

The incidence of presacral tumors is relatively rare. Jao et al. reported the incidence of presacral tumors to be 1 out of 40,000 admissions [1]. The vast majority of presacral lesions are asymptomatic. At present, most patient's pathology is incidentally identified when undergoing cross sectional imaging. In patients who do present with symptoms, the most common chief complaint is pain with sitting or lower back pain at rest, particularly after experiencing a fall on their buttocks/coccyx. Larger lesions can present with more vague abdominal or pelvic pain, or even obstructive symptoms, fecal or urinary incontinence, leg or gluteal symptoms, or sexual dysfunction. Pain is often vague and ill-defined and many patients may be referred to pain management or psychiatry for evaluation after inability to identify etiology or lack of improvement of symptom management [2].

Less commonly, patients may present with drainage in the perineum which are frequently misdiagnosed as an abscess, fistula, or pilonidal disease [3]. In recurrent or non-healing perineal wounds associated with drainage, presacral lesions should be considered in the differential diagnosis.

Retrorectal lesions have a female predilection, with about 75% of tumors occurring in women. Median age of onset is 45 years. Historically, a significant portion of patients with retrorectal tumors were considered to have malignant disease. In Uhlig and Johnson's case series, 58% of lesions were found to be benign and 42% malignant. However, more recent data now report approximately 82% of lesions are benign and 18% malignant [4]. The change in the ratio of benign to malignant lesions is thought to be due to the increasing number of lesions detected incidentally on cross sectional imaging in modern times.

Physical exam remains an important aspect of workup and care of presacral lesions. The main focus of the physical exam is the perineum and rectum. On an external exam of the perineum, a postanal dimple and a draining sinus may be present. On a digital rectal exam, a mass posterior to the rectum may be palpated, as well as anterior displacement of the rectum. Endoscopic evaluation should accompany work up to evaluate any anatomic or mucosal changes. Findings may include externally obstructing masses, potential decompression or erosion of the tumor, or evidence of infection.

1.1 Case presentations

Case 1: 50 year old female with complaint of worsening perianal and rectal pain radiating to upper buttocks, perineum and labia for 5 months. She denied history of trauma to the rectum or perineum. She denied changes in bowel habits or urinary incontinence or urgency. She has tried oral narcotic pain medications, ibuprofen, and topical lidocaine to the perianal region without significant improvement. On digital rectal exam, a 2 cm mass was felt posterior to the rectum. She underwent MRI of the pelvis which revealed a complex appearing multicystic mass with hemorrhagic components in the presacral space at the level of S5 abutting the posterior anal rectal wall and left ischial anal fat. Screening colonoscopy was normal. Endoscopic ultrasound was performed showing extraluminal, smooth, lobulated mass posterior to the rectum. Preoperative biopsy was not obtained as the mass was cystic in nature. As the presacral tumor was low in the pelvis, posterior approach with coccygectomy was performed to completely excise the tumor. Surgical pathology was consistent with a tailgut cyst with lymphohistiocytic inflammation. Her postoperative recovery was unremarkable. Patient had some improvement in the rectal pain postoperatively.

Case 2: 50 year old male, who was a retired veteran, who was referred to our service from another health system after workup and attempted percutaneous drainage of a cystic presacral mass. He had history of trauma resulting in rib fractures and a coccygeal fracture in the past. For a year, the patient developed worsening perirectal pain with sitting. Patient denied changes in bowel habits or bleeding per rectum. He underwent a pelvic MRI which diagnosed a cystic mass anterior to the coccyx which was unfortunately drained percutaneously. He then developed recurrent infections and recurrence of presacral cysts for which he was referred to a quaternary care center. Patient underwent a colonoscopy which revealed benign colonic polyps. Repeat MRI pelvis showed a 17 mm cystic anterior to the coccyx with thin peripheral enhancement and no soft tissue nodularity. As the presacral tumor was low in the pelvis, posterior approach with coccygectomy was performed to completely excise the tumor. Surgical pathology was consistent with cystic hamartoma. Patient's postoperative course was complicated by superficial wound dehiscence which required local wound care at follow up visits.

2. Classification system of presacral tumors

Presacral tumors are a heterogenous group of masses ranging from benign cystic lesions to large, complex invasive malignancies. Given this diversity, the differential diagnoses of presacral tumors is exceedingly broad. Symptomatic tumors are associated more frequently with malignancy. On imaging, purely cystic lesions are more likely to be benign, whereas solid or heterogeneous masses can be either benign or malignant. Large lesions or lesions invading other structures are often malignant.

These tumors exist in an anatomic location surrounded by multiple tissues derived from 3 different germ cell origins in close proximity- connective tissue, osseous tissue, and neural tissue, resulting in the wide differential diagnosis and often diagnostic dilemmas. Lesions may be classified into two groups- congenital or acquired. Congenital lesions are defined as those arising from an abnormality during embryologic development. Acquired lesions arise from residual embryologic tissue or differentiated tissue within the presacral space.

Multiple attempts have been made to develop a classification system which comprehensively encompasses all possible presacral lesions. First published in 1975, Uhlig and Johnson established a classification system based on a large cohort of patients over 30 years in Portland, Oregon [5]. This classification system remains the basis for more modern presacral classification systems. It is organized by tissue origin and categorized as congenital, inflammatory, neurologic, osseous, and miscellaneous.

The most important factor in the treatment of presacral tumors is the presence of malignancy. As such, the American Society of Colon and Rectal Surgeons (ASCRS) have further delineated Uhlig and Johnson's initial classification system further into benign and malignant entities (see **Table 1**) [6].

	Benign	**Malignant**
Congenital	Adrenal rest tumor	Chordoma
	Anterior sacral meningocele	Germ cell tumor
	Developmental cysts (dermoid, epidermoid [aka epidermal], enterogenous [aka rectal duplication], tailgut [aka cystic hamartomas/mucous secreting], teratoma)	Malignant developmental cysts
		Teratocarcinoma
Neurogenic	Ganglioneuroma	Ependymoma
	Neurofibroma	Ganglioneuroblastoma
	Schwannoma (aka neurilemoma)	Malignant schwannoma
		Neuroblastoma
		Peripheral nerve sheath tumors (aka neurofibrosarcoma)
		Primitive neuroectodermal
Osseous	Aneurysmal bone cyst	Chondrosarcoma
	Giant cell tumor	Ewing's sarcoma
	Osteoblastoma	Giant cell tumor
	Osteoma	Myeloma
	Simple bone cyst	Osteogenic sarcoma
		Plasmacytoma
		Reticulum cell sarcoma
		Spindle cell sarcoma

	Benign	Malignant
Miscellaneous	Aggressive angiomyxoma	Angiosarcoma
	Benign gastrointestinal stromal tumor	Carcinomasarcoma
	Benign hemagiopericytoma	Degenerated hamartoma
	Desmoid (aka fibromatosis)	Epithelioid sarcoma
	Ectopic kidney	Fibrosarcoma
	Endothelioma	Fibromyxoid sarcoma
	Fibroma	Histiosarcoma
	Hamartoma	Hydatid cyst
	Hemangioma	Leiomyosarcoma
	Leiomyoma	Liposarcoma
	Lipoma	Lymphoma
	Lipofibroma	Malignant desmoid
	Myelolipoma	Malignant hemagiopericytoma
	Pecoma	Malignant gastrointestinal stromal tumor
	Solitary fibrous tumor	Malignant solitary fibrous tumor
	Tuberculosis	Metastatic carcinoma
		Myeloliposarcoma
		Neuroendocrine tumors
		Rhabdomyosarcoma
		Small cell tumor
		Spindle cell tumor
		Squamous cell carcinoma
		Undifferentiated sarcoma

Table 1.
Classification system of presacral tumors. Benign and malignant presacral tumors based on by subtype. CC-BY 4.0: Used with permission from ASCRS Textbook of Colon and Rectal Surgery, Fourth Edition (2022) [2].

The majority of presacral tumors (55–65%) are congenital in tissue origin. Of the congenital lesions, about two-thirds are found to be benign [2]. These lesions include epidermoid, dermoid, and tailgut cysts, and teratomas. There remains a strong female predominance in congenital tumors with upwards of 75% of lesions diagnosed in women [5]. As these are the most common presentations, congenital lesions are discussed in further detail below.

2.1 Congenital lesions

2.1.1 Tailgut cysts

These lesions account for the majority of benign congenital lesions, with about 45% falling into this category. They may also be referred to as cystic hamartomas or mucin secreting cysts. Arising from normal primitive hindgut tissue which did not regress, they are lined with columnar epithelium resembling intestinal tissue [2].

2.1.2 Chordomas

Chordomas are the most common congenital, retrorectal malignant tumors. Found predominantly in men under the age of 30, they are derivatives of the embryologic notochord and can occur anywhere along the spinal cord. However, they are most commonly found at the base of the skull or presacral region [2]. Resection is the treatment modality of choice, with controversial efficacy of radiation therapy and relative resistance to chemotherapy. Unfortunately, even with wide local excision, sacral chordomas have local and distant recurrence rates of 42.6% and 22.4% despite treatment, and a 5-year survival rate of 73–86% and a 10-year survival rate of 49–71% [7].

2.1.3 Epidermoid/Dermoid cysts

Thought to result from defects of closure within the ectodermal layer. Histologically are found to have keratinized stratified squamous epithelium [2]. These cysts may communicate with the skin and are usually responsible for the characteristic "dimpling" on exam. These may be misdiagnosed as perianal or subcutaneous abscesses. Recurrent or persistent infection can result, albeit rarely, in malignant transformation to squamous cell carcinoma

2.1.4 Duplication cyst

Also known as enterogenous cysts, these cysts result from failure of regression of endodermal tissue. Squamous, columnar, cuboidal, or transitional epithelium may be noted histologically. The cyst must be attached to the alimentary tract, a mucous membrane similar to the attached gastrointestinal tract organ must be present, and it must possess a smooth muscular component [2].

2.1.5 Teratomas

Two to three germ cell layers must be present to be considered a teratoma. Sacrococcygeal teratomas are most common in the pediatric and female population. These lesions can harbor any number of tissue types, commonly nervous, skeletal, respiratory, and gastrointestinal etiologies.

2.1.6 Meningoceles

Another benign congenital lesion, anterior sacral meningoceles are unilocular (more common) or multilocular (rare) extension of the meninges into the presacral space through bony defects in the sacral foramina. These contain cerebrospinal fluid (CSF) contained by two the dura mater and the arachnoid mater. Incidence of these tumors is relatively rare with less than 300 reported cases in the last 200 years [8]. These lesions may be associated with anorectal abnormalities, gynecologic abnormalities, spina bifida or teratomas [8]. These also can be associated with bony abnormalities, classically the Scimitar sign seen on radiography (**Figure 1**). Given the communication with the central nervous system and risk of catastrophic central

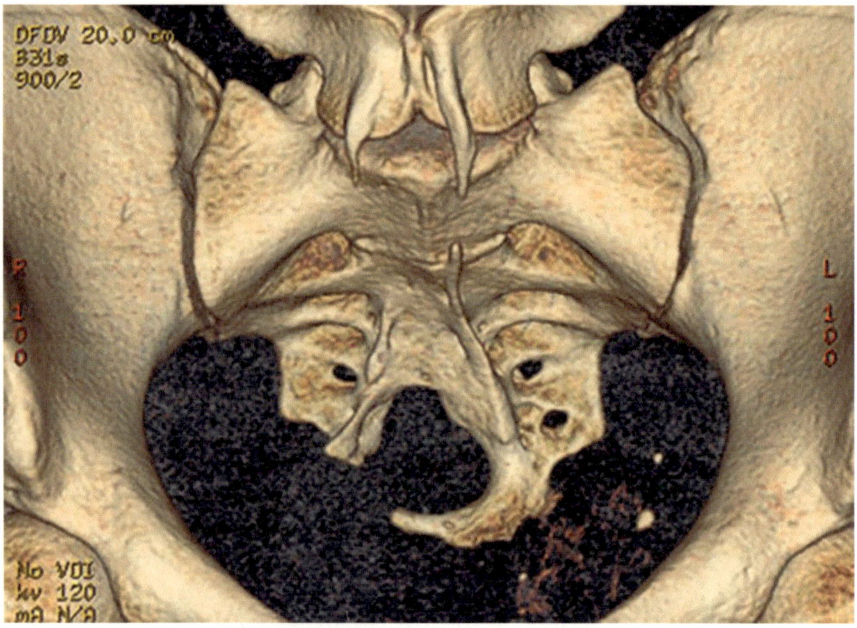

Figure 1.
Scimitar sign for meningocele. 3D CT reconstruction of sacrum resembling the shape of a scimitar, which is a characteristic imaging sign for a sacral meningocele. CC-BY-NC/ND 4.0 or copyrighted source: Used with permission from ASCRS Textbook of Colon and Rectal Surgery, Fourth Edition (2022) [2].

nervous system infection, these lesions should not be biopsied. MRI or myelogram should be used for diagnosis. Treatment for symptomatic lesions is surgical intervention with the goal to obliterate the communication between the spinal subarachnoid space and the meningocele [8]. In conjunction with a spine surgeon, surgery for meningocele involves detethering of the cord, laminectomy, ligation of the pedicle with excision of any associated lesions, and a watertight closure of the meningocele pedicle to prevent a CSF leak.

2.2 Neurogenic lesions

This group of tumors encompasses both malignant and benign lesions. Neurogenic tumors may include neurofibrosarcoma, ependymoma, neuroblastoma, neurofibroma, ganglioneuroma, or schwannoma. These represent about 10% of all presacral lesions, about 70% of which are benign and 30% are malignant [1]. Treatment for tumors is primarily surgical but some lesions may require radiation therapy. Patients with malignant tumors generally undergo more extensive resection resulting in higher morbidity, lower functional status and higher rates of local recurrence. For malignant tumors, Local recurrence rate of 40%, 5 year metastasis rate of 26%, and 5 year survival hovers around 50% [9]. Patients with benign disease have much better functional outcomes, likely secondary to less aggressive resection, nerve root resection, and lack of radiation.

2.3 Osseous lesions

Osseous tumors originate from the bone itself and are associated structures including cartilage, marrow, or fibrous tissues. This includes, but is not limited to osteosarcoma, chondrosarcoma, Ewing's sarcoma, and fibrosarcoma. Even if benign in etiology, these can be incredibly locally aggressive resulting in bony destruction [1]. There is a similar distribution between male and female patients [10]. About 50% of these tumors are malignant with a predilection for metastases to the lungs [11]. If sarcoma is the expected diagnosis, we recommend involving an orthopedic or spine surgeon to assist in excising the tumor.

2.4 Miscellaneous lesions

This encompasses a number of tumors which do not fit in the aforementioned tissue categories. These may include gastrointestinal stromal tumor, carcinoid, lymphoma, fibrosarcoma, lipoma, leiomyomas, or hemangiomas [1].

3. Diagnostic imaging modalities

Pelvic MRI (**Figure 2**) is traditionally the imaging modality of choice given its superior ability to characterize the intricacies of soft tissue lesions and evaluate involvement with adjacent structures such as neural involvement. CT imaging, however, has greater sensitivity for evaluating bony involvement and malignant bony lesions. When evaluating for possible malignant presacral tumors, obtaining both imaging modalities may offer critical information.

In patients with presacral tumors who present with persistent or recurrent draining sinuses, a fistulogram should also be considered.

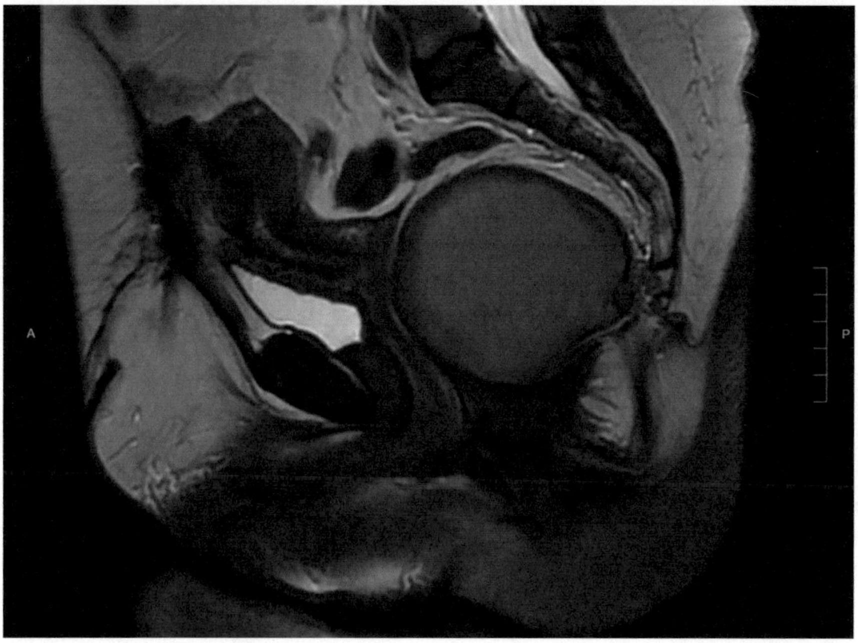

Figure 2.
Magnetic resonance imaging of presacral tumor. Pelvic magnetic resonance imaging in a female patient showing a large cystic presacral tumor displacing the rectum and vagina anteriorly.

4. Role of preoperative biopsy

Evaluation of malignant potential and involvement of surrounding structures on imaging is imperative for operative planning and further management. However, the role of preoperative biopsy continues to be of some debate. Historically, there have been reports of tumor seeding with biopsy and some experts have argued against preoperative biopsy given the potential risk of seeding the biopsy tract [12, 13]. However, more recent literature suggests that percutaneous biopsy, be it core needle biopsy or fine needle aspiration, are safe [14]. Preoperative biopsy should be reserved for solid tumors only.

Preoperative biopsy is effective and accurate. A retrospective review from the Mayo Clinic reviewed 73 patients over the course of 20 years. It further elucidated the diagnostic role of preoperative biopsy. Fifty three patients underwent percutaneous biopsy, 14 open, and 3 both. Of all comers, 63/73 patients (91%) had a correct diagnosis from percutaneous biopsy to final pathology post excision. Thirty-five patients received a preoperative diagnosis based on radiographic findings. Interestingly, 10 out of 35 patients (29%), had discordant findings between preoperative imaging diagnosis and final pathology. In this cohort, sensitivity, specificity, and positive and negative predictive values of imaging to diagnose malignant disease was 83%, 81%, 83%, and 81% respectively. With preoperative biopsy, the diagnostic sensitivity, specificity, and positive and negative predictive values were 96%, 100%, 100%, and 98% respectively [15].

Given that many malignant tumors are sarcoma in origin, preoperative biopsy should be considered when suspicion is high for malignancy. Tissue biopsy increases diagnostic certainty compared to imaging alone, which is important when counseling patients for neoadjuvant therapies. In the modern era of tumor profiling, performing next generation sequencing of the tumor specimen may also help identify potential actionable mutations for targeted therapy. Additionally, malignant tumors likely require wide margins, which depending on size and location may have significant morbidity for the patient and should be included in preoperative discussion and planning. Thus, in tumors that are indeterminate or likely malignant, we would recommend proceeding with biopsy to guide further treatment. Trans-perineal percutaneous biopsy can often be performed. Cystic lesions on the other hand should not be biopsied. Transvaginal or transrectal biopsy is also not recommended as this may result in fistula formation between the lesion and adjacent structure, further complicating resection [15].

Traditionally, resection of the biopsy tract was recommended if any biopsy was performed. However, this is controversial. Messick and colleagues have published their retrospective review on 87 presacral tumors, 24 patients underwent preoperative biopsy. Only 4 of these patients underwent biopsy site excision at the time of surgery and all were histologically negative for malignancy. The remaining 20 patients did not undergo excision and were followed clinically with any reported recurrences at the biopsy site [16]. At this time, no definitive recommendation is supplied by ASCRS regarding biopsy site excision. Commonly, the interventional radiologist team will be able to perform percutaneous biopsies of presacral tumors under imaging guidance. **Figure 3** illustrates common areas for potential biopsy. Multiple approaches for biopsy have been described which include anterior or lateral transabdominal, transgluteal/trans-sciatic, anterolateral extraperitoneal, trans-sacral, and trans-iliac approaches [15]. Complication rates after percutaneous biopsy are low and mainly include infection.

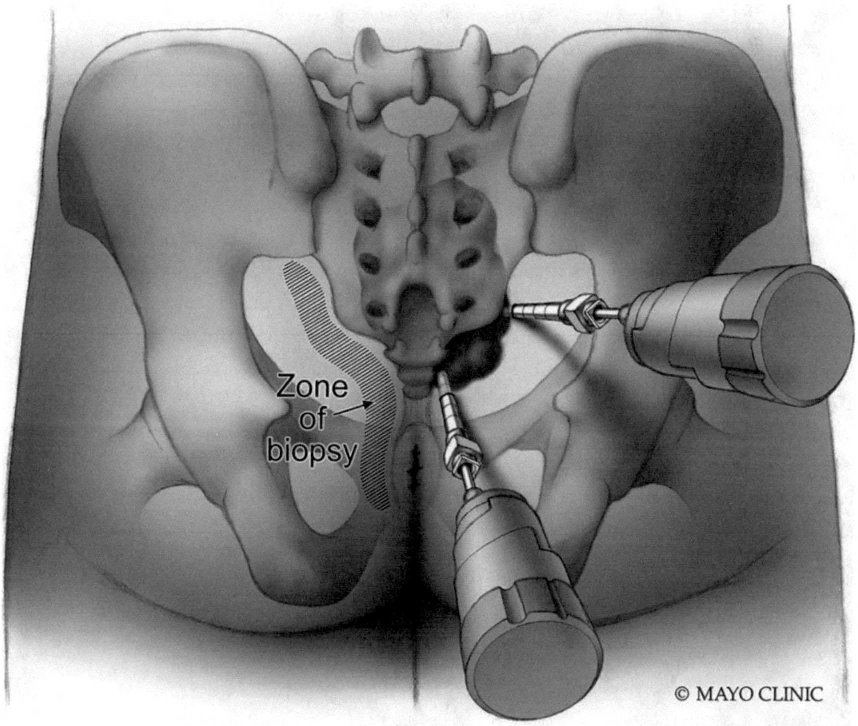

Figure 3.
Percutaneous biopsy of presacral tumors. Illustration of commonly approached target zones for percutaneous biopsy of presacral tumors. CC-BY-NC/ND 4.0 or copyrighted source: Used with permission from ASCRS Textbook of Colon and Rectal Surgery, Fourth Edition (2022) [2].

5. Role of multidisciplinary management/adjuvant therapy

Multidisciplinary care for these patients remains a cornerstone of treatment. Radiologic assessment and intervention with high-resolution cross-sectional imaging and image guided biopsy of malignant appearing lesions are essential in diagnosis and treatment planning. Moreover, due to the rarity of these tumors, we recommend presenting these cases in the institution's multidisciplinary tumor board to garner insight from providers across specialities to explore additional diagnostic modalities, consider neoadjuvant and adjuvant treatment strategies involving chemotherapy and/or radiation along with surgical resection. It is imperative to complete full staging workup for malignant tumors to assess the need to treat any metastatic lesions and provide prognostic information to the patient during treatment counseling. Given that these tumors can often be large and involve other critical organs, surgical resection may require multiple surgical teams including colorectal surgery, orthopedic oncology, neurosurgery, urology, gynecology and vascular surgery. Plastic surgery consultation should be considered preoperatively, particularly in the case of need for tissue coverage.

Most of the presacral lesions are benign in nature and can be excised while preserving other local structures by dissecting within the embryological tissue planes. However, when resecting a large malignant presacral tumor that's involving local structures, sometimes an en bloc resection of soft tissue, adjacent organs such as the ureter, rectum, reproductive organs or bone followed by reconstruction may be required which can lead to significant morbidity in certain situations. If the resection would lead to high morbidity, sometimes radiation or chemotherapy may be the definitive treatment. Although an R0 resection with upfront surgery may be possible for some lesions, many lesions do require further treatment in addition to surgery for optimal outcomes. Ewing's sarcoma or osteosarcoma for example, would be recommended to be treated with neoadjuvant chemotherapy followed by restaging and then be considered for a wide resection. Sarcomas that are sensitive to radiation should be considered for neoadjuvant radiation to downsize the tumor prior to wide resection in an attempt to achieve R0 resection and limit the morbidity of extensive surgery [17]. Given the multitude of potential pathologic diagnoses and different individualized therapies required, it is outside of the constraints of this chapter to discuss each treatment algorithm of malignant presacral tumors individually. However, it is noted that many of these lesions, particularly chondromas or sarcomas, may require radiation therapy, chemotherapy, and the role of immunotherapy should continue to be explored. Treatment guidelines published by the National Comprehensive Cancer Network may help outline a treatment plan based on the subtype of sarcoma.

6. Surgical approach

6.1 Anatomic considerations

The presacral space is a potential space with the peritoneal reflection as the superior border, levator muscles as the inferior border, ureter and iliac vessels as the lateral border, and the meosrectum and sacrum as the anterior and posterior borders, respectively. The presacral space contains totipotent cells and cells of hindgut and neuroectoderm origin. Therefore, a variety of tumors can arise from this space [18].

Surgery is the primary treatment of presacral tumors as it allows a tissue diagnosis, removes the lesion before malignant degeneration, and prevents morbidity from secondary infections. Due to the anatomic constraints of the pelvis, lesions below the S3 vertebrae (**Figure 4**) are commonly resected via a perineal approach whereas the lesions above this level are resected via a transabdominal approach. If malignancy is suspected, en bloc resection based on general surgical oncology principles should be followed.

6.2 Perineal approach (preferred for low lesions below S3)

Perineal approach is recommended for lesions below S3 vertebrae. Various perineal incision techniques have been described for the perineal approach [18, 19]. For the perineal approach, the patient is positioned in a prone jack-knife position and buttocks are taped apart for exposure of the coccyx and anus.

We prefer a trans-sacrococcygeal approach (**Figure 5**) by making an S shaped incision along the gluteal cleft from the lower sacrum past the coccyx to avoid a midline wound which has a higher risk of wound complications. Coccygectomy can be performed to improve exposure. For tumors that invade the sacrum, a distal sacrectomy should be considered. Lesion is then dissected from the surrounding tissue, taking care not to injure the rectal wall. Wound is then closed in layers.

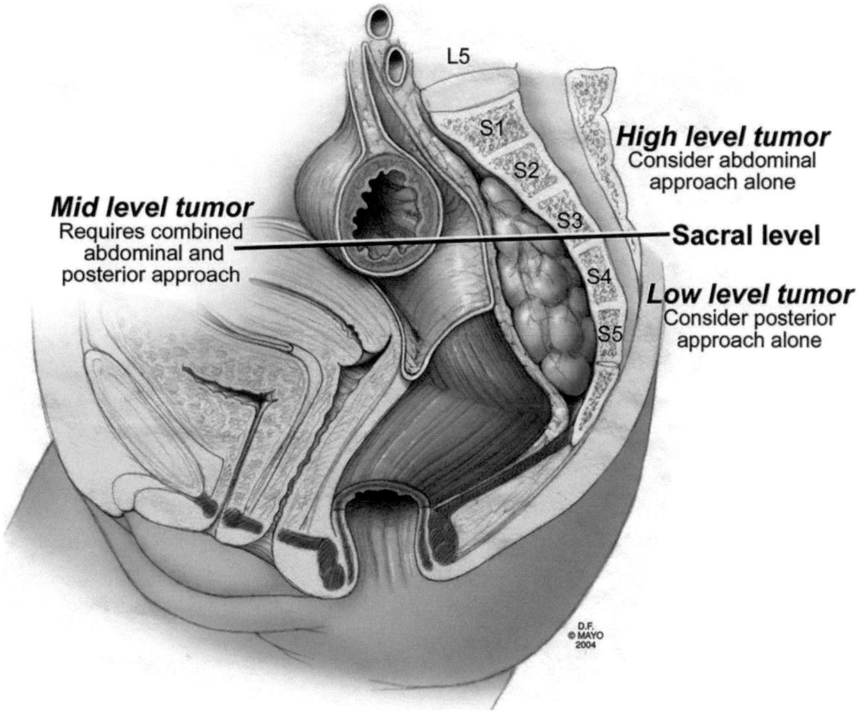

Figure 4.
Anatomic considerations by tumor location. Illustration highlights the clinical relevance of the location of presacral tumors with S3 being the landmark to consider abdominal versus posterior approach. CC-BY-NC/ND 4.0 or copyrighted source: Used with permission from ASCRS Textbook of Colon and Rectal Surgery, Fourth Edition (2022) [2].

6.3 Transabdominal approach (preferred for high lesions above S3)

Lesions above S3 vertebrae are easier to approach transabdominally. However, sometimes lower lesions (below S3 vertebrae) can involve the pelvic sidewall or visceral organs which may still require a transabdominal approach or a combination approach strategy as it provides better exposure of the iliacs and ureters [19, 20].

For open transabdominal approach, the patient is positioned supine and a lower midline incision is made and rectum is lifted anteriorly to dissect the presacral space to identify the lesion. Lesion is then sharply dissected out from the presacral fascia. The middle sacral artery sometimes supplies the lesion and must be taken.

Minimally invasive transabdominal approaches with laparoscopy or robot allow better visualization during the presacral dissection with the robotic approach providing improved surgeon dexterity and ergonomics. We prefer minimally invasive surgery as it has been shown to reduce postoperative pain, hospital length of stay, and overall patient recovery [19, 21, 22]. Recently, robotic transabdominal approach has been shown to be feasible in resecting lesions even below the S3 vertebrae, pushing the limits of traditional open approaches [21].

6.4 Operative considerations in complex tumors

For large tumors extending above and below the S3 level may require a combination of a transabdominal and perineal approach which could be performed by

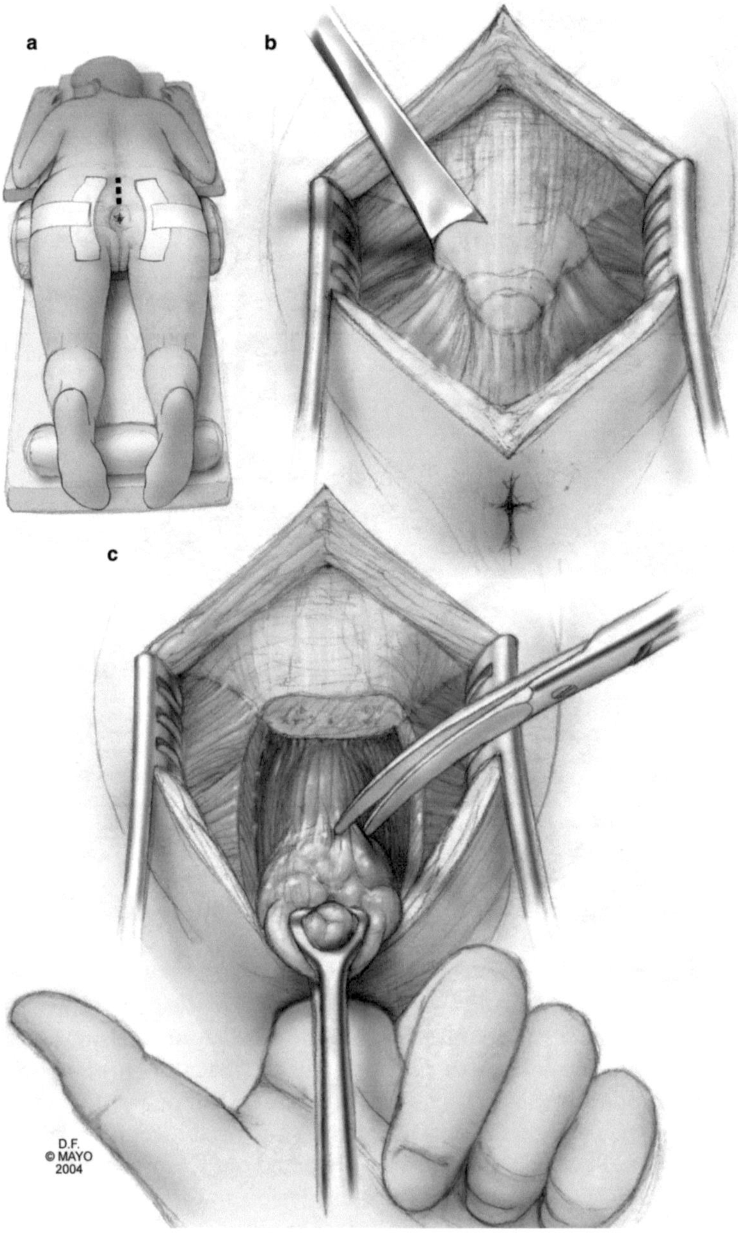

Figure 5.
Illustration of transperineal approach. (A) Patient positioned in prone jack-knife with buttocks taped apart for exposure. (B) Coccygectomy being performed to improve exposure. (C) Presacral mass is sharply excised from the rectal wall. CC-BY-NC/ND 4.0 or copyrighted source: Used with permission from ASCRS Textbook of Colon and Rectal Surgery, Fourth Edition (2022) [2].

repositioning the patient or performing this in dorsal lithotomy in trendelenberg position. Preoperative angioembolization of hypervascular tumors may be helpful in reducing intraoperative blood loss during resection and also reduce the size of the tumor. Tumors that are extending laterally may involve the ureters and we would recommend starting the case with ureteral stents to help identify the ureters during dissection. If a malignant tumor is inseparable from surrounding structures, it would be recommended to perform an en bloc resection. If this is involving the rectum, an en bloc partial or total proctectomy should be performed after separating the rectum anterior from the bladder, seminal vesicles, prostate, or vagina. In very large tumors, the median sacral artery, and branches from the internal iliac artery and vein may supply and drain the tumor. Blood loss can be minimized either by coil embolization preoperatively or by taking these vessels intraoperatively with the help of a vascular surgeon if needed. Close communication with the anesthesia team with adequate intravascular access, real-time hemodynamic monitoring and blood prepared on hold is vitally important for these cases. For malignant tumors that are invading the sacrum, an orthopedic surgeon can assist with a sacrectomy with resection of any involved nerve roots and the glutues and piriformis muscles. For lesions involving the spinal cord, such as a meningocele, work in conjuction with the neurosurgery or orthopedic surgery team to perform a laminectomy, obliteration of the meningocele pedicle and transdural closure.

7. Outcomes

Given the rarity and the multiple subtypes of presacral tumors, there is no well-defined recurrence or survival data on a patient with a specific presacral tumor.

Jao et al. and Messick et al. published the two largest case series of presacral tumors with 120 patients and 87 patients respectively, which may shed some light on the outcomes of rare subtypes of malignant tumors. 30 out of 120 patients had chordomas with a 5-year survival of 75%. 16/30 (53%) patients with chordoma were able to undergo complete resection and 7/30 (23%) ended up with a recurrence. 3 patients had Ewing sarcoma and only 1 patient with Ewing sarcoma survived up to 9 years [1]. In the 87 patients reported by Messick et al., the overall survival rate was 93% and survival was clearly better in the patients with benign tumors (99%) versus patients with malignant tumors (70%) [16]. Recurrence rate was 16% overall and higher 30% for malignant tumors. Interestingly, 7 out of 64 patients with benign tumors later developed distant recurrence. Patients with distal metastasis had a median survival of 47.5 months.

Systematic review of case reports that analyzed over 1700 patients with various presacral tumors who underwent resection showed that the overall mean postoperative hospital stay was about 7 days. Overall postoperative complication rate was 13.2% which included postoperative bleeding (28%), neurogenic bladder (23%), neurologic complication (18%), and wound infection (15%). Overall recurrence rate was 21.6% [19].

Postoperative mortality rates are extremely low and patients with a malignant presacral tumor had higher recurrence rates [10, 20].] As with most rectal surgeries, transient changes in urinary and sexual function were reported in a subset of patients [21].

8. Conclusion

Patients with presacral tumors will present with vague symptoms or no symptoms at all. Cross sectional imaging will help identify a presacral tumor. A variety of tissue types can form presacral tumors and a classification system organized by tissue origin helps categorize presacral tumors. Malignant tumors should be considered for percutaneous biopsy to determine appropriate adjuvant therapies. The surgical approach depends on the location of the tumor along the sacrum. Given the rarity and poor prognosis associated with malignant presacral tumors, a multi-disciplinary approach is recommended for these lesions.

Disclosures

The authors have no relevant conflicts of interest to disclose.

Author details

Jin K. Kim, Kaylee Smith and Jorge Marcet*
Division of Colon and Rectal Surgery, University of South Florida Morsani College of Medicine, Tampa, FL USA

*Address all correspondence to: jmarcet@usf.edu

References

[1] Jao SW, Beart RW, Spencer RJ, Reiman HM, Ilstrup DM, Retrorectal tumors. Mayo clinic experience, 1960-1979. Diseases of the Colon and Rectum. 1985;**28**(9):644-652

[2] Kelley SR. Presacral Tumors. In: Steele SR, Hull TL, Hyman N, Maykel JA, Read TE, Whitlow CB, editors. The ASCRS Textbook of Colon and Rectal Surgery. 4th ed. Charm: Springer; 2022. pp. 375-396

[3] Singer MA, Cintron JR, Martz JE, Schoetz DJ, Abcarian H. Retrorectal cyst: A rare tumor frequently misdiagnosed. Journal of the American College of Surgeons. 2003;**196**(6):880-886

[4] Otote J, Butnari V, Ravichandran PS, Mansuri A, Ahmed M, Pestrin O, et al. Presacral tumors: A systematic review of literature. Journal of Clinical Imaging Science. 2024;**14**:17

[5] Uhlig BE, Johnson RL. Presacral tumors and cysts in adults. Diseases of the Colon and Rectum. 1975;**18**(7):581-589

[6] Dozois EJ, Marcos MDH. Presacral Tumors. In: Beck DE, Roberts PL, Saclarides TJ, Senagore AJ, Stamos MJ, Wexner SD, editors. The ASCRS Textbook of Colon and Rectal Surgery. New York: Springer; 2011. pp. 359-374

[7] Kerekes D, Goodwin CR, Ahmed AK, Verlaan JJ, Bettegowda C, Abu-Bonsrah N, et al. Local and distant recurrence in resected sacral chordomas: A systematic review and pooled cohort analysis. Global Spine Journal. 2019;**9**(2):191-201

[8] Manson F, Comalli-Dillon K, Moriaux A. Anterior sacral meningocele: management in gynecological practice. Ultrasound in Obstetrics & Gynecology. 2007;**30**(6):893-896

[9] Alderete J, Novais EN, Dozois EJ, Rose PS, Sim FF. Morbidity and functional status of patients with pelvic neurogenic tumors after wide excision. Clinical Orthopaedics and Related Research. 2010;**468**(11):2948-2953

[10] Lev-Chelouche D, Gutman M, Goldman G, Even-Sapir E, Meller I, Issakov J, et al. Presacral tumors: A practical classification and treatment of a unique and heterogeneous group of diseases. Surgery. 2003;**133**(5):473-478

[11] Freier DT, Stanley JC, Thompson NW. Retrorectal tumors in adults. Surgery, Gynecology & Obstetrics. 1971;**132**(4):681-686

[12] Verazin G, Rosen L, Khubchandani IT, Sheets JA, Stasik JJ, Riether R. Retrorectal tumor: Is biopsy risky? Southern Medical Journal. 1986;**79**(11):1437-1439

[13] Cody HS, Marcove RC, Quan SH. Malignant retrorectal tumors: 28 years' experience at memorial sloan-kettering cancer center. Diseases of the Colon and Rectum. 1981;**24**(7):501-506

[14] Bommer KK, Ramzy I, Mody D. Fine-needle aspiration biopsy in the diagnosis and management of bone lesions: A study of 450 cases. Cancer. 1997;**81**(3):148-156

[15] Merchea A. Role of preoperative biopsy in the management of presacral tumors. Seminars in Colon and Rectal Surgery. 2020;**31**(3):100761

[16] Messick CA, Hull T, Rosselli G, Kiran RP. Lesions originating within

the retrorectal space: A diverse group requiring individualized evaluation and surgery. Journal of Gastrointestinal Surgery. 2013;**17**(12):2143-2152

[17] von Mehren M, Kane JM, Agulnik M, Bui MM, Carr-Ascher J, Choy E, et al. Soft tissue sarcoma, version 2.2022, NCCN clinical practice guidelines in oncology. Journal of the National Comprehensive Cancer Network. 2022;**20**(7):815-833

[18] Hassan I, Wietfeldt ED. Presacral tumors: Diagnosis and management. Clinics in Colon and Rectal Surgery. 2009;**22**(2):84-93

[19] Baek SK, Hwang GS, Vinci A, Jafari MD, Jafari F, Moghadamyeghaneh Z, et al. Retrorectal tumors: A comprehensive literature review. World Journal of Surgery. 2016;**40**(8):2001-2015

[20] Woodfield JC, Chalmers AG, Phillips N, Sagar PM. Algorithms for the surgical management of retrorectal tumours. The British Journal of Surgery. 2008;**95**(2):214-221

[21] Ferrari D, Violante T, Addison P, Perry WRG, Merchea A, Kelley SR, et al. Robotic resection of presacral tumors. Techniques in Coloproctology. 2024;**28**(1):49

[22] Yamauchi S, Matsuyama T, Tokunaga M, Kinugasa Y. Minimally invasive surgery for colorectal cancer. JMA J. 2021;**4**(1):17-23

Section 4

Anatomy, Emergencies, and Diagnostics

Chapter 10

Revisiting the Anatomy of the Rectum and the Anal Canal

Joyce El-Haddad

Abstract

The rectum and anal canal form the terminal regions of the gastrointestinal tract. They are essential for fecal storage and defecation. Situated within the pelvic cavity, the rectum transitions into the anal canal in the perineum, housing critical neurovascular structures vital for continence. Extensive knowledge of these structures is vital for surgical precision. This chapter examines the anatomy, histology, embryology, and clinical relevance of these structures. Key anatomical features such as rectal folds, curvatures, and the anal sphincter complex are described. Histological adaptations, including goblet cells for lubrication and M cells for immune defense, are reviewed alongside the structural transitions in the epithelium of the anal canal, which predispose certain zones to specific pathologies. The vascular and lymphatic networks, crucial for rectal cancer staging and hemorrhoidal disease, are detailed, alongside somatic and autonomic innervation critical to anorectal function. This overview emphasizes the anatomical and histological complexity of the anorectal region, its clinical significance in disease, and the implications for effective diagnosis, treatment, and surgical interventions.

Keywords: anatomy, histology, embryology, surgical anatomy, rectum, anal anatomy

1. Introduction

The rectum, anal canal, and anus contribute to the most distal end of the gastrointestinal tract. The rectum is situated within the pelvic cavity, while the anal canal and anus project into the perineum. When comparing quadrupedal and bipedal organisms, several evolutionary adaptations of the rectum and anal canal are noteworthy. In quadrupedal organisms, the rectum is more horizontally aligned with the gastrointestinal tract, functioning primarily as a conduit for fecal matter with minimal storage capacity or capacity for voluntary defecation [1]. On the other hand, bipedal species, including humans, have evolved a rectal ampulla, allowing for fecal retention and voluntary defecation control. This adaptation has been crucial in accommodating the pressures exerted by an upright posture, influencing factors such as continence, influence of gravity, pressure distribution, and defecatory mechanisms [1]. Thus, the anatomical evolution of the rectum and anal canal in humans reflects broader adaptations to locomotion, pelvic stability, and social behaviors surrounding appropriate settings for defecation.

Furthermore, many structures are intimately related to the rectum and the anus. Among these structures are delicate neurovascular networks which can present subtle clinical signs of rectal or anal involvement. In the same token, the proximity to such structures has severe implications during rectal or anal surgery if injured. Thus, knowledge of the anatomy of the rectum and the anus, including their relations is paramount for the effective management of rectal and anal pathology and disease.

There are several gaping holes in the literature that reflect our understanding of the anatomy of the rectum and anal canal relative to other regions and structures of the body. One of the compounding factors contributing to this is the cultural taboo surrounding discussions of defecation and anorectal function [2, 3]. Another factor is the mere complexity of studying these structures due to their deep pelvic location, intricate neurovascular supply, and involvement in both autonomic and voluntary control mechanisms [3–7]. The lack of detailed investigation has implications for clinical practice, as many rectal and anal conditions, including functional disorders and malignancies, remain poorly understood or are diagnosed late due to inadequate screening tools, accessibility to such tools, and public education [5–8].

The aim of this chapter is to outline the clinically relevant anatomy, relations, histology, and embryology of the rectum and anal canal, highlighting the complexity and importance of this underappreciated region of the human body. It will first cover the embryology and histology of the rectum and anal canal, followed by the extent, relations, and neurovascular supply of the rectum and anal canal.

2. Embryology

The rectum and the upper part of the anal canal are derived from the primitive gut tube; specifically, the hindgut. The hindgut is suspended dorsally by the mesorectum [9]. The mesorectum is a specialized layer of connective tissue that is similar to the peritoneum but differs slightly as the mesorectum itself is encased within the mesorectal fascia. The rectal epithelium is derived from the endoderm of the hindgut, while the surrounding tissue is derived from the splanchnic mesoderm [10]. The lower end of the anal canal is derived from the cloaca [9]. The cloaca around the 4th to 7th weeks of development partitions into the urorectal septum that keeps the anal canal and the urogenital sinus as separate structures. Failure to separate results in anorectal malformations such as imperforate anus or rectovaginal/rectourethral fistulas [10].

3. Histology of the rectum

The histology of the rectum is continuous with the histology of the hindgut with slight differences.

3.1 Mucosa

The mucosal layer of the colon is the most metabolically and immunologically active. The mucosa consists of epithelium, lamina propria, and the muscularis mucosae.

3.1.1 Epithelium

Rectal mucosa is covered with glycocalyx which contributes to the microbial ecosystem and acts as a protective barrier. Deep to the glycocalyx is simple columnar epithelium lining regularly spaced crypts (similar to a test-tube rack). The crypts are aligned perpendicular to and extend to the muscularis mucosae. Within the epithelium several types of cells are found many of which include absorptive enterocytes (colonocytes), goblet cells, and M cells [11].

Since the function of the rectal is for storage of feces the number of absorptive enterocytes is significantly less than that of the right side of colon. These cells where present in the rectal epithelium characterized by rigid, tightly packed apical microvilli with a lightly eosinophilic cytoplasm [11]. Relating the structure to function of the rectum again, the rectal mucosa is prone to abrasion from the friction pushing feces into the anal canal has potential to cause, thus a large number of goblet cells here would make sense. Goblet cell nuclei, appear hyperchromatic, dense, and irregular [11]. M cells in the rectum are integral to the gut's immune defense system, particularly in sampling and presenting luminal antigens to immune cells to trigger appropriate immune responses. Their role during inflammation may also reflect a protective mechanism or contribute to chronic inflammation, as seen in inflammatory bowel diseases [11, 12]. On histology, M cells appear with a reduced number of irregular microvilli, and have a basolateral membrane forms an intraepithelial pocket which provides a docking site for intraepithelial B and T cells [11, 12].

3.1.2 Lamina propria

The lamina propria of the colon, located between the crypts and muscularis mucosae, plays a critical role in immunologic, metabolic, proliferative, and motility functions. It is a highly organized structure housing inflammatory and mesenchymal cells within a loose connective tissue matrix, facilitating immune surveillance and response [11, 13].

3.1.3 Muscularis mucosae

The muscularis mucosae is external to the lamina propria. The muscularis mucosae is a thin layer of smooth muscle physically tethered to the mucosa. It receives innervation from the inner part of the submucosal plexus. Assessment of the integrity, invasion, and injury of the muscularis mucosae has diagnostic significance [14].

3.2 Submucosa

The submucosa of the rectum is composed of smooth muscle fibers, connective tissue, vasculature, lymphatic channels, and various neural networks. The submucosal neural plexuses are the inner plexus (Meissner's) which innervates the muscularis mucosae and the second is the outer submucosal plexus (Henle's) which contributes to the innervation of the muscularis layer.

Clear distinction between the mucosa and submucosa are crucial for rectal cancer staging. Tumor invasion into the submucosa (T1 stage in TNM staging) indicates an early stage of cancer spread beyond the mucosal layer, specifically beyond the muscularis mucosae [13]. Tumor invasion into the submucosa increases the likelihood of metastasis through lymphatic spread to regional lymph nodes or distant metastases [13].

3.3 Muscular externa

The muscularis externa layer of the rectum consists of two smooth muscle layers. The first is the inner circular layer which facilitates constriction and segmentation movements of the rectum. The next is the outer longitudinal layer which aids in shortening and propelling colonic contents from rectum into the anal canal. Between these two layers exists a myenteric plexus (Auerbach's) which innervates the two layers. Additionally, interstitial cells (of Cajal) which are specialized pacemaker cells that drive peristalsis are found throughout the muscularis propria. As mentioned above, distinction between the histological layers of the rectum is crucial for rectal cancer staging [13]. If the tumor is confined to the muscularis externa, it is classified as T2 in the TNM staging system. When the tumor breaches the muscularis externa and extends into the perirectal fat or mesorectal tissue, it is classified as T3. Further extension into adjacent organs or structures (such as the bladder, prostate, or peritoneum) is classified as T4 [13].

4. Anal canal

The anal canal is defined both anatomically and surgically. The anatomical anal canal extends from the anal verge to the dentate (pectinate) line. While the surgical anal canal extends from the anal verge to the anorectal line. The anatomical delineation aligns with its embryological origin from the cloaca, where the dentate line serves as a landmark where there is a change in the neurovasculature [15]. The anal canal has several important structures part of it and related to it as outlined below.

4.1 Internal anatomy and histology of the anal canal

The histology of the anal canal is continuous with the histological arrangement of the gastrointestinal tract i.e. mucosal, submucosal, muscularis, and serosa/tunica adventitia layers. The contents and composition of each of these layers corresponds to the location and function of the anal canal.

4.1.1 Mucosa of the anal canal

The mucous membrane of the anal canal has 10–15 permanent longitudinal folds called anal columns, joined at the bases to form anal valves at the level of the pectinate line. Histologically, there are four important transition zones in the epithelium of the anal canal – colorectal, anal transitional, squamous, and perianal zones (**Figure 1**) [11, 16].

i. The colorectal zone is approximately at the anorectal junction where a change in epithelium is seen from simple to stratified columnar epithelium. This zone is most susceptible to colorectal like adenocarcinomas (**Figure 2**) [11].

ii. The anal transitional zone (ATZ) features stratified columnar or stratified cuboidal epithelium. Here the epithelium begins to transition towards a stratified squamous appearance (**Figure 2**). The ATZ extends from the dentate line to the new squamous columnar junction at the pectineal line. On anoscopy, the SCJ is the most important and readily identifiable landmark, typically visible as a clear

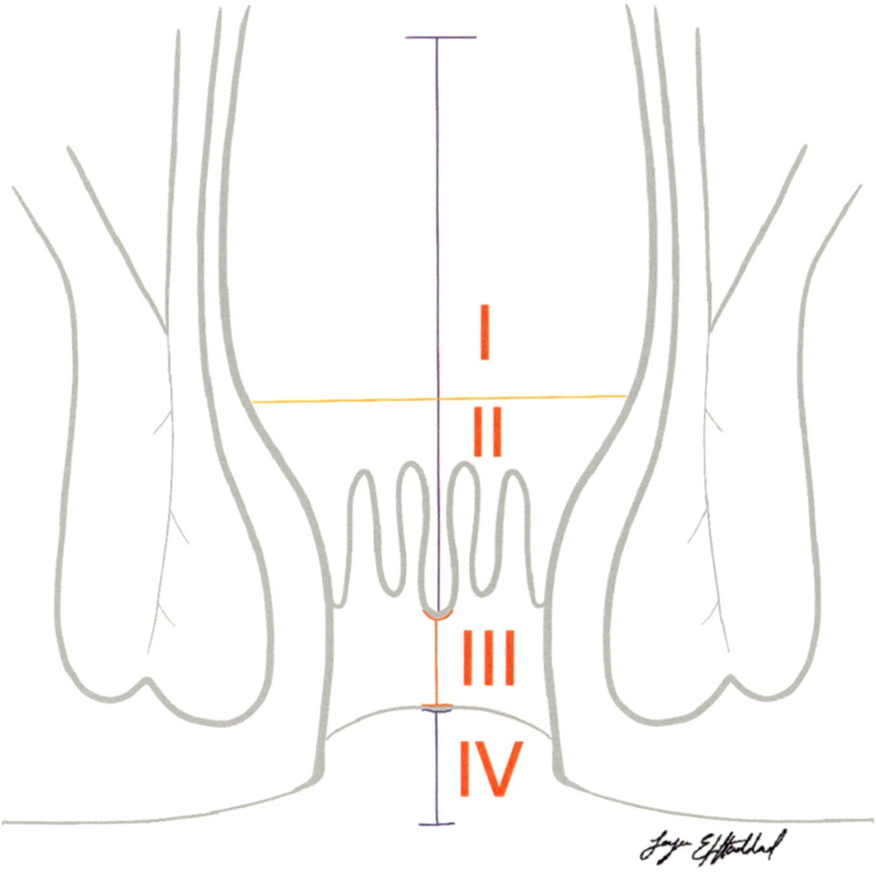

Figure 1.
Histological zones of the anal canal. Colorectal zone (I); Anal transitional zone (II), Squamous Junction (III), Perianal Zone (IV). Illustration by Joyce El-Haddad.

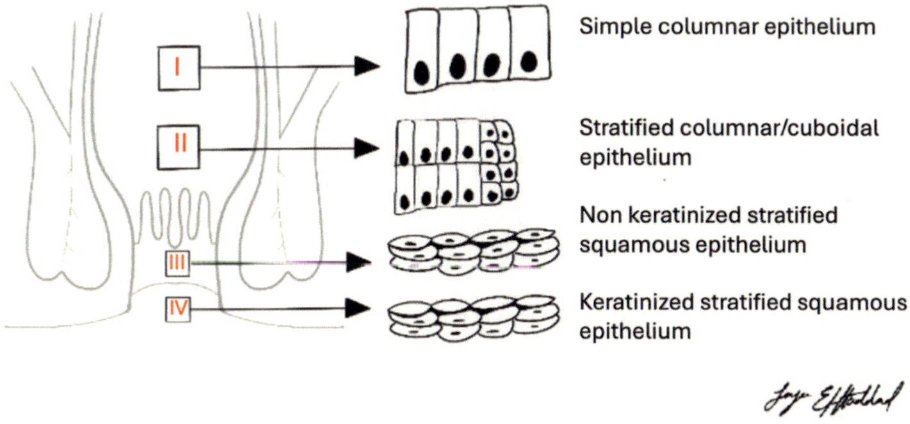

Figure 2.
Histological zones of the anal canal. Colorectal zone (I); Anal transitional zone (II), Squamous Junction (III), Perianal Zone (IV) and their respective epithelium. Illustration by Joyce El-Haddad.

line of tissue that is paler than the adjacent proximal rectal epithelium – this corresponds to the pectinate line. The boundaries between the colorectal and ATZ are not well demarcated. This zone, because of the volatile nature of transitioning cells, is susceptible to anal intraepithelial neoplasia and squamous cell carcinomas in the presence of oncogenic strains of HPV [11, 16, 17].

iii. The squamous zone is composed of uninterrupted, non-keratinized stratified squamous epithelium. This extends towards the white line (of Hilton) (**Figure 2**) [11, 16, 17].

iv. The perianal skin zone mirrors the histology of the skin - i.e., keratinized stratified squamous epithelium (**Figure 2**), with hair follicles, sebaceous glands, sweat glands, and apocrine glands (circumanal glands). Melanocytes are also seen in this zone. This extends from the white line towards the anal margin (i.e., perianal skin). Due to the nature of the histology, this zone is susceptible to hidradenitis suppurativa [18], melanomas [19], lichen planus [20], and benign fibroepithelial growths.

4.1.2 Submucosa of the anal canal

The submucosal layer of the anal canal houses the internal and external haemorrhoidal plexuses. These plexuses contain both tributaries of veins (superior and inferior rectal veins) and arterioles (superior and inferior rectal arteries) [15, 21]. The internal rectal (haemorrhoidal) plexus within the submucosa layer in the upper anal canal pushes the subepithelial tissue towards the mucosa and lumen of the anal canal. These expansions are known as the anal cushions and are most prominent in the 3, 7, 9 o'clock positions [15, 21].

Under normal physiological and mechanical conditions, the anal cushions help seal the anal canal and contribute to fecal and flatus continence [7]. The external rectal (haemorrhoidal) plexus is found in the submucosal layer of the perianal space beneath the perianal skin. The anatomy of the haemorrhoidal plexuses and anal cushions are contentious. Stelzner [22], describes their anatomy to be akin to erectile tissue (corpus cavernosum recti) [13], in that they possess deep vascular spaces that are engorged with arteriovenous blood to seal the anal canal. While some earlier studies suggested a connection between haemorrhoidal disease and portal hypertension, more recent evidence distinguishes anal varices secondary to portal hypertension as a separate entity from hemorrhoids [23–25].

It is important to reiterate, that that the term 'hemorrhoids' does not indicate pathology, but rather the prolapse and transformation of the anal cushions into anal nodules secondary to the engorgement of the respective plexus does. Consistent and accurate use of the terminology has potential to improve interdisciplinary communication and research, and patient education.

4.2 Muscularis layer of anal canal (anal sphincter complex)

The anal sphincter complex consists of both the internal and external anal sphincters which are separated by a conjoint longitudinal muscle layer. The anal sphincter complex plays a critical role in defecation and maintaining continence. This complex corresponds histologically to the muscularis layer of the anal canal.

4.2.1 Internal anal sphincter

The internal anal sphincter (IAS) is a continuation and thickening of the inner circular layer of the rectum. The IAS is smooth muscle and thus innervated by the autonomic nervous system. The IAS commences at the anorectal junction and ends above the anal verge [26]. At the intersphincteric groove, the lower margin of the IAS is palpable. Under normal, non-pathological conditions, the IAS is contracted and provides the resting anal tone felt during a digital anal examination. This function ensures that continence is maintained at rest. Cali et al. [16] reported normal variations of resting anal tone and noted that due to larger and thicker sphincteric muscle mass, males generally exhibit greater squeeze and resting pressures [27]. They also reported that females who have undergone vaginal deliveries had a decrease in maximum resting pressures which was exacerbated in multiparous females [27].

4.2.2 External anal sphincter

The external anal sphincter (EAS) is a skeletal muscle under somatic innervation. The EAS historically has been divided into 3 parts (deep, superficial and subcutaneous parts) however functionally these are irrelevant as the EAS along with the levator ani and puborectalis muscles function as a collective unit. The EAS and the levator ani work in concert during voluntary contraction to enhance continence [26, 27]. For example, during coughing or sneezing (i.e., increased intrabdominal pressure), the levator ani contracts reflexively to provide additional support, while the EAS tightens to prevent leakage. Anatomically and with respects to attachments, the EAS can be divided into an upper and lower part. The upper part of the EAS attaches posteriorly to the anococcygeal ligament and anteriorly to the perineal body [26, 28].

The lower portion of the EAS extends beneath the IAS and is penetrated by the terminal fibers of the conjoint longitudinal muscle (see below). Anteriorly, it connects to the bulbospongiosus and bulbocavernosus muscles [28] – this forms an '8' shaped figure that connects the urogenital and anal triangles.

4.2.3 Conjoint longitudinal muscle

The conjoint longitudinal muscle (CLM) is the continuation of the outer longitudinal muscle of the rectal wall. It originates at the level the rectal muscularis layer and is situated between the IAS and EAS and plays a role in anorectal stability. The CLM inserts into inserts into the perineal body anteriorly and the anococcygeal raphe posteriorly. The CLM is thought to be thicker in fetal life, and as IAS develops the CLM regresses eventually into connective tissue later in life [26]. The CLM fibers transverse the submucosa and connect to the mucosa of the anal canal to anchor the anal cushions. The anal cushions, composed of vascularized tissue, are crucial for maintaining continence. If the CLM weakens, the anchoring support diminishes, allowing the cushions to prolapse and form hemorrhoids [26]. Consequently, the downward movement of the anal cushions due to weakened CLM tension can disrupt venous return in the hemorrhoidal plexus, leading to engorgement of the arteriovenous plexuses, inflammation, and potentially symptomatic/prolapsed hemorrhoids [29].

The CLM and its extensions can also provide potential pathways for the spread of infection. The extensions of CLM between IAS and EAS create potential anatomical planes and pathways through which infections can spread between the rectum, anal canal, and adjacent spaces, such as the perineum or ischioanal fossae. Its insertion into the perineal body and anococcygeal raphe also provides a direct anatomical bridge for infections to travel in spaces such as the ischioanal fossae and/or presacral spaces. However, it should be noted that during early stages of infection and before the anatomical barriers are breached, the CLM plays a role in compartmentalizing infections in the abovementioned spaces [16, 26, 30].

5. Extent of the rectum and the anal canal

Knowledge and orientation of the extent of the rectum is essential to effective surgical precision, imaging interpretation, preoperative planning, patient positioning during clinical examinations, and education [15, 28]. However, as basic as defining the extent of the rectum and anal canal may seem, it remains controversial [13]. This section will provide an overview of the consensus in the literature regarding the extent of the anorectal area.

5.1 The upper limit of the rectum

The upper limit of the rectum begins at the rectosigmoid junction (RSJ). The RSJ serves as an important landmark for procedures such as total mesorectal excision (TME), resection margins in rectal cancer surgeries, and colostomy planning. This junction is characterized by the absence of taeniae coli and omental appendages (epiploic appendages). The RSJ is found at the level of the third sacral vertebrae. The RSJ is said to be 2.8 cm long in adults and 0.7 cm in neonates [30]. Histologically, the RSJ also marks the transition from sigmoid colon mucosa to rectal mucosa. The RSJ can be identified via an array of modalities. Some examples include:

5.1.1 Identifying the RSJ on CT and MRI

The sigmoid take off (STO) has been suggested as an imaging landmark to identify the RSJ on CT and MRI [31]. The STO is defined as the junction between the mesorectum and sigmoid mesocolon [13]. The STO has also been defined as the region where the fixed mesorectum ends and no longer tethers the rectum to the sacrum, and thus the rectum becomes mobile [28, 32]. The STO is seen on a sagittal view where the sigmoid colon moves horizontally away from the sacrum (**Figure 2**). Axially, the sigmoid colon moves ventrally (**Figure 3**). Identification of the STO allows for accurate classification of sigmoid or rectal tumors, above and below the STO, respectively [31].

While the STO is a promising landmark for defining the RSJ and improving the sensitivity of rectal cancer diagnoses, it is not without its limitations. For example, Hazen et al. [31], aimed to evaluate the use of the STO in clinical practice and found that in the presence of complex anatomy and pathology, and/or suboptimal and inconsistent imaging conditions identification of STO was not feasible and requires extensive training and expertise. The authors also highlighted that without adequately addressing the abovementioned challenges, the risk of misclassification of tumors would have a downstream effect on treatment plans and ultimately prognosis. Similar observations have been corroborated by other studies [13].

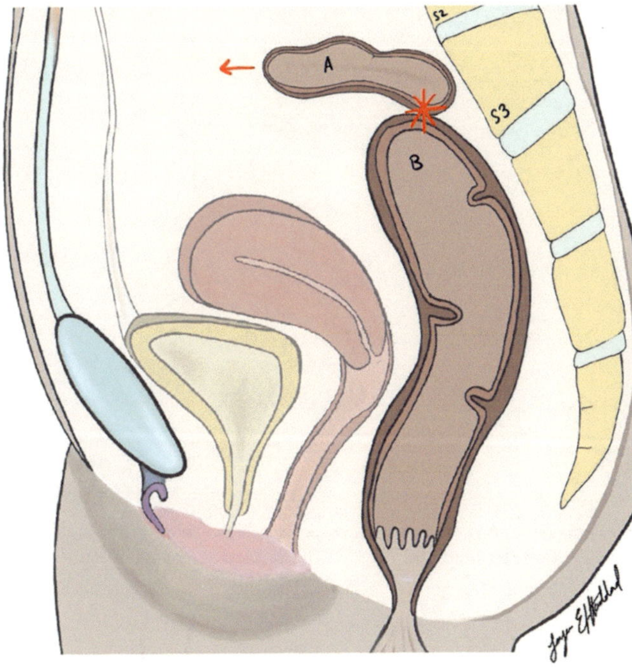

Figure 3.
Mid sagittal view of the female pelvis. A represents the sigmoid colon and B represents the rectum. Sigmoid colon from this view is seen to move horizontally away from the sacrum. The asterisk represents the sigmoid take off (STO) at the level of S3. Illustration by Joyce El-Haddad.

5.1.2 Identifying the RSJ on sigmoidoscopy

On sigmoidoscopy, various landmarks of the RSJ have been proposed [33]. The RSJ is said to be 12–17 cm proximal from the anal verge [34, 35]. However, it should be noted that the range of lengths seem to be based on a limited and narrow demographic group and likely do not consider age, sex, ancestral heritage, nor the presence or absence of various pathologies.

5.1.3 Identifying the RSJ on barium enema studies

To identify the RSJ reliably, Rubesin et al. [35] highlight that the patient should be positioned laterally to avoid sigmoid loops from obstructing the RSJ view. Rubesin et al. recommend that the overhead view obtained with the tube angled about 30° caudad and with the patient in the prone position is optimal to observe the rectosigmoid junction [35]. To the author's knowledge, no literature to date outlines landmarks to identify the RSJ that are specific to barium enema studies (**Figure 4**).

5.2 The lower limit of the rectum and upper limit of the anal canal

The lower limit of the rectum is even more controversial than the upper limit. The main classifications are anatomical and clinical (**Figure 5**).

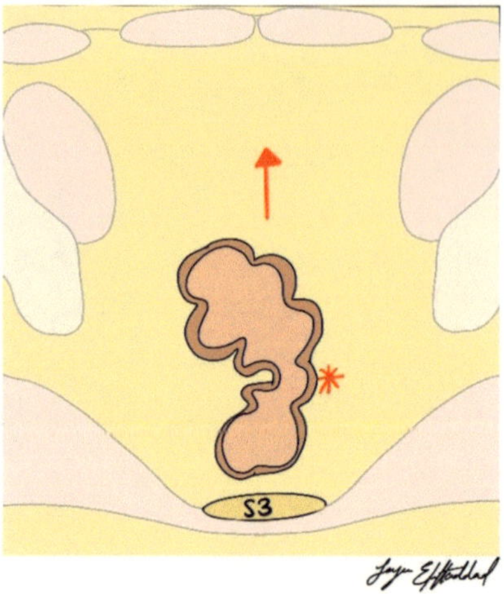

Figure 4.
Axial view of the pelvis at the level of S3. The sigmoid colon from this view is seen to move anteriorly away from the sacrum. Asterisks represents the sigmoid take off (STO). Illustration by Joyce El-Haddad.

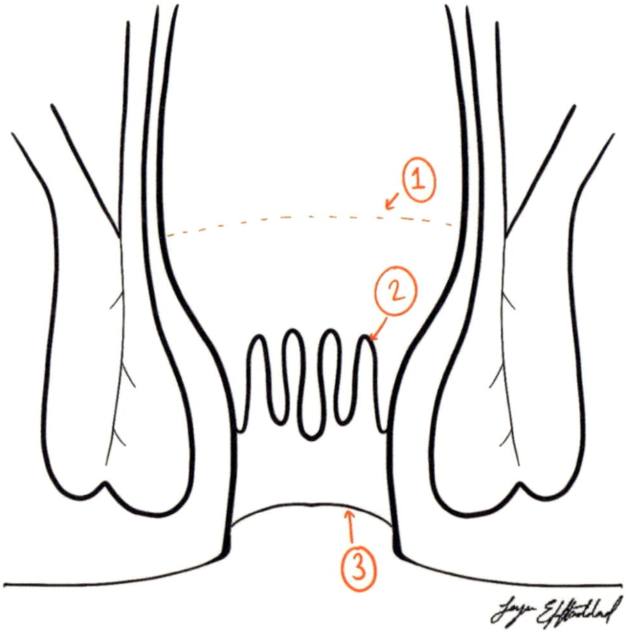

Figure 5.
Surgical vs. anatomical classification of anal canal. The lower limit of the rectum is clinically found at the anorectal line (1) which aligns with the anorectal muscle sling. Anatomical lower limit of the rectum is the dentate line (2). Lower limit of the anal verge (margin) (3) Illustration by Joyce El-Haddad.

5.2.1 Anatomical

The dentate (pectinate) line remains the most commonly referred to landmark to distinguish the end of the rectum and the start of the anal canal (**Figure 5**). This known as the start of the "anatomical anal canal". The dentate line used as the demarcation of the end of the rectum also aligns with its histology, as the dentate line is where the transition in the histology between columnar rectal mucosa to squamous anal mucosa occurs.

5.2.2 Surgical anal canal

Surgically, the lower limit of the rectum is said to be at the anorectal junction (ARJ). The ARJ is approximately 1 cm above the dentate line (**Figure 5**). The ARJ is in line with the level of the muscular anorectal ring and thus palpable on a digital rectal exam. The ARJ is also used as a surgical landmark to separate the rectum from the anus during low anterior resections or abdominoperineal resections [21]. Identification of the ARJ is important to use as a landmark to measure the height of a suspected tumor. From a sagittal view, the anorectal junction is situated at the level of an imaginary line between the lower margin of the sacral and pubic bone [14]. From a coronal view the ARJ aligns with an imaginary line along the upper edge of the puborectal sling [14].

5.3 Lower limit of the anal canal

The lower limit of the surgical anal canal is around the mucocutaneous junction of the non-keratinised squamous mucosa (anal verge) and the keratinised perianal skin in line with the intersphincteric groove [36]. The intersphincteric groove is approximately 2 cm below the pectinate line in adults. The anal margin, also referred to as the perianal skin extends radially for about 5 cm distal to the anal verge. This is the skin around the anus proper and is what is seen on clinical examination (**Figure 5**) [37].

6. Internal anatomy and relations of the rectum

When the rectum is empty, it possesses several temporary longitudinal folds that stretch when the rectum is full. The folds likely exist as a way to accommodate for volume changes and reduce risk of perforation. The rectum typically has 3 permanent semilunar folds which become more prominent when the rectum is distended [26]. The three folds (although the number can vary) are known as superior, middle and inferior rectal folds. The middle rectal fold in particular serves as a landmark during sigmoidoscopy or rectal surgery as it is lies immediately above the rectal ampulla. In addition, tumors below this valve are palpable on a digital rectal examination [38]. Externally, the rectum typically has two curvatures. The first is the sacral flexure – an anteroposterior curve with anterior concavity. The second is the anorectal flexure - an anteroposterior curve with anterior convexity that is maintained by the puborectalis muscle. Additionally, externally the rectum has several important relations that are noteworthy (**Figure 5**).

6.1 Peritoneal relations of the rectum

The rectum is both intra and extraperitoneal. The upper two thirds of the rectum is classified as intraperitoneal given that its anterior and lateral aspects are covered by peritoneum. Meanwhile, the lower third is classified as extraperitoneal. It should be noted that in the middle third of the rectum, only the anterior aspect of the rectum is covered by peritoneum [26] It is important to understand the peritoneal relations of the rectum, particularly in the context of rectal perforations. Any perforations through a part of the rectal wall that is covered by peritoneum means that the perforated matter has access to the peritoneum, potentially leading to sepsis [30].

6.2 Fascial relations of the rectum

The mesorectum covers the rectum and its surrounding fat. The mesorectum transmits the superior rectal artery (and its branches) and vein (and its tributaries), and lymphatics. Anterolaterally in the mesorectum, are branches of the inferior hypogastric plexus and the middle rectal arteries (where present). Dissection around the inferior hypogastric plexus must be carefully done to preserve urinary bladder and sexual functions [26]. There are suggestions that branches of the inferior hypogastric plexus and the middle rectal arteries are enclosed by the lateral ligaments, however, not much is known about the morphology, extent, and prevalence of these ligaments.

The mesorectum, with its fatty tissue predominantly deposited posteriorly, provides not only a protective role but also supplies vascular, lymphatic, and neural elements crucial for rectal function. The mesorectum itself is encased within the mesorectal fascia (fascia propria of the rectum). The mesorectal fascia covers the rectum down to the level of levator ani muscle [26] Surgically, the mesorectal fascia provides the resection plane for total mesorectal excision (TME). Posterior to the mesorectal fascia is the presacral space (retrorectal space). This space itself is anterior to the presacral fascia which some texts suggest is synonymous with Waldeyer's fascia. The exact definition of Waldeyer's fascia remains debated, with two predominant interpretations: (1) it is considered the presacral fascia, which forms the base of the

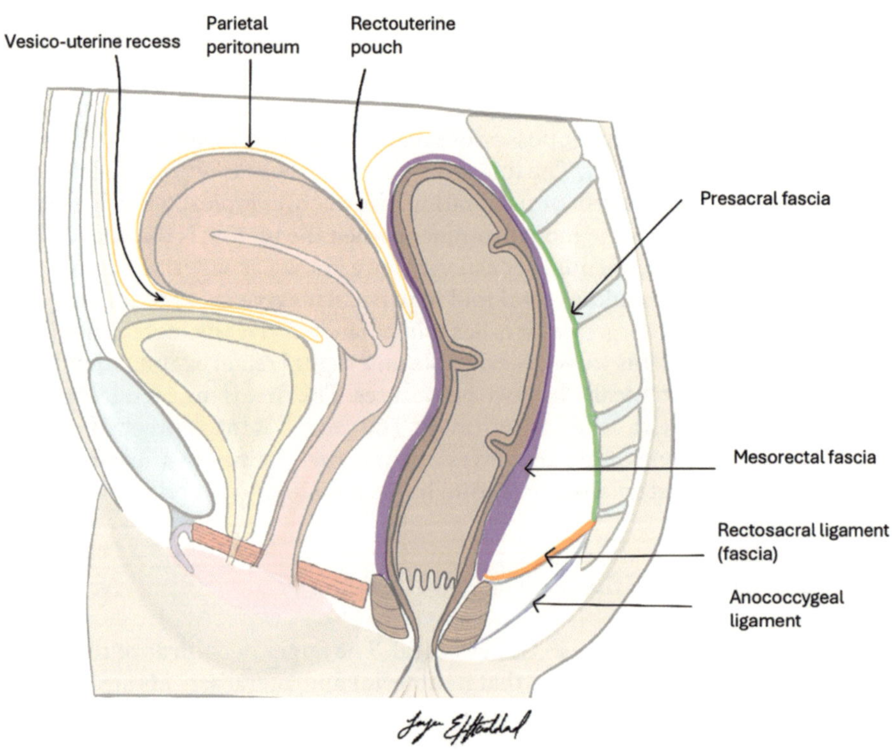

Figure 6.
Fascial relations of the rectum in the female pelvis. Illustration by Joyce El-Haddad.

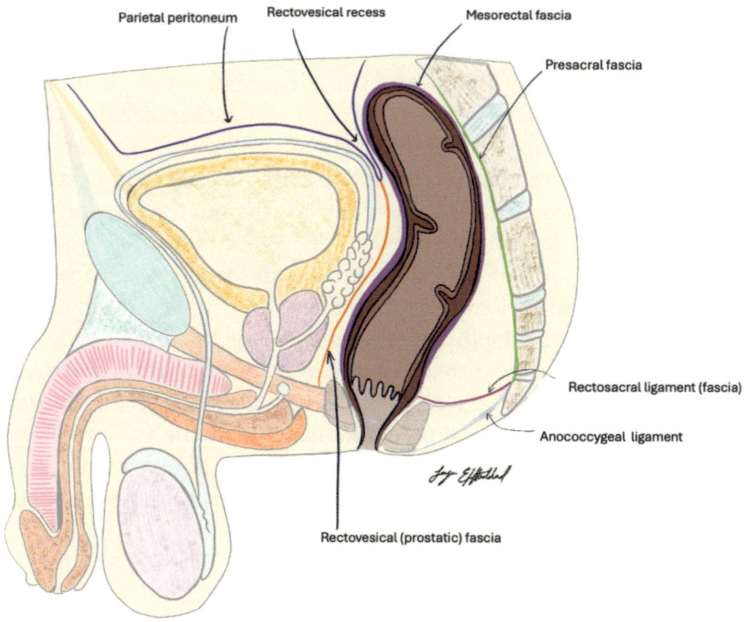

Figure 7.
Fascial relations of the rectum in the male pelvis. Illustration by Joyce El-Haddad.

retrorectal space and condenses into the rectosacral ligament; or (2) it is described as the rectosacral fascia, a dense connective tissue layer extending from the periosteum of the fourth sacral vertebra to the posterior rectal wall (**Figure 6**) [39]. Waldeyer's fascia, however, remains a critical landmark during posterior rectal mobilization. It is suggested that improper blunt dissection may compromise the mesorectum, increasing the risk of cancer metastasis. Additionally, tearing of Waldeyer's fascia from the sacrum can lead to significant bleeding from the presacral veins [39].

Anteriorly, in males the mesorectal fascia becomes coalesced with the rectoprostatic (rectovesical) fascia (Denonvilliers fascia), which is anterior to the rectovesical pouch. In females, the mesorectal fascia anteriorly combines with rectovaginal fascia (Denonvilliers fascia) to form the rectovaginal septum which is anterior to the rectouterine pouch (of Douglas). It has been suggested that the merging of the respective fascia potentially limits the spread of malignancy from one adjacent organ to the other (**Figure 7**) [40].

7. Arterial supply of the rectum and anal canal

The rectum is supplied by three arteries - the superior, middle (bilateral), and inferior rectal (bilateral) (hemorrhoidal arteries). Sometimes, the median sacral artery from the abdominal aorta can contribute to the supply of the posterior wall of the rectum and the anal canal.

7.1 Superior rectal artery

The inferior mesenteric artery (IMA) branches from the aorta at the level of L3 anterolaterally to the left. It gives off branches to the distal segments of the colon and its pelvic continuation is the superior rectal artery (SRA). The SRA commences at the level of the pelvic brim and crosses the left common iliac vessels with the inferior hypogastric nerves on both sides. It pierces the mesorectum and gives off branches to the rectosigmoid junction, an upper rectal branch which then divides into right and left terminal branches (**Figure 8**) [41]. At the level of S3 the SRA enters the upper mesorectum and the right and left terminal branches that descend posterolaterally [1]. The right terminal branch of SRA is usually larger than the left and is considered the true continuation of the SRA (**Figure 8**) [41]. The left terminal branch of SRA is considered a collateral branch of IMA and supplies the anterior surface of the rectum [41]. The perforating arteries of the SRA branches enter the rectal submucosa and anastomose with branches of the middle and inferior rectal arteries. The SRA is the main artery that supplies the rectum and contributes significantly to the arterial supply of the internal hemorrhoids [26] The branches of SRA terminate usually above the anal valves [41]. The SRA also supplies two muscles of the anal sphincter complex i.e., the IAS and CLM. The SRA is closely associated with lymph nodes serving as the primary pathway for lymphatic drainage from the rectum and upper anal canal.

7.2 Middle rectal artery

The prevalence rate of the middle rectal artery (MRA) ranges from 12 to 97% [42]. The MRA is a direct branch off the anterior division of the internal iliac artery (**Figure 8**). The MRA is thought to provide the anatomical basis for lateral spread of rectal cancer [42]. The blood supply territories of the MRA are not clear.

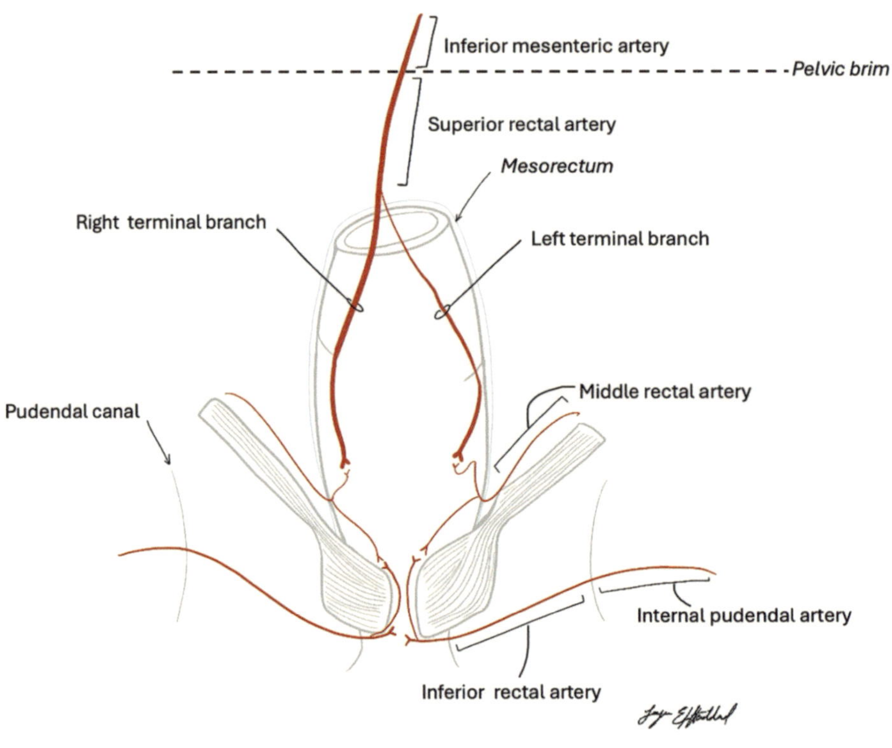

Figure 8.
Blood supply of the rectum. Illustration by Joyce El-Haddad.

The MRA is thought to contribute to the supply of the lower rectum and anal canal and thought to provide a collateral pathway with SRA and IRA. This thought process comes from the fact that the MRA perfuses the rectal stump significantly post ligation of the SRA [43]. Careful consideration should be taken when near the vicinity of the MRA to reduce risk of bleeding and consequently impairment of the surgical field [43]. The MRA perforates the inferior hypogastric plexus and the mesorectal fascia laterally.

Heinze et al., aimed to evaluate the anatomy of the middle rectal artery to facilitate surgical management. Out of 22 body donor dissections, they found the MRA to have originated from the internal pudendal artery in 45.5%, the gluteal artery in 22.7%, a common gluteal-pudendal trunk in 22.7%, or formed a trifurcation with these arteries in 9.1% of cases [42]. Where present, the MRA also gives off branches to the surrounding pelvic organs. The MRA perforating branches enter the rectal submucosa and anastomose with branches of the superior and inferior rectal arteries.

7.3 Inferior rectal artery

The inferior rectal artery (IRA) is the terminal branch of the internal pudendal artery. The internal pudendal arteries on the left and right sides enter the pudendal (Alcock's canal) (**Figure 8**). The IRA then exits medially into the ischioanal fossae to supply the distal third of the rectum to supply the internal and external anal sphincters, anal canal, and perianal skin [26] There is bilateral communication between the pair of IRAs which leaves a watershed area in the dorso-caudal area of the rectal ampulla [26, 44, 45]. The watershed area potentially provides an anatomical rationale as to why anastomotic leaks are observed in the dorso-caudal rectal ampulla post low anterior resection of the rectum [44, 45].

Similar to the SRA and MRA, the IRA perforating branches enter the rectal submucosa and anastomose with branches of the middle and superior rectal arteries. Klosterhalfen et al. [45], outlined two main anatomical variants of the IRA. The first variant of the IRA gives no branches to the posterior commissure of the anal canal, whilst the second variant which is less common, supplies the posterior commissure. The authors concluded that where there is less perfusion to the posterior commissure (as seen in the first type of variant), makes the region more prone to ischemia and slower at healing if an injury such as anal fissure occurs [45].

8. Venous drainage of the rectum and anal canal

The rectum and anal canal are drained by two main veins – the inferior mesenteric vein and the internal iliac vein.

8.1 Rectal venous plexus

The rectal venous plexus surrounds the rectum and has direct connections to local venous plexuses such as the vesical venous plexus in males and uterovaginal venous plexus in females [26]. The rectal venous plexus is divided into 2 parts based on the orientation relative to the histological layers of the rectum. The internal veins are found deep to the mucosa of the rectum and upper anal canal [26]. The external veins are found outside the muscularis layer.

8.2 Superior rectal vein

The unilateral superior rectal vein (SRV) drains the upper two-thirds of the rectum and the upper anal. The SRV eventually drains into the portal system via the inferior mesenteric vein. The superior rectal vein forms from the rectal plexus. The SRV runs along the upper mesorectum and the root of the sigmoid mesocolon. The SRV runs to the left of the SRA [26]. The SRV continues as the inferior mesenteric vein at the pelvic brim once the SRV crosses the left common iliac vessels. The pelvic brim is also the site where the abdominal ureter becomes the pelvic ureter. This close relationship is clinically significant because procedures involving the ligation or manipulation of the SRV, may pose a risk of inadvertent injury to the ureter.

8.3 Middle and inferior rectal veins

The lower third of the rectum and lower anal canal are drained by the middle and inferior rectal veins which enter the systemic venous circulation via the internal iliac veins. The venous drainage of the rectum provides several areas of hematogenous metastasis of cancer. For example, although rare, tumors in the lower rectum and anal canal can first metastasize to the lungs via systemic circulation without the involvement of hepatic metastases [44, 46]. In addition, the connection between systemic veins and the portal venous system provides a site for development of varicosities due to portal hypertension secondary to advanced liver disease.

9. Innervation of the rectum and anal canal

The rectum, the upper anal canal, along with the rest of the hindgut receives autonomic innervation.

9.1 Visceral afferents

The visceral afferent pathway for most of the hindgut corresponds to the levels of the sympathetic motor division. While most of the hindgut afferents follow the sympathetic pathway, the rectum's location below the peritoneal reflection (i.e., pelvic pain line), means that majority of its visceral afferents may travel via parasympathetic routes typically associated with pelvic viscera below the pelvic pain line. However, although minor, the upper aspect of the rectum which straddles the pelvic pain line, may have its visceral afferents follow the levels of sympathetic motor division. This may account for the blended sensory input seen in rectal distension and pain, where both noxious and innocuous stimuli are processed across different spinal levels [47, 48]. The convergence of these afferents within the spinal cord may explain the broad and poorly localized nature of rectal pain, as well as its tendency to mimic somatic or pelvic pathologies. Thus, afferent signals from the hindgut are received by afferent neurons from L1–L3 (via lumbar splanchnic nerves) and S2–S4 (via pelvic splanchnic nerves) dorsal root ganglia (**Figure 9**) [47, 48].

Visceral afferents in the rectum convey the sensation of rectal filling and are involved in reflex propulsive activity - a coordinated effort between the rectum, relaxation of pelvic floor, and anal sphincter complex that pushes feces through the rectum to the anal canal, into the external environment [26]. Feng and Guo [49] suggested

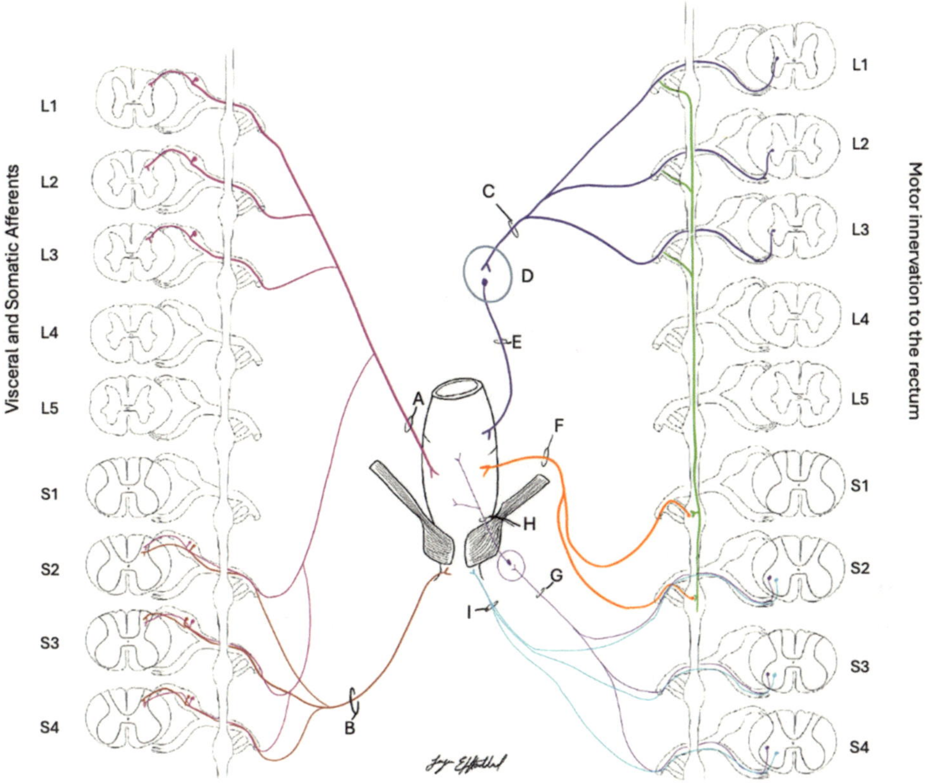

Figure 9.
Innervation of the rectum and the anal canal. On the left-hand side is a schematic representation of visceral and somatic afferent innervation. (A) represents visceral afferents from L1–L3 (via lumbar splanchnic nerves) and S2–S4 (via pelvic splanchnic nerves), which convey pain and distension from the rectum to their respective dorsal root ganglia. (B) represents somatic afferent fibers of the pudendal nerve (S2–S4), which transmit fine touch, pain, and temperature from the perianal skin and anal canal below the pectinate line. On the right-hand side is a schematic representation of the motor innervation to the rectum and anal canal. (C) represents preganglionic sympathetic fibers from L1–L3 spinal cord levels projecting via lumbar splanchnic nerves to the (D) inferior mesenteric ganglion, where they synapse. (E) shows the postganglionic sympathetic fibers that travel via the inferior hypogastric plexus to the rectal wall. Preganglionic fibers may also descend through the sympathetic chain to the sacral levels and exit via (F) sacral splanchnic nerves, which also contribute postganglionic fibers to the superior and inferior hypogastric plexuses. (G) and (H) represent the preganglionic and postganglionic parasympathetic fibers, respectively, arising from the pelvic splanchnic nerves (S2–S4), which synapse in ganglia near or within the target organ. (I) represents the somatic motor fibers of the pudendal nerve (S2–S4) that innervate the external anal sphincter and perianal muscles, facilitating voluntary control. Note: Both afferent and efferent innervation to the rectum is bilateral. Illustration by Joyce El-Haddad.

that the lumbar splanchnic nerves predominantly carry high-threshold nociceptive signals, likely involved in detecting significant mechanical stress (e.g., distension) in the rectum and adjacent areas. They also suggested that the sacral nerves, in contrast, encode both nociceptive and innocuous sensations, which can contribute to a more complex pain presentation [48]. The diffuse nature of visceral and referred pain makes it challenging to pinpoint its exact source without additional diagnostic methods. Furthermore, the complex referral pattern of pain from the rectum (proctalgia fugax) and the overlap with innervation of adjacent structures in the pelvis might mimic conditions like lower back pain, pelvic pain syndromes, gynecological conditions, and/or biopsychosocial factors and should be considered accordingly.

9.2 Sympathetic motor innervation

The sympathetic preganglionic motor portion is conveyed from the lumbar splanchnic nerves (L1-L2/3) via the sacral splanchnic nerves (S1-S2). The cell bodies of the preganglionic sympathetic motor neurons originate from the intermediolateral columns L1-L2/3 and synapse in the inferior mesenteric plexuses. The preganglionic neurons also reach the sacral splanchnic nerves which then go onto to contributing to the superior (aka presacral nerve) and inferior hypogastric plexuses (**Figure 9**). The postganglionic neurons reach the rectal wall via neural networks that are intertwined along the corresponding arteries. The postganglionic sympathetic neurons from both sources release noradrenaline (norepinephrine) and thus, sympathetic innervation of the rectum results in inhibition of peristalsis by acting on the muscularis layer of the rectum [26].

9.3 Parasympathetic motor innervation

The hindgut receives parasympathetic motor innervation from the pelvic splanchnic nerves (S2-S4). The cell bodies of the preganglionic neurons originate from the lateral intermediate substance, found in S2, S3 and S4 segments of the spinal cord (i.e., the sacral parasympathetic nucleus). The preganglionic axons enter the inferior hypogastric plexus where they will either go directly to the rectum or ascend via the right and left hypogastric nerves to the superior hypogastric plexus to innervate some proximal segments of the hindgut or innervate adjacent pelvic organs (**Figure 9**). Parasympathetic stimulation via the release of acetylcholine causes colonic propulsion and the relaxation of the internal anal sphincter, both functions essential in defecation [26].

9.4 Somatic innervation of the anal canal

Of significance to pain perception and patient presentations of anorectal pathologies, is the change at the pectinate line in innervation from visceral afferent via superior rectal nerve (proximally) to somatic afferents via the pudendal (pelvic) nerve (distally) (**Figure 9**). The pudendal nerve also provides somatic motor innervation to the EAS.

10. Lymphatic drainage of the rectum and anal canal

The lymphatic drainage of the rectum and anal canal corresponds to the arterial supply. However, it should be noted that the lymphatic drainage of the rectum and anal canal is complex, not fully clear, and not fully agreed upon [44, 50, 51]. Population, anatomical variation, and imaging-based studies are likely to prove useful here.

The rectum and the upper anal canal (above pectinate line) eventually drains into the preaortic nodes (inferior mesenteric nodes) (**Figure 10**). The lower anal and EAS drains via the superficial inguinal nodes to the paraaortic nodes (via the common iliac nodes) (**Figure 9**). The lymphatic drainage of the rectum ultimately drains to cisterna chyli, and eventually to the thoracic duct.

Lymphatic drainage of the rectum and upper anal canal can be divided via two intertwined groups: intramural, intermediate, and extramural lymphatic groups.

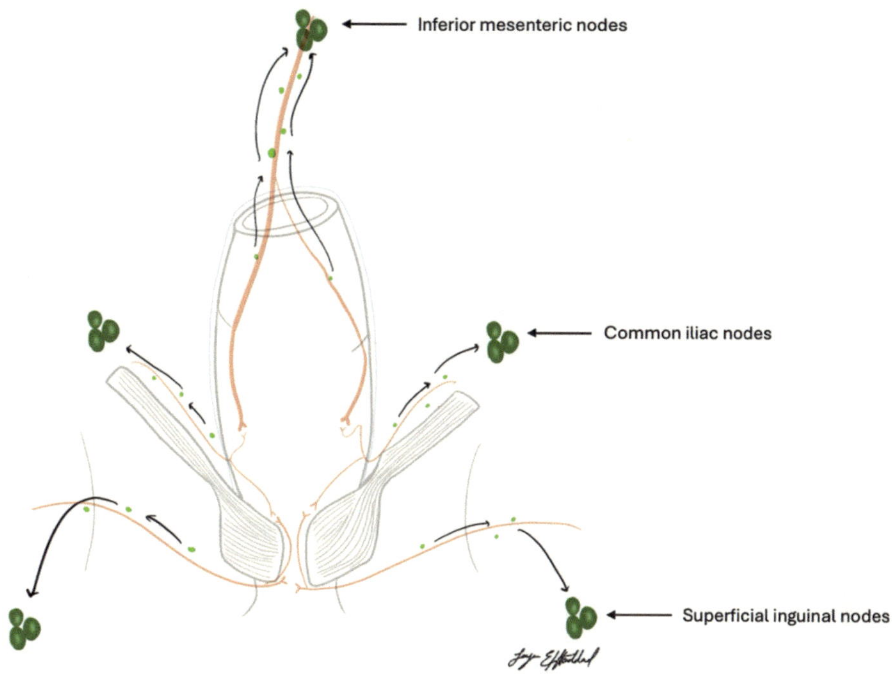

Figure 10.
Lymphatic drainage of the rectum. Illustration by Joyce El-Haddad.

The intramural nodes are found within the submucosal layer of the rectum and upper anal canal and drain into the extramural group. These nodes are significant as the extramural nodes are often the first site of metastatic spread of rectal cancers. The extramural group i.e., superior, middle, and inferior rectal nodes are located outside the rectal wall and correspond to the arteries [50].

In terms of the intermediate group – from the literature, it is not clear what layer of the rectal wall they are confined to [26, 50]. However, from the name it likely suggests that it would be the muscularis layer. Understanding the role of the intermediate nodes is important as tumors or other space occupying lesions can obstruct proximal pathways and redirect lymphatic drainage/spread laterally or distally. For example, some rectal cancers may spread laterally to internal iliac nodes, bypassing proximal pathways [50].

11. Conclusion

The anatomy of the rectum and the anal canal is often overlooked or shied away from. More often than not, the rectum and anal canal are reduced to pipes 'down there'. However, the importance of their normal function is quintessential to life. Only those with dysfunction of the rectum and/or anal canal, and those who treat such patients can truly appreciate the profound significance of the aforementioned sentiment.

The anatomy of the rectum and anal canal is complex and of significant clinical relevance, particularly in colorectal surgery, oncology, and functional disorders of the lower gastrointestinal tract. Understanding the intricate anatomical and histological features of the rectum and anal canal is crucial for accurate diagnosis, surgical precision, and effective treatment of conditions such as colorectal cancer, haemorrhoidal disease, and congenital anorectal malformations. Despite extensive research, there remains several gaps and controversies in the understanding of the anatomy of the rectum and anal canal. A significant challenge lies in the variability of anatomical structures, and the inconsistent identification of key landmarks such as the recto-sigmoid junction and anorectal junction, both of which influence and potentially complicate surgical planning and diagnostic accuracy. The precise role of the middle rectal artery in the lateral spread of rectal cancer is also still debated, and variations in lymphatic drainage patterns add to the complexity, with differing interpretations of how tumor cells seed and spread through these networks.

Moreover, the terminology surrounding conditions like hemorrhoids and anal cushions can be misleading, often conflating normal anatomical features with pathological states. Further, the mesorectal fascia's role in rectal cancer surgery, particularly in total mesorectal excision, remains an area of ongoing investigation. These unresolved anatomical questions highlight the need for further research and refined imaging techniques to better clarify these structures and their clinical significance. Future research, including imaging-based and body donor-based studies, may help clarify these ambiguities and contribute to improved clinical outcomes.

Author details

Joyce El-Haddad
Department of Anatomy, School of Biomedical Sciences, Medicine and Health, The University of New South Wales, Sydney, Australia

*Address all correspondence to: j.el-haddad@unsw.edu.au

References

[1] Nakashima J, Zulfiqar H. Embryology, rectum and anal canal. In: StatPearls. Treasure Island (FL): StatPearls Publishing; 2023. p. 2025

[2] Arthur R. You Will Die: The Burden of Modern Taboos. Port Townsend (WA): Feral House; 2012

[3] Lee JM, Kim NK. Essential anatomy of the anorectum for colorectal surgeons focused on the gross anatomy and histologic findings. Annals of Coloproctology. 2018;**34**(2):59-71. DOI: 10.3393/ac.2017.12.15. Epub 2018 Apr 30

[4] Regadas FS, Murad-Regadas SM, Lima DM, Silva FR, Barreto RG, Souza MH, et al. Anal canal anatomy showed by three-dimensional anorectal ultrasonography. Surgical Endoscopy. 2007;**21**(12):2207-2211. DOI: 10.1007/s00464-007-9339-0. Epub 2007 May 4

[5] Moskowitz DA, Rahman M, Li DH. Exploring anal self-examination as a screening tool for women at risk for anal cancer: Awareness, interest, and barriers to behavioral uptake. Cancer Causes and Control. 2019;**30**:559-568. DOI: 10.1007/s10552-019-01175-1

[6] Hiller DJ, Chadi SA, Rosen L, Wexner SD. Consequences of increasing complexity in anorectal surgery performed at an academic center. Diseases of the Colon and Rectum. 2019;**62**(3):343-344

[7] Burns EM, Quyn A, Lexicon Collaboration of UKPEN and the ACPGBI Advanced Cancer Subcommittee, Al Kadhi O, Angelopoulos G, Armitage J, et al. The 'pelvic exenteration lexicon': Creating a common language for complex pelvic cancer surgery. Colorectal Disease. 2023;**25**(5):888-899

[8] Liss DT, Baker DW. Understanding current racial/ethnic disparities in colorectal cancer screening in the United States: The contribution of socioeconomic status and access to care. American Journal of Preventive Medicine. 2014;**46**(3):228-236

[9] Netter FH, Cochard LR. Netter's Atlas of Human Embryology. Teterboro, NJ: Icon Learning Systems; 2002

[10] Sivakumar S, Thirunavukarasu K, Veerappan M. Anorectal embryology and anatomical structure. Journal of Basic and Clinical Reproductive Sciences. 2024;**13**(1):Article 12101

[11] Mills SE. Histology for Pathologists. 4th ed. Philadelphia (PA): Lippincott Williams and Wilkins; 2012

[12] Bennet SM, Polster A, Törnblom H, Isaksson S, Capronnier S, Tessier A, et al. Global cytokine profiles and association with clinical characteristics in patients with irritable bowel syndrome. The American Journal of Gastroenterology. 2016;**111**(8):1165-1176

[13] Bogveradze N, Snaebjornsson P, Grotenhuis BA, van Triest B, Lahaye MJ, Maas M, et al. MRI anatomy of the rectum: Key concepts important for rectal cancer staging and treatment planning. Insights Into Imaging. 2023;**14**(1):13

[14] Nakadoi K, Oka S, Tanaka S, Hayashi N, Terasaki M, Arihiro K, et al. Condition of muscularis mucosae is a risk factor for lymph node metastasis in T1 colorectal carcinoma. Surgical Endoscopy. 2014;**28**:1269-1276

[15] Brennan PA, Standring S, Wiseman S. Gray's Surgical Anatomy

[E-Book]. Edinburgh (UK): Elsevier Health Sciences; 2019

[16] Cali RL, Blatchford GJ, Perry RE. Normal variation in anorectal manometry. Diseases of the Colon and Rectum. 1992;**35**:1161-1164

[17] Shafik A, Shafik IA, el-Sibai O. Physioanatomical relationship of the external anal sphincter to the bulbocavernosus muscle in the female. International Urogynecology Journal and Pelvic Floor Dysfunction. 2007;**18**:851-856

[18] Mitchison M, Novelli MR. Inflammatory disorders of the anal region. In: Shepherd NA, Warren BF, Novelli MR, editors. Morson and Dawson's Gastrointestinal Pathology. 6th ed. Hoboken (NJ): Wiley-Blackwell; 2024. pp. 1009-1016

[19] Ceylan C. Perianal region malignancies. International Journal of Health Sciences. 2023;**22**:222-230

[20] Fundarò S, Spallanzani A, Ricchi E, Carriero A, Perrone S, Giusti G, et al. Squamous-cell carcinoma developing within anal lichen planus: Report of a case. Diseases of the Colon and Rectum. 1998;**41**:111-114

[21] Beck DE. Handbook of Colorectal Surgery. In: Beck DE, editor. New York, NY: Marcel Dekker; 14 May 2003

[22] Stelzner F. The corpus cavernosum recti. Diseases of the Colon and Rectum. 1964;7:398-399. DOI: 10.1007/BF02616852

[23] Heaton ND, Davenport M, Howard ER. Symptomatic hemorrhoids and anorectal varices in children with portal hypertension. Journal of Pediatric Surgery. 1992;**27**(7):833-835

[24] Misra SP, Misra V, Dwivedi M. Effect of esophageal variceal band ligation on hemorrhoids, anorectal varices, and portal hypertensive colopathy. Endoscopy. 2002;**34**(03):195-198

[25] Al Khalloufi K, Laiyemo AO. Management of rectal varices in portal hypertension. World Journal of Hepatology. 2015;7(30):2992-2998

[26] Standring S, Ellis H, Healy J, Johnson D, Williams A, Collins P, et al. Gray's anatomy: The anatomical basis of clinical practice. American Journal of Neuroradiology. 2005;**26**(10):2703

[27] Andromanakos N, Filippou D, Karandreas N, Kostakis A. Puborectalis muscle and external anal sphincter: A functional unit? The Turkish Journal of Gastroenterology. 2020;**31**(4):342

[28] Abcarian H, Barrett JA. Complications of surgery for trauma to colon and rectum. In: Ferrari ET, Ray JE, Gathright JB Jr, editors. Complications in Colon and Rectal Surgery. Philadelphia: WB Saunders; 1985. pp. 143-155

[29] Madoff RD, Fleshman JW, Clinical Practice Committee, American Gastroenterological Association. American Gastroenterological Association technical review on the diagnosis and treatment of hemorrhoids. Gastroenterology. 2004;**126**(5):1463-1473

[30] Liguori P, Reginelli A, Sparano A, Ruggiero G, Pinto A. Pneumoretroperitoneum associated with "dirty mass": An unusual case of rectal perforation. Radiology Case Reports. 2016;**2**(1):22

[31] Hazen SJA, Sluckin TC, Horsthuis K, Lambregts DMJ, Beets-Tan RG, Tanis PJ, et al. An updated evaluation of the implementation of the sigmoid take-off landmark 1 year after the official

introduction in the Netherlands. Techniques in Coloproctology. 2023;**27**(12):1243-1250

[32] D'Souza N, Lord A, Shaw A, Patel A, Balyasnikova S, Tudyka V, et al. The sigmoid take-off: An anatomical imaging definition of the rectum validated on specimen analysis. European Journal of Surgical Oncology. 2020;**46**(9):1668-1672

[33] Massalou D, Moszkowicz D, Mariage D, Baqué P, Camuzard O, Bronsard N. Is it possible to give a single definition of the rectosigmoid junction? Surgical and Radiologic Anatomy. 2018;**40**:431-438

[34] Sobin LH, Gospodarowicz MK, Wittekind C. TNM Classification of Malignant Tumours. 7th ed. Oxford (UK): Wiley-Blackwell; 2011

[35] Rubesin SE, Levine MS, Laufer I, Herlinger H. Double-contrast barium enema examination technique. Radiology. 2000;**215**(3):642-650

[36] Yang E, Palefsky JM. Diseases of the anus. In: Crum CP, Nucci MR, Lee KR, editors. Diagnostic Gynecologic and Obstetric Pathology. 3rd ed. Amsterdam (Netherlands): Elsevier; 2018. pp. 224-257

[37] Sands DR, Mahmoud NN. Anal cancer. In: Steele SR, Hull TL, Hyman N, Maykel JA, Read TE, Whitlow CB, editors. The ASCRS Textbook of Colon and Rectal Surgery. 4th ed. Cham (Switzerland): Springer; 2022. pp. 263-278

[38] Wang FG, Jiang Y, Liu C, Qi H. Comparison between endoscopic submucosal dissection and transanal endoscopic microsurgery in early rectal neuroendocrine tumor patients: A meta-analysis. Journal of Investigative Surgery. 2023;**36**(1):2278191

[39] Beddy D, Stocchi L, Pemberton JH. Anatomy and physiology of the rectum and anus including applied anatomy. In: Yamada T, editor. Shackelford's Surgery of the Alimentary Tract. 7th ed. Philadelphia (PA): WB Saunders; 2013. pp. 1703-1727

[40] Zhai LD, Liu J, Li YS, Yuan W, He L. Denonvilliers' fascia in women and its relationship with the fascia propria of the rectum examined by successive slices of celloidin-embedded pelvic viscera. Diseases of the Colon and Rectum. 2009;**52**(9):1564-1571

[41] Ayoub SF. Arterial supply to the human rectum. Acta Anatomica (Basel). 1978;**100**(3):317-327

[42] Heinze T, Fletcher J, Miskovic D, Stelzner S, Bayer A, Wedel T. The middle rectal artery: Revisited anatomy and surgical implications of a neglected blood vessel. Diseases of the Colon and Rectum. 2023;**66**(3):477-485

[43] Nano M, Marchisio F, Ferronato M, et al. Vascular anatomy of the rectal stump after total mesorectal excision. Diseases of the Colon and Rectum. 2006;**49**:1897-1904

[44] Sakorafas GH, Zouros E, Peros G. Applied vascular anatomy of the colon and rectum: Clinical implications for the surgical oncologist. Surgical Oncology. 2006;**15**(4):243-255

[45] Klosterhalfen B, Vogel P, Rixen H, Mittermayer C. Topography of the inferior rectal artery: A possible cause of chronic, primary anal fissure. Diseases of the Colon and Rectum. 1989;**32**(1):43-52

[46] Riihimäki M, Hemminki A, Sundquist J, et al. Patterns of metastasis in colon and rectal cancer. Scientific Reports. 2016;**6**:29765

[47] Song XY, Chen BN, Zagorodnyuk VP, et al. Identification of medium/high threshold extrinsic mechanosensitive afferent nerves to the gastrointestinal tract. Gastroenterology. 2009;**137**:274-284

[48] Feng B, Pierce DM. The biomechanics of distal colon and rectum and its relevance to visceral pain. In: Gebhart GF, Bielefeldt K, editors. Visceral Pain. Cham (Switzerland): Springer; 2023. pp. 81-103

[49] Feng B, Guo T. Visceral pain from colon and rectum: The mechanotransduction and biomechanics. Journal of Neural Transmission. 2020;**127**(4):415-429

[50] Bell S, Sasaki J, Sinclair G, Chapuis PH, Bokey EL. Understanding the anatomy of lymphatic drainage and the use of blue-dye mapping to determine the extent of lymphadenectomy in rectal cancer surgery: Unresolved issues. Colorectal Disease. 2009;**11**(5):443-449

[51] Budamagunta V, Foster TC, Zhou D. Cellular senescence in lymphoid organs and immunosenescence. Aging (Albany NY). 2021;**13**(15):19920-19941

Chapter 11

Anorectal Emergencies

Luisa Berto and Marcos Marton

Abstract

Anorectal conditions, mostly benign, can cause significant symptoms that impact patients' quality of life, often requiring urgent interventions. Early diagnosis is challenging due to severe pain and patient embarrassment, resulting in delays in medical care. The anorectal abscess, a common condition characterized by pus formation in the perianal region, may progress to fistulas and has a high recurrence rate, especially when inadequately drained. Necrotizing fasciitis, a rare and highly fatal infection, demands immediate treatment with surgical debridement and antibiotics. Complicated hemorrhoids, frequently associated with factors such as obesity and chronic constipation, may require surgical treatment, including hemorrhoidectomy or rubber band ligation. Anorectal varices, related to portal hypertension, pose a risk of severe bleeding and require hemodynamic stabilization followed by sclerotherapy, embolization, or surgery. Rectal prolapse, common in women—typically due to pelvic floor weakness—can progress to severe complications, such as strangulated prolapse, necessitating emergency surgery. Treatment may involve perineal or abdominal approaches, with options like laparoscopic-assisted sigmoid resection, which reduces recurrence rates. In complicated cases, antimicrobial therapy is indicated. Anorectal foreign bodies, more prevalent in adult men and often linked to erotic stimulation or psychiatric disorders, require prompt diagnosis and removal, frequently through minimally invasive methods. In cases of perforation, emergency surgery is mandatory. Lastly, anal fissures, usually caused by constipation or local trauma, may initially be managed with conservative measures. Surgery, such as lateral internal sphincterotomy, is reserved for refractory chronic fissures, demonstrating high cure rates and low complication rates. The management of these conditions should be individualized, taking into account symptom severity and each patient's clinical profile.

Keywords: anorectal, hemorrhoids, fissure, fistula, abscess

1. Introduction

Most anorectal conditions are benign; however, many of them provoke uncomfortable symptoms that affect patients' quality of life. They may require urgent treatment and can often be managed clinically or resolved in the emergency department. Accurate diagnosis in the early stages is frequently challenging, as severe pain can hinder a complete and thorough physical examination. Additionally, the embarrassment associated with the affected area leads many patients to postpone seeking medical attention. Treating such conditions based on the best evidence can reduce symptom duration and the number of complications resulting from overly invasive procedures.

2. Anorectal abscess

An anorectal abscess is a common condition defined as a localized collection of pus, either subcutaneously or submucosally, in the area surrounding the anus. Its origin is cryptoglandular, resulting from an infectious process caused by the obstruction of the crypt opening of one or more anorectal glands, leading to the accumulation of septic material within. Other possible causes include inflammatory bowel diseases, infections, trauma, and neoplasms, although they represent only a small fraction of cases.

The condition is more frequent in males, with a higher incidence between the ages of 20 and 40, and is often associated with the development of anorectal fistulas. According to Skovgaards [1], the incidence of fistula formation after an anorectal abscess is approximately 15.5% in idiopathic cases but can be as high as 41.6% in patients with inflammatory bowel disease, with Crohn's disease being a significant risk factor. Another study reported a fistula formation rate of 33.7% following anal abscess drainage [2, 3].

Symptoms include perianal pain, edema, local warmth, and possibly the drainage of purulent secretion, as can be seen in **Figure 1**. When located in deeper tissues, pain may radiate to the buttocks, back, and abdomen. Additionally, the patient may present systemic signs, such as fever, tachycardia, and leukocytosis, potentially evolving into a septic condition. Additional examinations, such as complete blood count, inflammatory markers, and creatinine levels, are useful for evaluating the clinical picture and guiding appropriate management.

The differential diagnosis of necrotizing fasciitis, or even the evolution to this condition, should be considered in the decision-making process, as deep tissue involvement is possible.

Risk factors for the development of cryptoglandular anorectal abscess include recent smoking, obesity, and diabetes mellitus, particularly in individuals with inadequate glycemic control. Due to the high association between anorectal abscesses and diabetes, the World Society of Emergency Surgery recommends evaluating serum glucose and glycated hemoglobin levels in these patients to detect possible cases of undiagnosed diabetes mellitus.

Radiological studies are not necessary for the diagnosis of anorectal abscess, but they may be useful in atypical cases or when there is suspicion of complications, such as supralevator abscesses or perianal Crohn's disease. Imaging techniques such as magnetic resonance imaging (MRI) and anal endosonography have good accuracy, although the former has access limitations in emergency settings, and the latter depends on the operator's experience. Computed tomography (CT) offers advantages in terms of speed and availability, but its accuracy is limited, especially in immunocompromised patients. Transperineal ultrasound is gaining prominence as a diagnostic tool in emergencies. The choice of the appropriate examination should consider the patient's history, clinical setting, and availability of resources (**Table 1**).

The treatment of choice for anorectal abscesses remains surgical drainage. The incision should be made as close as possible to the anal verge to minimize the length of a potential fistula while ensuring effective drainage and reducing the risk of sphincter

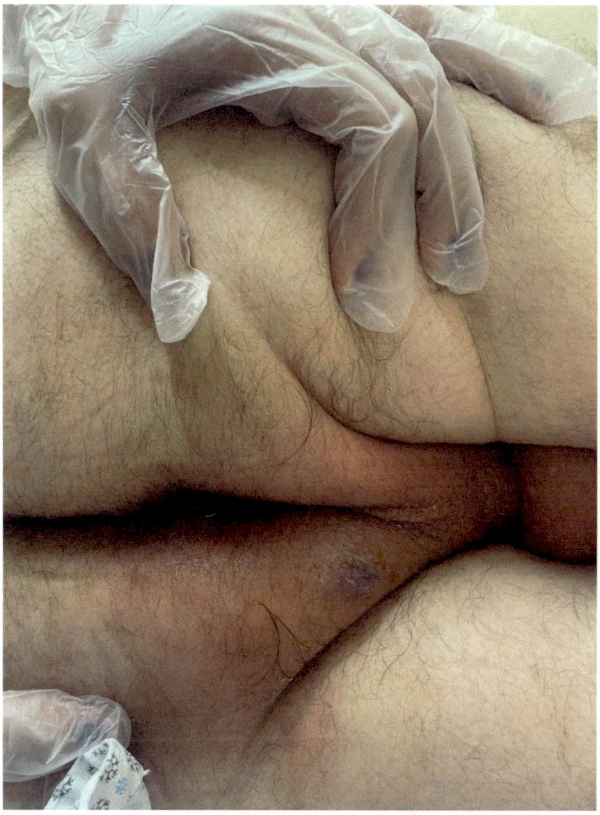

Figure 1.
Anorectal Abscess. Inflammatory signs associated with a necrotic point with fluctuance.

Type of Procedure	Technique/Procedure
Perineal Techniques	Anal circumference (Thiersch procedure)
	Mucosal sleeve resection (Delorme procedure)
	Perineal proctosigmoidectomy (Altemeier procedure)
Abdominal Procedures	Rectopexy by suture
	Mesh rectopexy: Rectopexy with posterior fixation and anterior mesh sling (Ripstein procedure)
	Rectopexy with posterior fixation and posterior mesh sling (Wells procedure)
	Rectopexy with ventral fixation and double anterolateral mesh sling and modified ventral sling (Orr-Loygue procedure)
	Resection rectopexy with or without mesh

Table 1.
Summary of key diagnostic tests, their benefits, and limitations.

injury. It is important to note that recurrence rates after drainage are significant, reaching up to 44%. Factors such as inadequate drainage, loculated abscesses, horseshoe abscesses, and delayed incision after symptom onset are associated with a higher risk of recurrence [4, 5].

The timing of surgery depends on the patient's clinical condition and comorbidities. Emergency drainage is required in cases of sepsis, immunosuppression, diabetes mellitus, or diffuse cellulitis. If these factors are absent, surgical drainage should ideally be performed within 24 hours.

Drainage can be performed in an outpatient setting under local anesthesia, particularly for perianal and small ischiorectal abscesses. Larger abscesses, septic patients, or those on anticoagulation should undergo drainage in the operating room for better infection control. The drainage technique varies by location: perianal and ischiorectal abscesses are drained near the anus, while intersphincteric abscesses require drainage into the rectal lumen. Supralevator abscesses may be drained transrectally or externally, depending on their origin. For horseshoe abscesses, deep postanal space drainage with seton placement is necessary.

In patients with anorectal abscess and an obvious fistula, fistulotomy during abscess drainage is recommended only for low fistulas not involving the sphincter muscle (e.g., subcutaneous fistulas). If the fistula involves any sphincter muscle, a loose draining seton should be placed. However, in patients without a visible fistula, probing should be avoided to prevent iatrogenic complications [4, 6].

Post-drainage antibiotics are indicated in cases of sepsis, surrounding tissue infection, or immunocompromised. Pus cultures should be obtained in high-risk patients or those predisposed to multidrug-resistant infections. A meta-analysis suggested that post-drainage antibiotics may reduce fistula formation, though evidence quality is limited. Additionally, the American Heart Association guidelines recommend antibiotic prophylaxis for patients with prosthetic valves, prior bacterial endocarditis, congenital heart disease, or cardiac transplant recipients with valvular pathology [7].

2.1 Take-home messages

- Anorectal abscess is an infection characterized by pus accumulation around the anus.
- Symptoms include pain, swelling, and possible purulent drainage.
- Risk factors include smoking, obesity, and diabetes.
- Treatment involves surgical drainage, preferably near the anal verge.
- Antibiotics may be required post-drainage to prevent complications.

3. Necrotizing fasciitis: Fournier's gangrene

According to the guidelines from the Association of Coloproctology of Great Britain and Ireland (ACPGBI), necrotizing fasciitis is a rare, rapidly progressive necrotizing infection with a high mortality rate (7–16%), particularly if treatment is delayed [6]. It primarily affects the fascia and subcutaneous tissues of the genital or perineal region and can lead to severe complications such as septic shock and multiorgan failure. Men are predominantly affected (42:1 ratio compared to women), with a mean age of 51 years. Comorbidities such as diabetes, obesity, and conditions impairing cellular immunity (e.g., alcoholism, HIV) increase the risk, with mortality rates as high as 88% in these groups [6].

The infection typically begins at a site of skin breakdown in the perineum, allowing commensal bacteria (e.g., *Streptococcus*, *Staphylococcus*, *Escherichia coli*) to invade, triggering intense inflammation and local vascular thrombosis. This leads to tissue ischemia, necrosis, and anaerobic bacterial proliferation. Clinically, patients present with severe pain, swelling, erythema, purulent discharge, and, in advanced cases, subcutaneous emphysema (crepitus). Systemic manifestations (e.g., fever, tachycardia) are common.

Diagnosis is primarily clinical, supported by imaging (ultrasound, CT, MRI). Bedside ultrasound is useful for assessing infection extent in unstable patients, while contrast-enhanced CT helps map disease spread and identify underlying causes. MRI, though highly sensitive for soft tissue evaluation, is limited by acquisition time. Risk stratification tools such as the LRINEC (Laboratory Risk Indicator for Necrotizing Fasciitis) and FGSI (Fournier Gangrene Severity Index) aid in predicting mortality and guiding treatment [5].

Emergent surgical debridement is the cornerstone of treatment. All necrotic tissue must be excised; radical surgery may suffice in some cases. Severe cases may require orchiectomy, colostomy, or suprapubic cystostomy, with decisions made after 48 hours of observation to assess inflammation and sphincter integrity. Broad-spectrum antibiotics covering Gram-positive, Gram-negative, aerobic, and anaerobic organisms (including MRSA) should be initiated promptly, with adjustments based on microbiological cultures [8].

Negative-pressure wound therapy promotes exudate removal, vascularization, and granulation tissue formation but may be challenging in perianal regions due to frequent dressing changes.

Hyperbaric oxygen therapy may be considered, particularly for Clostridium infections, though evidence of benefit remains unclear [9].

3.1 Take-home messages

- Necrotizing fasciitis is a life-threatening infection with high mortality, primarily affecting men with comorbidities.

- It is a polymicrobial infection causing rapid tissue necrosis.

- Diagnosis is clinical, supported by imaging and risk stratification scores (e.g., LRINEC).

- Treatment requires emergency surgical debridement and broad-spectrum antibiotics.

- Negative pressure wound therapy (NPWT) and hyperbaric oxygen (HBO) may serve as adjunctive therapies.

4. Complicated hemorrhoids

Hemorrhoidal plexuses are vascular structures that become symptomatic when enlarged, causing pain and discomfort in the anal and perianal regions. The condition is highly prevalent, with risk factors including obesity, low-fiber diets, excessive straining, chronic constipation, and portal hypertension. The highest incidence occurs in individuals aged 45–65 years [10].

Prolonged prolapse and excessive straining can lead to venous stasis and endothelial damage, resulting in thrombosis—especially in external hemorrhoids. This causes swelling and severe pain, a hallmark of acute thrombosed hemorrhoids (see **Figures 2** and **3** for examples with necrosis and significant edema). However, anorectal masses may mimic other conditions (e.g., abscesses, fissures), complicating diagnosis. Complicated hemorrhoids are also associated with inflammatory bowel disease (IBD).

A thorough history, physical exam, and anoscopy are essential for diagnosis. Anoscopy effectively identifies hemorrhoidal bleeding, but severe pain from thrombosis or strangulation may require sedation. Importantly, bleeding should not be attributed solely to hemorrhoids without ruling out colorectal cancer or IBD. High-risk patients should undergo colonoscopy for further evaluation [4, 11].

Several pharmacological approaches have been investigated for the treatment of complicated hemorrhoids. Fiber-based laxatives and venotonic agents are commonly employed, demonstrating favorable outcomes in reducing symptoms such as bleeding and pruritus, although their effect on postoperative pain remains limited.

Muscle relaxants, including topical nitrates and calcium channel blockers, have shown efficacy in the management of thrombosed hemorrhoids, with topical nifedipine being particularly effective. However, challenges persist due to side effects (e.g., headache associated with nitrate use) and limited evidence regarding antithrombotic therapies.

Prolonged use of topical steroid creams is not recommended due to the risk of anal and perianal mucosal thinning, which may lead to tissue injury. Furthermore,

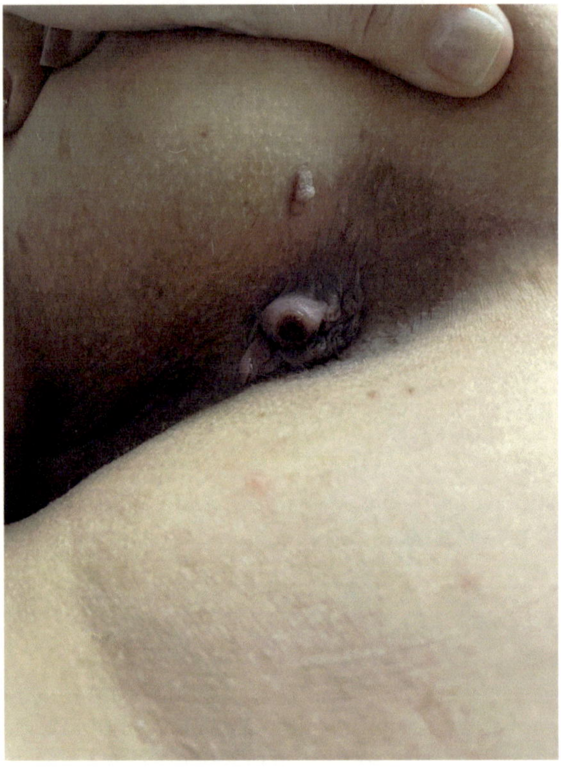

Figure 2.
Thrombosed external hemorrhoid. A necrotic point is observed at the center.

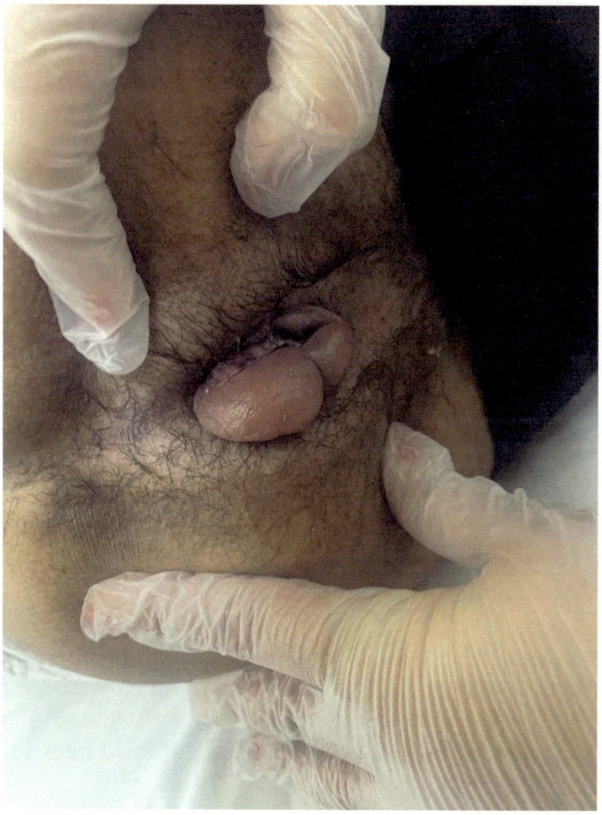

Figure 3.
Thrombosed internal hemorrhoid causing significant edema in the anoderm.

insufficient evidence exists to support the use of nonsteroidal anti-inflammatory drugs (NSAIDs), corticosteroids, or local anesthetics in the treatment of complicated hemorrhoids (**Table 2**) [4, 10].

The degree of hemorrhoids is a determining factor in deciding the need for and type of surgical intervention. However, the European Society of Coloproctology recommends that surgical treatment should be based on patient preferences, availability of therapeutic options, and suitability of procedures for each specific case. In patients

Exam	Benefits	Limitations
Magnetic Resonance Imaging	High accuracy	Limited access in emergencies
Anal Endosonography	High precision in experienced hands	Depends on the operator's experience
Computed Tomography	Fast and widely available	Limited accuracy, especially in immunocompromised patients
Transperineal Ultrasound	Promising for emergency diagnosis	Still being consolidated as a main tool

Table 2.
Summary of main pharmacological treatments for hemorrhoids.

whose conservative treatments have not resulted in satisfactory symptom improvement, other approaches should be considered. As some treatments are less invasive, have lower complication rates, and are more cost-effective, physicians should initially consider outpatient procedures such as rubber band ligation (RBL), sclerotherapy (SCL), or infrared coagulation (IRC) [12, 13].

Patients with circular prolapse grade III, or especially grade IV hemorrhoids, may require surgical interventions such as hemorrhoidectomy, stapled hemorrhoidopexy (SH), or Doppler-guided hemorrhoidal artery ligation with mucopexy (DG-HAL). However, rubber band ligation is acceptable for grade III prolapsed hemorrhoids, recognizing that in some cases, surgery will be necessary for patients whose symptoms are not relieved by these less invasive techniques, or for those with circular prolapse [13, 14].

Similarly, outpatient procedures may be indicated for patients with grade III and IV hemorrhoids when primary surgery is contraindicated or if the patient chooses not to undergo surgical intervention. The choice of outpatient procedure should be made jointly between physician and patient, taking into account patient preferences, technique availability, and clinical suitability for each case [13].

5. Surgical treatment

In cases where conservative treatment or outpatient procedures have not been effective—or in patients with grade III and IV hemorrhoids—surgical options may be indicated. Among these, the most notable are hemorrhoidectomy, stapled hemorrhoidopexy, and mucopexy, with or without Doppler-guided hemorrhoidal artery ligation.

According to European guidelines, for grade I and II hemorrhoids, rubber band ligation is considered the treatment of choice, as it yields significantly superior results compared to sclerotherapy or infrared coagulation, including a lower recurrence rate. Infrared coagulation, in turn, may be used as a first-line option for grade I hemorrhoids with bleeding, as it causes less pain and fewer complications.

For grade III and IV hemorrhoids, hemorrhoidectomy remains the most effective approach. Although stapled hemorrhoidopexy is an alternative, its efficacy tends to be lower, especially in more advanced cases. Doppler-guided hemorrhoidal artery ligation combined with mucopexy may be considered in patients with grade II and III hemorrhoids [12–14].

5.1 Take-home messages

- Risk factors: Obesity and constipation increase the risk of hemorrhoids.
- Diagnosis: Physical examination and anoscopy are essential.
- Pharmacological treatment: Laxatives and muscle relaxants may help but have side effects.
- Outpatient treatment: Rubber band ligation is effective for grade I and II hemorrhoids.
- Surgical treatment: Hemorrhoidectomy is required for grade III and IV hemorrhoids.

6. Anorectal variceal bleeding

Anorectal varices are submucosal collateral veins that form primarily in patients with portal hypertension, affecting about 89% of these individuals. Although bleeding from rectal varices is uncommon, it can be severe, occurring in a small percentage of the population, ranging between 0.05 and 5% of cases [4].

The initial evaluation of patients with hematochezia should follow the protocol for lower gastrointestinal bleeding. The severity of bleeding should be determined and risk stratified, with laboratory tests including complete blood count, electrolytes, and coagulation studies.

For diagnosis, investigation may begin with endoscopy. When inconclusive, endoscopic ultrasound may be useful, as it is more effective in detecting deep rectal varices, identifying 85% of cases, compared to 45% with conventional endoscopy [6].

Other modalities such as computed tomography may be employed, offering high sensitivity for detecting bleeding sources, with the advantage of being rapid and able to identify other potential causes of bleeding. Studies show that CT, in combination with early colonoscopy, improves detection of vascular lesions, providing significant additional diagnostic value.

Management of rectal variceal bleeding involves hemodynamic stabilization and identification of the bleeding source. In mild cases, intravenous fluid resuscitation, blood transfusion, and correction of coagulopathies are generally effective. In severe cases, tamponade devices such as the Sengstaken-Blakemore tube may be used to control bleeding until stabilization or transfer to a specialized center.

Treatment of rectal variceal bleeding aims to reduce portal pressure, using medications such as terlipressin, vasopressin, and somatostatin, which are effective for esophageal varices. Nonselective beta-blockers may be used for prevention but are contraindicated in hypotensive patients. Antifibrinolytic therapies, such as tranexamic acid, may be administered for persistent bleeding. Additionally, prophylactic antibiotics are recommended to prevent infections in cirrhotic patients with gastrointestinal bleeding.

Radiologic embolization, alone or combined with TIPS, controls rectal variceal bleeding and when combined with TIPS reduces rebleeding rates by decompressing the portal system. Balloon-occluded retrograde transvenous obliteration (BRTO) is a less invasive alternative. Another option is anterograde transvenous sclerotherapy, which provides good results. Surgery is considered only when interventional treatments fail.

Invasive surgery, such as suture ligation, inferior mesenteric vein occlusion, and portocaval shunt, is rare due to patients' clinical condition. Suture ligation is technically difficult and has high rebleeding rates, while stapled anopexy shows good results in refractory cases but is not feasible in severe bleeding. The optimal approach involves stepwise treatment, with endoscopic procedures and, in severe cases, TIPS or liver transplantation. Studies show that mortality is high in cirrhotic patients with anorectal variceal bleeding, primarily due to liver failure.

6.1 Take-home messages

- Etiology: Anorectal varices affect 89% of patients with portal hypertension

- Diagnosis: Endoscopy and Doppler ultrasonography to identify deep varices

- Initial management:
  - o Mild cases: Fluid resuscitation and blood transfusion
  - o Severe bleeding: Balloon tamponade (e.g., Sengstaken-Blakemore tube)
- Medical therapy: Nonselective beta-blockers (propranolol, nadolol) and vasoactive drugs (octreotide, terlipressin) for portal pressure reduction
  - o Interventional options:
  - o First-line: Embolization or TIPS (transjugular intrahepatic portosystemic shunt)
  - o Surgery: Rare, reserved for refractory cases

7. Complicated rectal prolapse

Rectal prolapse is a complex colorectal condition, known for its high recurrence rate after surgical intervention, with an annual incidence of 2.5 cases per 100,000 population. Its prevalence is notably higher in women, accounting for 80 to 90% of cases, which may be related to the pathophysiology of the disorder involving pelvic floor weakness. Factors such as multiple pregnancies and vaginal deliveries are additional factors that may exacerbate this weakness, increasing women's risk of developing the condition [4].

Incarcerated (strangulated) rectal prolapse refers to a condition where the full-thickness prolapsed rectum cannot be manually reduced. Unlike reducible prolapse, which can be manually repositioned, incarcerated prolapse remains outside its normal position, causing mucosal ischemia or even full-thickness intestinal wall ischemia, potentially leading to necrosis and perforation. This condition requires urgent surgical treatment [15, 16].

Diagnosis of rectal prolapse is typically made through detailed history, symptom assessment, and clinical examination. In practice, it is essential to differentiate this condition from prolapsed hemorrhoids: while rectal prolapse presents with concentric protrusion, prolapsed hemorrhoids are characterized by radial bulging and discrete prolapse of anal cushions.

The main symptoms include lower abdominal pain, constipation, and hematochezia. History and physical examination are usually sufficient for diagnosis, but depending on severity, additional tests such as complete blood count and inflammatory markers may be needed. In female patients, pregnancy must always be ruled out.

After assessing the patient's hemodynamic status, if clinical stability is confirmed, contrast-enhanced abdominopelvic computed tomography is recommended to investigate possible conditions associated with complicated rectal prolapse, such as acute intestinal obstruction, perforation signs and peritonitis, as well as prolapse of other pelvic organs. The exam is also crucial to rule out colorectal malignancy. CT findings may guide the choice between nonoperative treatment and surgery, as well as the optimal surgical approach (perineal vs. abdominal). It is important to emphasize that the decision to perform CT should be based on the patient's clinical condition and resource availability, without delaying immediate treatment of complicated rectal prolapse (**Figure 4**).

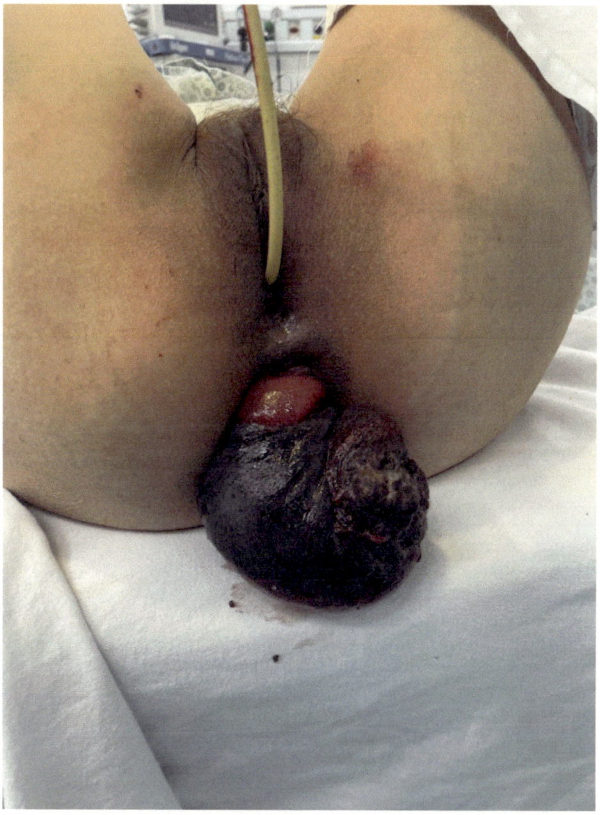

Figure 4.
Rectal prolapse with signs of ischemia.

For irreducible rectal prolapse without signs of ischemia, gentle manual reduction may be attempted with the patient in Trendelenburg position under intravenous sedation and analgesia, deferring surgery to an elective time. It is essential to attempt manual reduction of an incarcerated rectal prolapse to prevent complications such as strangulation and perforation. However, nonoperative management is not indicated in strangulated rectal prolapse with signs of gangrene, perforation, or in unstable patients.

Among nonoperative treatment techniques, the application of granulated sugar is notable, creating a hyperosmolar environment to reduce edema, though with low efficacy. Other options include hypertonic solutions of sugar or mannitol and hyaluronidase infiltration to reduce edema. Continuous elastic compression is also used to help drain fluid. Despite these approaches, the failure rate of nonoperative treatment is high, and surgery should be performed when manual reduction is unsuccessful to avoid serious complications.

The definitive approach for treatment of rectal prolapse is surgical, with various procedures described in the literature, each presenting its own advantages and disadvantages. When performed in an elective setting, repair may be done through the anus (perineal approach) or abdomen, depending on symptom severity, the patient's overall condition, and individual preferences. There is no proven superior technique, and approaches may be classified as perineal or abdominal according to the method used for correction (**Table 3**) [17].

Therapeutic Approach	Description	Effects	Considerations
Fiber-based laxatives	Used to improve bowel movements and reduce symptoms such as bleeding and itching.	Good reduction of symptoms like bleeding and itching.	Limited effect on post-operative pain.
Phlebotonics	Medications that enhance vein tone, commonly used to relieve symptoms.	Relief of symptoms such as bleeding and itching.	No significant effect on post-operative pain.
Muscle relaxants	Includes topical nitrates and calcium channel antagonists, such as topical nifedipine.	Effective in treating thrombosed hemorrhoids.	Side effects like headaches (nitrates) and lack of data on antithrombotic therapies.
Steroid creams	Used to reduce inflammation, but with prolonged use.	Reduction of inflammation.	Prolonged use is discouraged due to the risk of thinning of the anal and perianal mucosa, which may cause lesions.
Non-steroidal anti-inflammatory drugs (NSAIDs)	Not commonly recommended for treating complicated hemorrhoids.	No sufficient evidence of efficacy.	Not recommended for use in complicated hemorrhoids.
Cortisone	Corticosteroids used to reduce inflammation.	Reduction of inflammation.	Questionable efficacy and not recommended for prolonged use in complicated hemorrhoids.
Local anesthetics	Used for pain relief.	Temporary pain relief.	No sufficient evidence to support their use in the treatment of complicated hemorrhoids.

Table 3.
Main techniques associated with surgical correction of rectal prolapse.

A recently proposed approach has been the combined technique, which involves laparoscopic-assisted perineal sigmoid resection followed by coloanal anastomosis. Al-Ameen et al. described this technique in a case report, emphasizing the role of laparoscopy in the Altemeier procedure for strangulated prolapse. Laparoscopy allows detailed assessment of sigmoid length, facilitates proper colon mobilization, and ensures complete removal of redundant bowel. The authors concluded that this approach may reduce recurrence rates and the need for additional surgical interventions.

In cases of complicated rectal prolapse, the presence of strangulation or intestinal obstruction increases the risk of bacterial translocation, making empirical antimicrobial therapy recommended. For uncomplicated intra-abdominal infections where the source is definitively controlled, postoperative antibiotic therapy is unnecessary. In complicated intra-abdominal infections, a short course of antibiotics (3–5 days) is recommended after adequate source control. If signs of persistent peritonitis or systemic infection remain after 5–7 days of treatment, further investigation is warranted. Empirical antibiotic selection should consider the patient's clinical condition, risk of resistant pathogens, and local resistance patterns [14].

7.1 Take-home messages

- Epidemiology: Rectal prolapse predominantly affects women and has high postoperative recurrence rates

- Diagnosis: Clinical history, physical examination (including defecography), and CT imaging guide treatment planning
- Initial management: Manual reduction may be attempted first-line
- Definitive treatment: Surgical correction remains gold standard, with either perineal (Altemeier/Delorme) or abdominal (rectopexy) approaches
- Complications: Surgical site infections may require antibiotic therapy and wound management

8. Anorectal foreign bodies

The incidence of rectal foreign bodies (FB) varies by age and sex, with men peaking in their fifth decade and women in their second decade. The primary cause of rectal FB is anal erotic stimulation, followed by assault, accidents, ingestion of bones or foreign bodies, psychiatric disorders, drug trafficking, and attempts at self-treatment of fecal impaction in elderly patients. Many patients, due to embarrassment, attempt self-removal through digital or instrumental manipulation before seeking medical help. Retained FBs vary in size and material, being identified on imaging or, in some cases, palpated on digital rectal exam. The wide variety of objects leads to different clinical presentations related to varying degrees of damage to local rectal and distal colon tissues.

Reducing the time between object insertion and emergency department presentation is essential to prevent complications. The most common foreign bodies include sex toys, bottles, caps, jars, cans, drugs, balls, fruits, and vegetables.

Male predominance in retained anal foreign bodies is high, with a male-to-female ratio up to 37:1. They are very uncommon in children and typically result from assault or child abuse, which must be carefully and thoroughly investigated [4].

In up to 20% of cases, patients do not initially report retained foreign body as their chief complaint. Common complaints include rectal or abdominal pain, constipation or obstipation, bright red rectal bleeding, or incontinence.

Initial evaluation of patients with rectal foreign bodies should include detailed history and physical exam, focusing on signs of peritonitis, fever, tachycardia, and hypotension. Digital rectal exam, essential for determining object position and local injuries, should be performed cautiously, preferably after radiography to avoid injury to the surgeon. All findings (perianal lesions, anal sphincter status) should be documented, especially in suspected sexual assault cases. Laboratory tests are unnecessary except in perforation cases, when CBC, creatinine, inflammatory markers, and serum toxicology are useful.

Contrast-enhanced CT is typically the next diagnostic step, being essential for locating non-radiopaque objects, identifying perforation or abscess without intestinal involvement, and diagnosing bowel obstruction. This exam allows visualization of the foreign body and assessment of potential associated complications.

Management of retained rectal foreign bodies depends on the patient's clinical condition. In the presence of peritonitis or pneumoperitoneum, bedside extraction is contraindicated, and urgent surgical intervention is required after stabilization with fluids and antibiotics. If the patient is unstable, emergency laparotomy is mandatory. The use of anesthesia, such as pudendal nerve block or sedation, facilitates manual removal and improves visualization during physical examination [18].

The need for proctosigmoidoscopy after extraction is debated. Although expert opinions vary, many recommend it to identify possible injuries or retained fragments. Given the relative safety of the procedure, post-extraction endoscopy is suggested. For foreign bodies located distal to the rectum, techniques such as rigid or flexible sigmoidoscopy, polypectomy snares, and even fluoroscopy may be used for removal.

In cases involving drug-containing foreign bodies, such as in body packers, manipulation is contraindicated due to the high risk of overdose if the packaging ruptures.

In stable patients requiring surgery, a stepwise approach is recommended, beginning with laparoscopy to assess peritoneal contamination. If no perforation is found, laparoscopy-assisted transanal extraction with transmural pressure is preferred. Colostomy is reserved for cases where previous methods fail. If laparoscopy is not feasible, a minilaparotomy may be performed. If perforation is present, treatment depends on the extent of contamination and bowel wall conditions. Small, recent perforations may undergo primary repair if tissues are viable. The Hartmann procedure is indicated in cases of generalized peritonitis, particularly in critically ill patients or those with multiple comorbidities, serving as a safe option for emergency colectomy.

Regarding antibiotic use, there is still no clear consensus. Given the increasing risk of antimicrobial resistance, they should be avoided in patients without signs of infection or perforation. If perforation or septic complications occur, established guidelines for intra-abdominal infection management should be followed.

8.1 Take-home messages

- Epidemiology: Rectal foreign bodies predominantly affect adult male patients
- Clinical evaluation: Requires detailed history, digital rectal exam, and CT imaging for localization and complication assessment
- Emergent management: Immediate surgical intervention indicated for perforation, ischemia, or obstruction
- Stable cases: Transanal/endoscopic extraction preferred when feasible
- Antimicrobial therapy: Reserved for confirmed infection or perforation (broad-spectrum coverage recommended)

9. Acute anorectal fissure

Anal fissures are linear tears in the anal mucosa below the pectinate line, caused by trauma or other conditions. They may be acute (<4–6 weeks) or chronic (persisting longer), with 90% occurring in the posterior region. Contributing factors include constipation, straining, local trauma, and inflammatory bowel diseases. The primary pathogenic theory involves increased internal anal sphincter tone. Posterior anal canal vascular scarcity also favors fissure formation [4].

Anal fissure diagnosis is primarily clinical, based on history and complete physical exam. Patients typically report intense, prolonged anal pain, especially during/after defecation. Other symptoms include spasms and intermittent bleeding. When the internal sphincter tone is elevated, a digital rectal exam may be painful, requiring an exam under anesthesia to rule out associated conditions like abscesses or fistulas [11, 19].

When fissure diagnosis is unclear or physical exam inconclusive, especially in significant bleeding or high-risk colorectal cancer patients (>50 years), imaging may be needed. Techniques like endoanal ultrasound, endoscopy, CT, or MRI can confirm fissure presence or identify associated conditions [4].

Initial fissure treatment is predominantly conservative. Studies show ~50% of patients recover in 10–14 days with sitz baths, increased fiber intake, and topical agents. To prevent recurrence, a combination of dietary/lifestyle changes and medical treatment is recommended. The primary treatment goal is internal sphincter relaxation, pain relief, trauma minimization, and improved blood flow. Approaches include stool softeners, sphincter muscle relaxants, and agents like nitrates, calcium channel blockers, and botulinum toxin injection. Calcium channel blockers (nifedipine/diltiazem) show high cure rates and good cost-effectiveness [4, 11].

Effective pain control is essential in acute fissure treatment, reducing internal sphincter tone and promoting proper bowel habits to prevent defecation pain. Analgesics like topical lidocaine, paracetamol, ibuprofen, and perianal anesthetic infiltration are commonly used for severe pain relief.

Surgery is indicated only in the chronic phase after 6–8 weeks of failed medical treatment. Lateral internal sphincterotomy is the preferred technique, with high cure rates (>90%), lower recurrence, and greater patient satisfaction. Though open and closed approaches have similar outcomes, open sphincterotomy has been associated with more postoperative pain and delayed healing. Both techniques are more effective than fissurectomy or posterior sphincterotomy, with better results in terms of healing, pain, and fecal incontinence.

9.1 Take-home messages

- Etiology: Trauma, chronic constipation, and inflammatory bowel disease are predominant causes

- Diagnostic approach: Clinical examination (visual inspection + digital rectal exam) supplemented by imaging when complications suspected

- First-line management: Conservative treatment with fiber supplementation, stool softeners, and warm sitz baths

- Pain control: Topical analgesics (lidocaine 5% ointment) + oral NSAIDs for acute episodes

- Surgical indication: Lateral internal sphincterotomy demonstrates highest efficacy for chronic refractory cases

Author details

Luisa Berto[1] and Marcos Marton[2*]

1 Bauru State Hospital, Bauru, Brazil

2 University of São Paulo, Bauru, Brazil

*Address all correspondence to: marcos.marton@usp.br

References

[1] Skovgaards DM et al. Fistula development after anal abscess drainage—A multicentre retrospective cohort study. International Journal of Colorectal Disease. 2023;**39**(1):19-26

[2] Crook DL, Padfield O. A systematic review and meta-analysis of the use of packing in the management of perianal abscesses. Annals of the Royal College of Surgeons of England. 2025;**107**(1):29-34. DOI: 10.1308/rcsann.2023.0108. Epub 2024 Apr 2

[3] Sahnan K et al. Natural history of anorectal sepsis. British Journal of Surgery. 2017;**104**(13):1857-1865

[4] Tarasconi A et al. Anorectal emergencies: WSES-AAST guidelines. World Journal of Emergency Surgery. 2021;**16**(1):48

[5] Gaertner WB, Burgess PL, Davids JS, Lightner AL, Shogan BD, Sun MY, et al. Clinical practice guidelines for the Management of Anorectal Abscess, fistula-in-Ano, and rectovaginal fistula. Diseases of the Colon and Rectum. 2022;**65**(8):964-985. DOI: 10.1097/DCR.0000000000002473. Epub 2022 Jul 5

[6] Miller AS, Boyce K, Box B, Clarke MD, Duff SE, Foley NM, et al. The Association of Coloproctology of Great Britain and Ireland consensus guidelines in emergency colorectal surgery. Colorectal Disease. 2021;**23**(2):476-547. DOI: 10.1111/codi.15503

[7] Kata A, Abelson JS. Abscesso anorretal. Clinics in Colon and Rectal Surgery. 2023;**37**(6):368-375. DOI: 10.1055/s-0043-1777451

[8] Bowen D, Hughes T, Juliebø-Jones P, Somani B. Gangrena de Fournier: Uma revisão dos sistemas de pontuação preditiva e guia prático para o gerenciamento de pacientes. Therapeutic Advances in Infectious Disease. 2024;**11**:20499361241238521. DOI: 10.1177/20499361241238521

[9] Allaw F, Wehbe S, Kanj SS. Necrotizing fasciitis: An update on epidemiology, diagnostic methods, and treatment. Current Opinion in Infectious Diseases. 2024;**37**(2):105-111. DOI: 10.1097/QCO.0000000000000988. Epub 2023 Nov 30

[10] Zagriadskiĭ EA, Bogomazov AM, Golovko EB. Conservative treatment of Hemorrhoids: Results of an observational multicenter study. Advances in Therapy. 2018;**35**(11):1979-1992. DOI: 10.1007/s12325-018-0794-x. Epub 2018 Oct 1. Erratum in: Adv Ther. 2018;35(11):1993. DOI: 10.1007/s12325-018-0817-7

[11] Akinmoladun O, Oh W. Management of hemorrhoids and anal fissures. Surgical Clinics of North America. 2024;**104**(3):473-490. DOI: 10.1016/j.suc.2023.11.001

[12] van Tol RR, Kleijnen J, Watson AJM, Jongen J, Altomare DF, Qvist N, et al. Sociedade Europeia de ColoProctology: diretriz para a doença hemorroidária. Cor Dis. 2020;**22**(6):650-662. DOI: 10.1111/codi.14975

[13] Hawkins AT, Davis Bradley R, Bhama Anuradha R, Fang Sandy H, Dawes Aaron J, Feingold Daniel L, et al. Diretrizes de Prática Clínica da Sociedade Americana de Cirurgiões de Cólon e Desafio para o Gerenciamento de Hemorróidas. Doenças do Cólon e Reto. 2024;**67**(5):614-623. DOI: 10.1097/DCR.0000000000003276

[14] Samalavicius NE et al. Global treatment of haemorrhoids—A worldwide snapshot audit conducted by the International Society of University Colon and Rectal Surgeons. Colorectal Disease. 2024;**26**(10):1797-1804

[15] Emile SH, Wignakumar A, Horesh N, et al. Revisão sistemática da literatura e meta-análise do tratamento cirúrgico do prolapso retal completo em pacientes do sexo masculino. Techniques in Coloproctology. 2024;**28**:158. DOI: 10.1007/s10151-024-03039-6

[16] Fuschillo G, Selvaggi L, Cuellar-Gomez H, Pescatori M. Comparison between perineal and abdominal approaches for the surgical treatment of recurrent external rectal prolapse: A systematic review and meta-analysis. International Journal of Colorectal Disease. 2025;**40**(1):26. DOI: 10.1007/s00384-024-04771-z

[17] Mantzoros I, Brenta A, Bourtzinakou A-A, Kontaxi O, Gemousakakis G, Antoniou N, et al. Perineal rectosigmoidectomy (Altemeier's procedure) in the treatment of strangulated rectal prolapse: A case series and literature review. Journal of Personalized Medicine. 2024;**14**(11):1095. DOI: 10.3390/jpm14111095

[18] Tian J et al. Better out than in: A case series of retained rectal foreign bodies in a New York community hospital. International Surgery Journal. 2024;**11**(6):953-960

[19] Cirilo O et al. Emergências anorretais. JBMEDE - Jornal Brasileiro de Medicina de Emergência. 2024;**4**(3)

Chapter 12

Diagnostic Modalities in Anorectal Conditions

Hadeel Helmi, Atheer Alotaibi and Ayyob Alqarni

Abstract

The clinical picture of anorectal conditions has overlapping manifestations, with rectal bleeding, altered bowel motion, and anal pain or discomfort being the commonest complaints. Hence, diagnosis may be challenging. Furthermore, disorders of defecation are becoming increasingly common and have a significant effect on quality of life. Understanding the basis of diseases and the application of the various available diagnostic tools is essential. Furthermore, access to advanced diagnostic modalities may be limited. Proctoscopy and sigmoidoscopy, available as rigid or flexible, are simple tools used for diagnostic and therapeutic purposes in both benign and malignant conditions. Essential radiological investigations include magnetic resonance imaging (MRI) and endorectal ultrasound. While conventional MRI can diagnose anatomical abnormalities such as anorectal fistulae, sphincter injuries, and tumors, dynamic imaging in MRI defecography allows the diagnosis of pelvic floor disorders. Anal manometry is another dynamic modality used to assess sphincter function using transducers and pressure recording. Endorectal ultrasound is used to assess the anatomy and function of the anal sphincters. It aids in identifying abscesses, fistula tracts, and sphincter defects with high accuracy in the local staging of rectal tumors. This chapter will focus on a systematic approach to anorectal conditions and describe the physiology and indications of each diagnostic modality.

Keywords: anorectal diseases, radiology, diagnostic tools, endorectal ultrasound, anal manometry

1. Introduction

Diseases of the anorectum are common and may present with various symptoms. The clinical picture may include alteration in bowel habits, rectal bleeding, anal pain, tenesmus, difficulty in defecation, and fecal incontinence. Symptoms of such anorectal conditions commonly overlap; hence, diagnosis may be challenging. In addition, patients may experience concomitant urinary or sexual symptoms. The impact of these conditions affects patient's quality of life, making it imperative to diagnose and manage them promptly and appropriately. Understanding the basic pathological etiology of these conditions and the use of various advanced diagnostic tools are essential to reach an accurate diagnosis. This chapter will give an overview of the indications and interpretation of anal manometry, endorectal ultrasound, and other investigations used for assessing anorectal function.

IntechOpen

2. Anoscopy, rigid proctosigmoidoscopy, and flexible sigmoidoscopy

To perform a comprehensive physical examination of the anorectum, anoproctoscopy and sigmoidoscopy are often used for direct inspection of the lumen through the anal verge. Many types exist, ranging from disposable to reusable anoscopies and flexible and rigid sigmoidoscopies. They also vary in length. In addition, supplementary equipment for diagnostic and therapeutic purposes may be used, such as biopsy, banding, and sclerotherapy.

These tests are primarily performed in the left lateral decubitus position. Lighting is crucial for adequate visualization. While bright headlights or illuminating stand lamps have traditionally been used, newer models are often integrated with a built-in light. The bed height is imperative for adequate visualization and comfort of the physician. Although fleet enema is not routinely administered prior to anoscopy, studies have reported enhanced adequacy of examination following fleet enema or, in some instances, complete mechanical bowel preparation [1, 2]. Generous lubrication, particularly using anesthetic lubricants, is essential for better tolerability by the patient. Effective communication and asking the patients to take deep breaths during insertion are also helpful [3].

Various anoscopes exist, but mostly, they come in a tapered distal end for better tolerability. The tip may be straight or pivoted. A slanted or pivoted tip allows better visualization of specific quadrants and the identification of larger hemorrhoids. Upon insertion, the obturator is removed, allowing visualization of the lower rectum and anal canal. To visualize the entire circumference, rotation of the anoscope is performed, often with re-insertion of the obturator. Removal and re-insertion may sometimes be necessary to avoid mucosal injury. Additionally, sliding of the mucosa during rotation of the tool may impair the visualization and appropriate localization of pathologies. Inspection of the mucosa is the first step of the exam, noting any abnormalities, including vascular abnormalities, lesions, and/or fistula openings. In addition, hemorrhoidal cushions are inspected and graded when pathological. Patients may be asked to strain to inspect for rectal prolapse. Abnormalities may be documented at each quadrant, for example, anterior or posterior, right or left. Alternatively, the clock system can be used. Relation to the dentate line should also be noted. The physician may observe the expression of pus, blood, or mucus throughout the exam [3, 4].

Rigid proctosigmoidoscopies are similar but have longer scopes allowing inspection further into the anal canal and rectum. The average length of a proctosigmoidoscope is 25 cm, although it may vary based on the manufacturer. A pump is used for air insufflation. After complete insertion, the assessment is done upon withdrawal of the scope. Indications are similar to anoscopy in patients with anorectal complaints but allowing deeper lesions to be identified. Furthermore, it is considered the most accurate modality for the localization of rectal tumors, determining the distance of the pathology from the anal verge more accurately than flexible sigmoidoscopy or imaging modalities.

Flexible sigmoidoscopies are 60 cm long and connected through fiberoptic light and cable to a display screen, similar to a colonoscopy. Air insufflation and suctioning are used throughout the procedure. Furthermore, biopsies may be obtained through forceps passed from within the scope. While colonoscopy requires complete mechanical bowel preparation, flexible sigmoidoscopies may be carried out following an enema alone. Indications are similar to colonoscopy; however, they may be used in situations where complete bowel preparation is contraindicated. The scope may be advanced as far as the splenic flexure in some patients. The distal colonic and rectal mucosa is observed for abnormalities such as proctitis, pseudomembranous colitis, or lesions such as polyps or masses. While a complete colonoscopy offers a more comprehensive screening modality for colorectal cancer, flexible sigmoidoscopy combined with fecal testing may be used in the screening for colorectal cancer. Retroflexion within the rectum at the end of the procedure allows inspection of hemorrhoids. Because it is an invasive procedure, complications such as perforation may occur [5, 6].

2.1 High-resolution anoscopy

High-resolution anoscopy is a special type of scope that utilizes microscopic views and special dyes for the detection and diagnosis of anal intra-epithelial neoplasms. Like the abovementioned diagnostic tools, this is an office-based procedure. Inspection is carried out after 3% acetic acid or Lugol's solution is applied by using a soaked gauze. Dysplastic cells become more prominent when exposed to acetic acid, giving them a characteristic aceto-white appearance. On the other hand, dysplastic cells are unable to absorb the iodine-based Lugol's solution like normal cells do, allowing them to become more prominent [7–9].

3. Anal manometry

3.1 Introduction

Anal manometry is an advanced diagnostic modality utilizing sequences of pressure measurements to assess the anorectal sensorimotor function and mechanisms behind continence and defecation. It is also used to determine rectal sensitivity and capacity. This dynamic test records the resting and squeezing anal tones reflecting the involuntary and voluntary functions of the internal and external anal sphincter muscles, respectively. In addition, anorectal sensation and the rectoanal inhibitory reflex (RAIR) are assessed [10, 11]. However, various techniques exist, which may influence the interpretation of the result and create a lack of standardization. Furthermore, the integration of newer modalities, such as 3-dimensional and high-resolution manometry, may not be widely available [10]. The patient's position and cooperation, in addition to the study set-up, may influence results [11]. Gender may impact the normal values of test results, with men commonly having higher squeezing and resting pressures than women. In addition, nulliparous women have been found to have different normal values compared to parous women, with higher resting pressures observed among nulliparous women [12].

3.2 Indications

Although the most common utility of anal manometry is in fecal incontinence and defecatory disorders, it can also be used in other clinical settings. For example, it may be beneficial in patients who have chronic constipation, anal fissure or fistula, chronic anorectal pain (levator ani syndrome), Hirschsprung disease, as well as those with megarectum or megacolon. Less common uses include before and during biofeedback training and in surgical planning. Manometry can predict continence in pre-operative patients undergoing anal surgery, pelvic floor, or pouch reconstructions. It can also be used in patients with very low prior anastomoses before reversal of a diverting stoma [11, 13–16].

In patients with a history of obstetric injury, anal manometry results, along with other diagnostic modalities such as MRI, the anatomical and functional assessment of the anal sphincter may influence informed decisions regarding future pregnancies and modes of child delivery [11]. In cases of anal fissure, the evaluation of the anal pressure may influence the management options, whereas the decision to perform lateral internal sphincterotomy versus botox injection may be avoided in patients with low anal sphincter pressures. Visual biofeedback sessions allow better patient understanding and coordination of muscle contractions during this therapy. In addition, the baseline test prior to therapy initiation provides for improved quality of patient counseling and education. Furthermore, it can be compared to repeated testing done throughout their session, evaluating improvement and identifying targets during subsequent sessions [11, 16].

3.3 Testing modalities

The balloon-filled system is the earliest out of the various available modalities. Two latex balloons, which may be air- or water-filled, are connected to transducers through catheters. Each balloon is positioned per rectally at the level of the internal anal sphincter proximally and the lower edge of the external sphincter distally. Balloon inflation elicits RAIR, allowing subsequent measurement of resting and squeezing pressures. The mean resting and squeezing pressures are calculated from multiple readings. Despite its being a simple and affordable method, result interpretation has few concerns. The exact method, whether air- or water-filled balloon, may yield slightly different values. Furthermore, balloon size and rapid balloon distention may also influence results [14, 17, 18].

Water-perfused systems are based on catheters connected to gas or air pumps that infuse water through side holes in the catheters. Anal canal pressures are measured through water flow and yield or resistance pressures. The number and orientation of transducers may vary based on the production company. Therefore, rotation or pull-through maneuvers may be necessary to measure the pressures throughout the entire anal canal. Transducers may be arranged in a spiral or radial manner and contain as few as two transducers or up to 12 in some systems. One limitation of this modality is that it can only be performed in a lateral decubitus position [18].

Solid-state systems consist of pressure channels spaced onto transducers that do not require manipulation, making them more straightforward and less of a technical challenge compared to water-infused systems. Furthermore, this test can be performed in a sitting position, mimicking the physiological state of defecation [18].

High-resolution anorectal manometry (HRAM) and high-definition 3D anorectal manometry (HDAM) are newer modalities that have been introduced with advancements in medical technology. When compared to more traditional manometry setups, these modalities are easier to use and operate in a stationary manner, requiring minimal to no manipulation throughout the study, hence reducing operator-dependent results. Furthermore, the higher number and configuration of the sensors provide more continuous and dynamic measurements. However, they are more costly, and catheter durability may be limited [19]. With slight variations based on the manufacturer, HRAM consists of catheters with eight to 12 circumferential sensors spaced at 6 to 10 mm intervals. This technique utilizes water-perfused or solid-state systems. While HDAM also consists of circumferential sensors, the probe is rigid, wider in diameter, and consists of 256 sensors. HRAM and HDAM sensors are temperature-sensitive. Thermal drift, or alterations in pressure due to changes in temperature, may be observed throughout the study. In addition, thermal compensation is applied to correct for alterations in these pressures due to temperature changes. Based on the manufacturer, a digital software is used to analyze and display results in plots. Most software has the ability to configure numerical data into color topography, providing a display of pressures that is easier to interpret and understand, whether by physicians or patients [15, 19, 20].

3.4 Technique

3.4.1 Preparation

Anal manometry is a simple test that does not require much preparation. However, patients are advised to defecate at least 30 minutes before the study. Mechanical bowel preparation is not indicated but may be adopted by some centers. Other center protocols may advocate for enemas, particularly when stool is appreciated on digital rectal examination prior to initiation of the procedure. The procedure should be explained in full to the patient to ensure an adequate understanding of the process, enhancing the cooperation and efficacy of the study. Most manometry setups are done with the patient in the left lateral decubitus position with the knees and hips flexed at 90 degrees. Performing a digital rectal examination prior to study initiation may affect rectal function and, hence, is not routinely done. However, some advocate that its advantages include assessing for any local pathologies and ensuring the absence of impacted stools or loading. In addition, assessing the patient's understanding of the manometry requirements of squeezing and pushing may be helpful. However, if done, the patient should be given adequate time before study initiation to allow for relaxation. Upon starting the study, adequate lubrication of the probe allows for better patient tolerance. However, the use of non-anesthetic lubrication is essential for study accuracy [11, 16, 19].

3.4.2 Measurements

3.4.2.1 Resting pressure

The resting anal sphincter pressure is mostly by the internal anal sphincter, but the external anal sphincter and hemorrhoidal plexuses also contribute. It is measured at rest and over a period of 20–60 seconds, depending on hospital protocols. A period of adaptation is allowed for the patient to relax following probe insertion rectally and before testing initiation. There is a normal variation in the normal resting anal tone based on age and gender, with old age and female gender having a physiologically lower resting tone. Furthermore, nulliparous women were found to have higher resting pressures compared to parous women. However, pathologically low resting pressures are observed in patients with fecal incontinence secondary to sphincter injury following anal surgery or obstetric injuries. On the other hand, high resting anal pressure may be present in patients with spastic muscles. This may be induced by anal pain or an anal fissure at the time of exam. **Figure 1** demonstrates the resting anal pressure during anal manometry in normal individuals (A), compared to increased (B) and decreased resting pressures [11, 12, 18, 21].

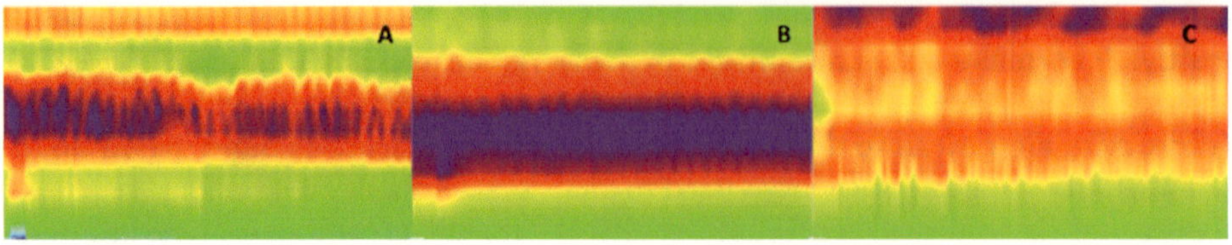

Figure 1.
Normal resting pressure on anal manometry (A), compared to increased (B) and reduced (C) anal pressures, respectively. (Reprinted from Continence, 10, Tanzeela Gala, Liam Johnston, Deepa Solanki, Ugo Grossi, Alexis Schizas, Alison Hainsworth, Linda Ferrari, Anorectal manometry—How to perform and interpret manometry, 101,214, Copyright (2024), with permission from Elsevier.)

3.4.2.2 Squeezing pressure

This is assessed while the patient is voluntarily contracting the anal sphincter by measuring the increase in pressure from the resting pressure at the level of the anal canal. The maximum pressure achieved is also recorded. During this test, the pressure is recorded during three attempts of squeezing for 5-second increments with 30-second relaxation periods in between (**Figure 2A**). In some protocols, a sustained squeezing pressure may also be measured. Squeeze pressure is a measure of the external anal sphincter function. It should not be confused with any change in pressure at the level of the rectal sensors, as these may be influenced by increased abdominal pressure. Anal sphincter injury causes reduced squeezing pressure, as demonstrated in **Figure 2B**, while impaired sphincter function may lead to high squeezing pressures. It is important to note that the normal interpretation of these two values varies based on gender, with men having higher squeezing and resting pressures than women. High squeezing pressure may be observed among patients with dyssynergia defecation secondary to spastic puborectalis muscle [11, 12, 16, 18, 21].

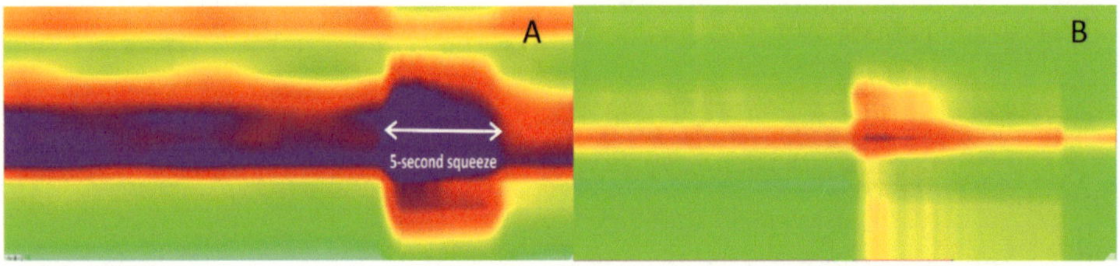

Figure 2.
Normal appearance of squeezing pressure measured by anal manometry (A). Reduced amplitude of squeezing pressure, as often observed among patients with sphincter injury (B). (Reprinted from Continence, 10, Tanzeela Gala, Liam Johnston, Deepa Solanki, Ugo Grossi, Alexis Schizas, Alison Hainsworth, Linda Ferrari, Anorectal manometry—How to perform and interpret manometry, 101,214, Copyright (2024), with permission from Elsevier.)

3.4.2.3 Cough reflex

Measurement of the involuntary squeezing pressure reproduced by a contracted pelvic floor muscle during maximum coughing. This is a natural response of the anal sphincter to increased intra-abdominal pressure *via* the sacral reflex arch. For accuracy of the measurement, two recordings during two single coughs separated by a 30-second interval for recovery are documented. The measurement with the highest achieved rectal pressure is considered. A normal cough reflex is shown in **Figure 3A**,

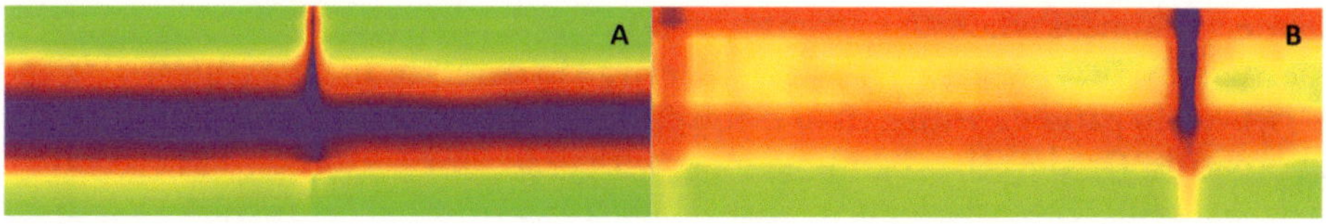

Figure 3.
Normal cough reflex with anal canal pressure that exceeds the intra-abdominal pressure (A), compared to (B) demonstrating appropriate contraction of the anal sphincter with simultaneous increase in intra-abdominal pressure. (Reprinted from Continence, 10, Tanzeela Gala, Liam Johnston, Deepa Solanki, Ugo Grossi, Alexis Schizas, Alison Hainsworth, Linda Ferrari, Anorectal manometry—How to perform and interpret manometry, 101,214, Copyright (2024), with permission from Elsevier.)

where the anal sphincter pressure is maintained higher than the intra-abdominal pressure produced during the test. Spinal cord injuries below the sacral level, cauda equina, and pudendal neuropathy lead to weak or absent cough reflex and may be demonstrated by higher intra-abdominal pressure despite anal sphincter contraction, as seen in **Figure 3B** [11].

3.4.2.4 Rectoanal inhibitory reflex (RAIR)

Mediated by the myenteric plexus, rectal distention causes temporary involuntary relaxation of the internal anal sphincter, as observed in **Figure 4**. This reflex is absent in patients with fecal incontinence, acquired myenteric neuropathies, Hirschsprung's disease, Chagas' disease, scleroderma, and dermatomyositis, and may be affected by anorectal surgeries. To perform this test, the rectal balloon is instilled with 30 ml of air while observing for decreasing anal pressure. Higher volumes of air may be needed to achieve a response in patients with large-volume rectums. Furthermore, voluntary contraction of the anal sphincter by the patient should be avoided during testing to produce proper results [11, 21].

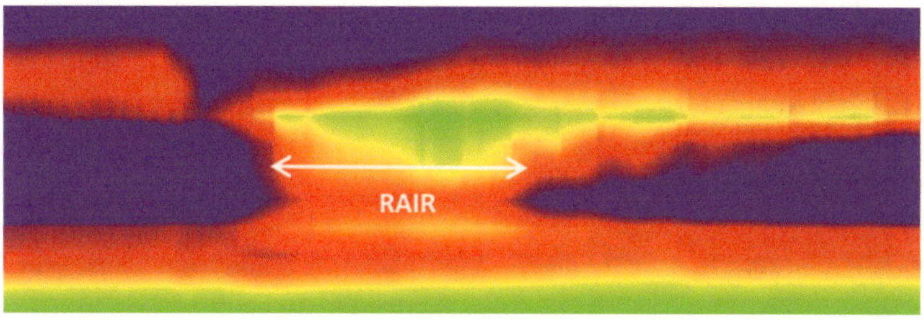

Figure 4.
Demonstration of RAIR with involuntary relaxation of the anal sphincter in response to balloon distention within the rectum. (Reprinted from Continence, 10, Tanzeela Gala, Liam Johnston, Deepa Solanki, Ugo Grossi, Alexis Schizas, Alison Hainsworth, Linda Ferrari, Anorectal manometry—How to perform and interpret manometry, 101,214, Copyright (2024), with permission from Elsevier.)

3.4.2.5 Rectal sensation

Three patient-reported sensory thresholds are recorded. The first is the first sensation volume, the volume at which the balloon pressure causes the patient a constant feeling. The desire-to-defecate volume or first urge volume is the pressure at which the patient feels a persistent urge to defecate. Finally, the maximum tolerated volume is when an uncomfortable or intolerable feeling is achieved. Rectal hypersensitivity is described as having the urge to defecate at lower thresholds and is observed in patients with irritable bowel syndrome, urge fecal incontinence, and proctitis. On the other hand, patients with defecatory disorders have rectal hyposensitivity. These patients require much larger thresholds to achieve a desire to defecate. In these patients, the reduced rectal sensation may improve with biofeedback training [11, 16, 19].

4. Pudendal nerve terminal motor latency (PNTML)

The pudendal nerve innervates the external anal sphincter muscle. Patients with fecal incontinence may be further investigated by PNTML, particularly when the integrity of the external anal sphincter is confirmed and other causes of incontinence are investigated thoroughly. PNTML refers to the time necessary for transmitting an impulse following stimulation of the pudendal nerve using electrodes passed transrectally. The electrodes are positioned along the examiner's gloved finger using an adhesive. Following a digital rectal examination in the left lateral decubitus position, the finger is directed toward the ischial spine. Impulses are then delivered through the electrodes, and the contraction of the external sphincter muscle is observed. This step is repeated on the contralateral side. Prolonged PNTML is suggestive of pudendal nerve injury or neuropathy. This may be a result of stretch injury during pregnancy or vaginal delivery [22–24].

5. Endorectal ultrasound (ERUS)

5.1 Introduction

ERUS provides detailed information about the anatomy of the rectum, anal canal, and pelvic floor muscles. In addition, it is one of the important diagnostic tools in assessing anorectal function among patients with fecal incontinence. Besides benign disorders, ERUS can aid in the initial staging of rectal cancer. However, for patients who underwent chemoradiation for rectal cancer, results have been poor in detecting recurrence using ERUS [25].

ERUS is a noninvasive imaging modality that uses sound waves emitted from a transducer. The ultrasonic sound waves, depending on tissue densities, will reflect back to the transducer, generating the images. ERUS carries no radiation risk and, therefore, can be used safely among various patient populations, including children and pregnant women. However, because the probe is applied in direct contact with the skin, it might be challenging to use in postoperative patients with wounds or in patients with anal fissures and anal stenosis.

5.2 Equipment and technique

The patient is placed in the left lateral decubitus position to start the procedure. Prior to ERUS, patients receive an enema to empty the rectum of stool. A digital rectal examination is performed prior to introducing the probe. To achieve optimal rectal distension, a lubricated water-filled balloon (typically containing 30–60 mL of water) is introduced per rectally, allowing direct contact between the probe and the rectal wall, [26] Ensuring that the ERUS probe is inserted into the rectum with the correct orientation is crucial for result interpretation and accuracy. The proper orientation should ensure that anterior structures are visualized at the 12 o'clock position, represented superiorly on the viewing screen, while the 3 and 9 o'clock positions represent the left and right sides of the patient, respectively. Finally, the posterior structures are seen at the 6 o'clock position.

The ERUS probe is slowly introduced to the anal canal until the identification of the puborectalis muscle. The transrectal probe rotates 360° mechanically and operates at an ultrasound frequency range of 5–15 MHz, depending on the lesions being examined [27]. Higher frequencies offer better resolution and a more precise definition of the rectal wall layers, while lower frequencies are crucial for evaluating other structures, such as the perirectal fatty tissue, and inspection for enlarged lymph nodes. Most ERUS machines have a 3D acquisition system in which the ERUS probe can generate an image reflecting a distance of 6 cm while remaining stationary [26]. The 3D image acquisition process is automated, with the movement from within the probe. The patient does not appreciate this movement externally, avoiding disrupting the testing process.

5.3 Interpretation

ERUS will clearly show the five different anatomical layers of the rectal wall, as shown in **Figure 5**. The first innermost hyperechoic layer is the interface caused by direct contact between the transducer balloon and rectal mucosa. The second layer is mucosa and muscularis mucosa, which is a hypoechoic layer. The middle layer is the submucosa, which is shown as a hyperechoic layer. Then, the fourth layer is a hypoechoic layer, representing the muscularis propria. The fifth and outermost layer is hyperechoic and signifies the perirectal fatty tissue. When ERUS is used to stage rectal lesions, it is crucial to identify the previously mentioned layers in order to obtain accurate staging.

ERUS has an important application in rectal cancer staging as it allows the assessment of the depth of tumor invasion, the involvement of the sphincter, and the lymph node status. Rectal cancer appears on ERUS as a hypoechoic lesion within the five normal rectal wall layers. T1 tumors are located at the submucosa, and do not go beyond

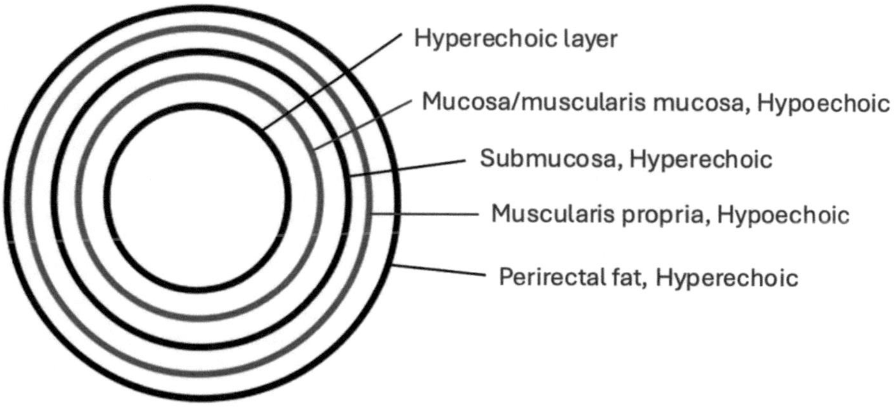

Figure 5.
Distinct layers of the rectal wall are shown by ERUS.

the first three echogenic layers seen on ERUS. T2 tumors are situated in the muscularis propria. If the lesion goes beyond the muscularis propria into the perirectal fatty plane, it is considered as T3, whereas T4 tumors involve invasion of adjacent organs such as the vagina, prostate, seminal vesicles, urinary bladder, or pelvic sidewall. The accuracy of ERUS in T staging of rectal cancer has been reported to range from 69 to 94% [28]. ERUS is considered superior to magnetic resonance imaging (MRI) and computed tomography (CT) scans in staging early rectal cancer because of its ability to visualize all the rectal wall layers [29]. Ghoneem et al. reported a higher sensitivity, specificity, and accuracy of ERUS in staging early rectal cancer compared to MRI. In fact, ERUS had a sensitivity of 95% compared to 78% by MRI and a specificity of 84% in ERUS compared to 68% in MRI [30]. Nevertheless, MRI remains the modality of choice in staging T3-T4 rectal tumors [31].

The normal anal canal is divided into upper, middle, and lower sections with distinct appearances of the musculature at each level (**Figure 6**). The puborectalis is seen in the upper part of the anal canal as a U-shaped hyperechoic sling. Whereas the middle anal canal will show a hypoechoic band is seen that represents the internal anal sphincter which has a thickness of 2-4 mm [33]. It has been found that older women may have a 33% thicker internal anal sphincter [34]. At the lower anal canal, there is a hyperechoic layer that represents the external anal sphincter.

Given its ability to accurately assess the anatomy of the anal sphincter complex, ERUS has been used to diagnose conditions with anatomical abnormalities, such as those seen in patients with anal fistulae and incontinence. The use of ERUS for the localization of anal sphincter defects in patients with fecal incontinence can aid in

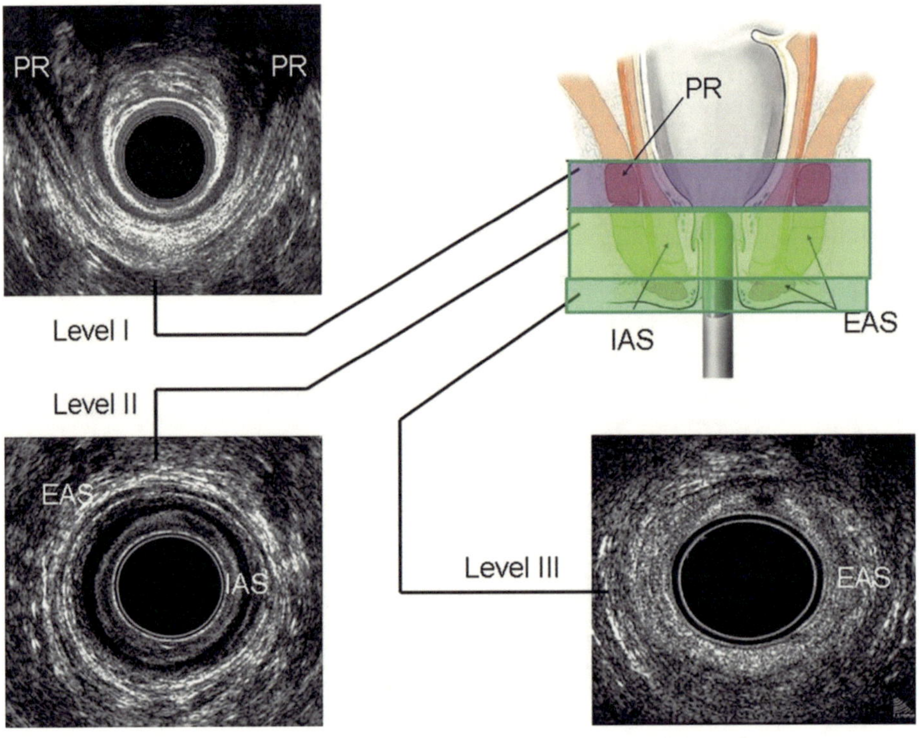

Figure 6.
Normal ultrasonographic anatomy of the anal canal. EAS, external anal sphincter; IAS, internal anal sphincter; PR, puborectalis muscle. (Reproduced with permission of Ref. [32] via *Copyright Clearance Center.)*

surgical planning. ERUS can accurately evaluate the size and exact site of sphincter injury. In addition, the measurement of perianal body thickness (PBT) is important in assessing patients with fecal incontinence. To measure the PBT, digital pressure is applied to the posterior vaginal wall, which appears hyperechoic in the image, facilitating the measurement of the distance. The normal thickness of PBT is usually more than 12 mm [35]. An abnormal measurement of less than 10 mm is associated with anterior sphincter defects [36]. The accuracy of ERUS in diagnosing sphincter disruption has been reported to be nearly 95% [37]. However, studies have shown that MRI is more sensitive in detecting sphincter injuries [38].

Additionally, ERUS has a role in the assessment of anal fistulae anatomy and any associated sphincter defects prior to surgery. A perianal fistula appears as a hypoechoic tract, which may contain fluid-like material or, if inactive, could demonstrate only a fibrotic band. A meta-analysis comparing MRI and ERUS in the diagnosis of anal fistula revealed similar sensitivities, but MRI had a higher specificity [39].

6. MRI defecography

6.1 Introduction

Pelvic floor dysfunction is common among female adults, particularly among the aging population. Pelvic floor dysfunction includes a wide range of functional disorders that affect the ligaments, fascia, and muscles supporting the pelvic floor organs. Patients may present with pelvic pain, dyspareunia, pelvic organ prolapse, incomplete emptying, and urinary and/or fecal incontinence. Clinical evaluation of patients with pelvic floor disease is challenging. Imaging has an important role in the diagnosis of different pelvic floor conditions. MRI defecography has emerged as a valuable technique to assess pelvic floor disorders. While anal manometry can be used to diagnose these conditions, MRI is noninvasive and can provide helpful information about the anatomy of the anal sphincter complex, pelvic floor compartments, along with muscles and ligaments.

6.2 Technique

The patient is placed in the supine position with knees slightly bent in a standard T1.5 or T3 scanner. Before imaging, 100-180 ml of rectal ultrasound gel is inserted to assess rectal evacuation [40]. The dynamic portion of MRI defecatory consists of a cycle of rest, squeeze, strain, and defecation. MRI defecography protocol starts with static single-shot fast spin echo T2-weighted images in the sagittal, axial, and coronal planes [40]. For dynamic MRI sequences, the steady-state free precession sequence in the sagittal plane (squeezing, straining, and defecation) [40].

6.3 Interpretation

Important reference lines are placed on MRI defecography, as observed in **Figure 7**. The pubococcygeal line (PCL), corresponding to the level of the pelvic floor, is drawn from the inferior part of the symphysis pubis to the most distal part of the coccyx [42]. The H line is measured by drawing a line from the inferior part of the symphysis pubis to the anorectal junction. This line represents the anteroposterior width of the levator hiatus and normally measures 6 cm or less [42]. The M line is

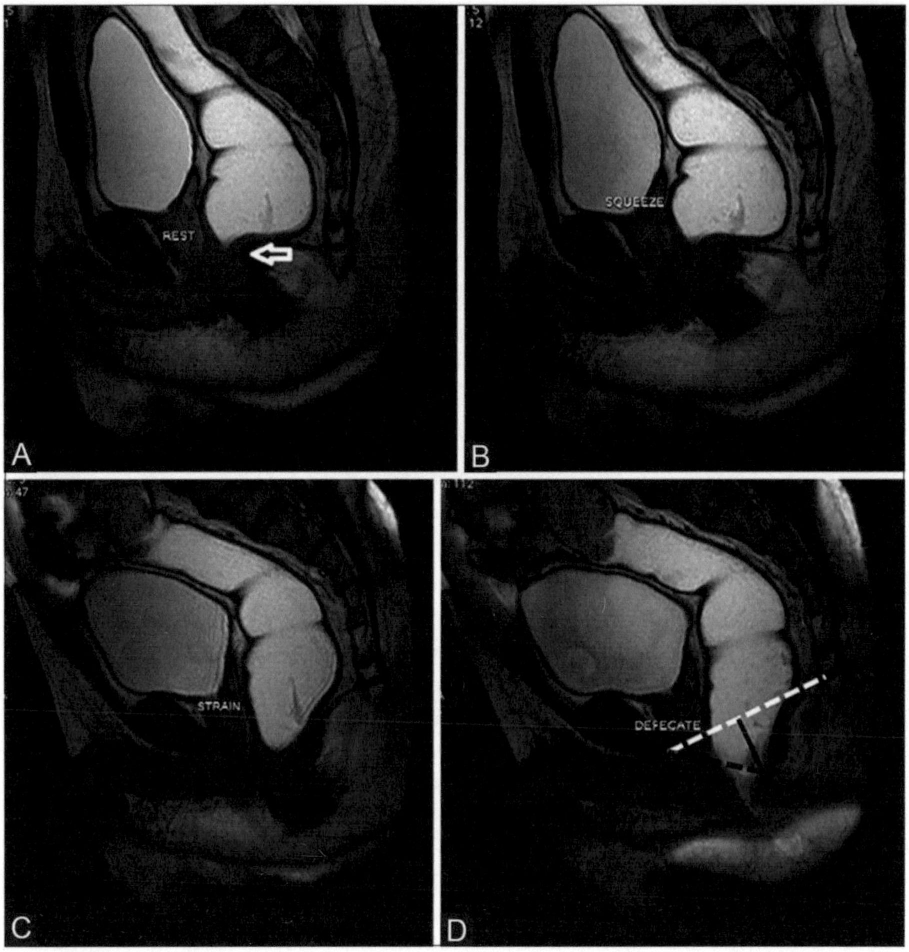

Figure 7.
(A-D): MRI defecography in a normal patient (A-D). The arrow in (A) shows the normal anorectal junction at rest. Mild descent of the anorectal junction can be appreciated with squeezing (B) followed by straining (C) and defecation (D). During defecation (D), the PCL is shown as the broken white line, and the H-line is represented by the broken black line. The M line is shown as a solid black line that is drawn perpendicularly from the PCL line to the posterior aspect of the H line. (Reproduced with permission of *Ref. [41]* via Copyright Clearance Center.)

drawn perpendicularly from the PCL line to the posterior aspect of the H line and should measure less than 2 cm [42]. Lastly, the anorectal angle is calculated by drawing a line from the posterior aspect of the rectal wall in relation to the long axis of the anal canal, which is approximately 104–127° at rest and normally increases by 15–20° with evacuation [40, 42].

Pelvic organ prolapse grading is based on European society of urogenital radiology/european society for gastrointestinal and abdominal radiology recommendations and the "rule of three" depending on the PCL line: mild prolapse if organ descent is 3 cm or less below the PCL line, moderate grade is between 3 and 6 cm, severe is more than 6 cm [43]. Rectal intussusception is the telescoping of the rectal wall within itself, as observed in **Figure 8**. Rectal intussusception can be categorized as intrarectal, without protrusion beyond the rectum; intra-anal, with protrusion limited to within the anal canal; and

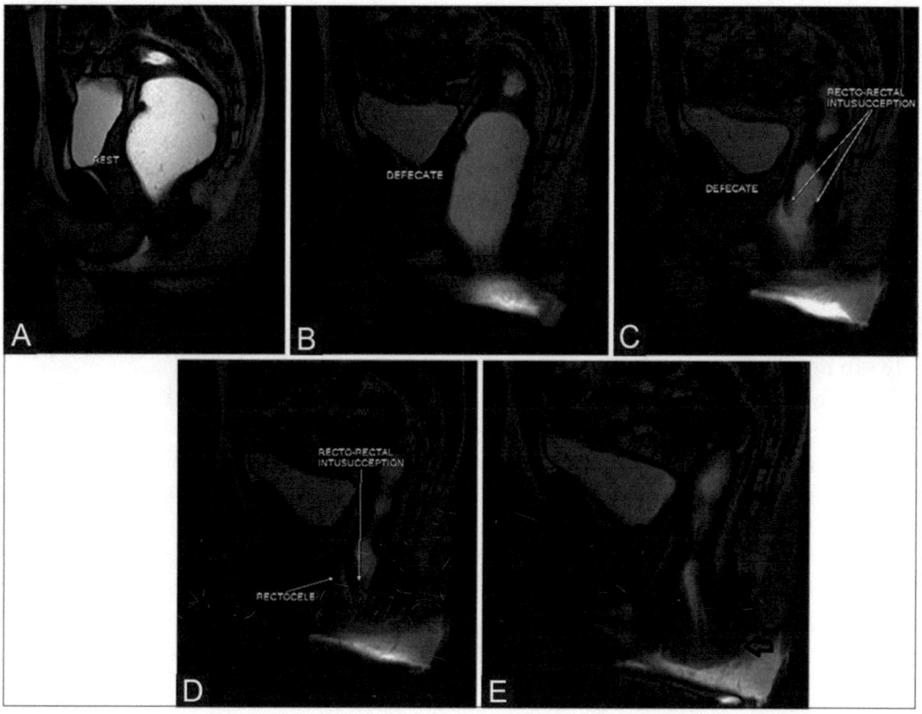

Figure 8.
(A-E): MRI defecography in a patient with rectal prolapse showing the normal appearance of the rectum at rest (A). During defecation, progressive rectal prolapse is seen (B-E). Initially, intrarectal intussusception is seen in C and D, followed by full-thickness rectal prolapse beyond the anal verge in E, represented by an arrow. (Reproduced with permission of *Ref. [41]* via Copyright Clearance Center.)

finally external, where it protrudes beyond the anal verge, also known as rectal prolapse [43]. Patients may report a feeling of incomplete emptying or obstructed defecation with rectal intussusception. A rectocele is defined as a bulge of the rectal wall during defecation due to weakness in supporting pelvic floor structures and laxity of fascia [43]. On MRI defecography, a rectocele can be graded as mild bulge of less than 2 cm, which is usually asymptomatic, moderate 2-4 cm, and large if more than 4 cm [42, 43].

MRI defecography can help in the assessment of fecal incontinence prior to surgical intervention, as MRI provides information about the anal sphincter anatomy. Thinning of the anal sphincter complex, sphincter defect, and fatty atrophy can be seen in such patients.

Pelvic floor dyssynergia, also known as anismus, is defined as an involuntary and paradoxical contraction of the puborectalis muscle during defecation, resulting in constipation and unsuccessful evacuation. In these patients, MRI defecography during defecation will show no widening of the anorectal angle, no descent in pelvic floor organs, hypertrophied puborectalis, and inability to evacuate [42].

7. Defecography

Evacuation defecography is a fluoroscopic imaging during defecation. It can help assess patients with obstructed defecation syndrome and pelvic organ prolapse.

Before the examination begins, a thick barium contrast of about 150-300 mL is inserted into the rectum to mimic stool [44]. Then, the patient is asked to sit on a commode and evacuate the barium, which is correlated with real-time fluoroscopic imaging from straining until defecation.

After images are acquired, reference lines are drawn for result interpretation, including the anorectal angle, puborectalis length, and extent of perineal descent [44]. The anorectal angle, similar to that assessed by MRI defecography, is measured by drawing a line from the posterior border of the rectum and the long axis of the anal canal. The puborectalis length is the minimal distance between the anterosuperior border of the symphysis pubis and the puborectalis. This length changes from rest between 14 and 16 cm, decreases to 12-15 cm during squeezing, and increases to 15-18 cm during the push phase [43]. Lastly, the extent of perineal descent is assessed by drawing a perpendicular line from the pubococcygeal line to the anorectal junction; a descent of more than 3 cm is considered abnormal [45]. A normal evacuation defecography will show an increase in anorectal angle, lengthening of puborectalis, and blunting of the puborectalis notch. This technique remains a reliable and cost-effective imaging modality despite the advancement of MRI defecography.

This chapter provides an overview of the various diagnostic modalities used to investigate common anorectal complaints. Anatomical abnormalities may be identified by direct inspection using anoscopy and/or proctosigmoidoscopy or imaging modalities, such as ERUS. While scopes allow direct visualization of luminal conditions within the anorectum, they may be utilized for therapeutic purposes as well. ERUS is an important diagnostic tool for assessing all layers of the anorectum and pelvic floor. On the other hand, functional abnormalities, as seen in conditions like fecal incontinence and obstructed defecation syndrome, are evaluated by dynamic studies. Anal manometry, defecography, and MRI defecography are essential in investigating such patients and may provide insight into therapeutic management options in these cases. A thorough understanding of these advanced diagnostic tools, as well as the normal and abnormal interpretations, is crucial for physicians treating anorectal conditions.

Author details

Hadeel Helmi[1]*, Atheer Alotaibi[2] and Ayyob Alqarni[1]

1 King Abdulaziz Medical City, Ministry of National Guard Health Affairs, Riyadh, Saudi Arabia

2 Security Forces Hospital, Riyadh, Saudi Arabia

*Address all correspondence to: hadeelhelmi@gmail.com

References

[1] Arnold GL, Norton RA, Faison ME. Preparation for proctosigmoidoscopy. Gastrointestinal Endoscopy. 1979;**25**(2):79

[2] Sajid MS, Caswell JF, Abbas MA, Baig MK, McFall MR. Improving the view during flexible sigmoidoscopy: A systematic review of published randomized, controlled trials comparing the use of oral bowel preparation versus enema bowel preparation. Updates in Surgery. 2015;**67**(3):247-256

[3] Ponka D, Baddar F. Anoscopy. Canadian Family Physician. 2013;**59**(5):510

[4] Rajab TK, Bordeianou LG, von Keudell A, Rajab H, Zhou H. Digital rectal examination and anoscopy. The New England Journal of Medicine. 2018;**378**(22):e30

[5] Aboulian A, Kumar RR. Diagnostic evaluations. In: Bailey HR, Billingham RP, Stamos MJ, Snyder MJ, editors. Colorectal Surgery. Philadelphia: W.B. Saunders; 2013. pp. 17-40

[6] Zuber TJ. Flexible sigmoidoscopy. American Family Physician. 2001;**63**(7):1375-1380, 83-8

[7] Cho SD, Groves E, Lao VV. History of high-resolution anoscopy. Clinics in Colon and Rectal Surgery. 2018;**31**(6):336-346

[8] O'Connor JJ. The study of anorectal disease by colposcopy. Diseases of the Colon and Rectum. 1977;**20**(7):570-572

[9] Gudur A, Shanmuganandamurthy D, Szep Z, Poggio JL. An update on the current role of high resolution anoscopy in patients with anal dysplasia. Anticancer Research. 2019;**39**(1):17-23

[10] Carrington EV, Heinrich H, Knowles CH, Rao SS, Fox M, Scott SM. Methods of anorectal manometry vary widely in clinical practice: Results from an international survey. Neurogastroenterology and Motility. 2017;**29**(8):e13016

[11] Gala T, Johnston L, Solanki D, Grossi U, Schizas A, Hainsworth A, et al. Anorectal manometry—How to perform and interpret manometry. Continence. 2024;**10**:101214

[12] Cali RL, Blatchford GJ, Perry RE, Pitsch RM, Thorson AG, Christensen MA. Normal variation in anorectal manometry. Diseases of the Colon and Rectum. 1992;**35**(12):1161-1164

[13] Bharucha AE, Basilisco G, Malcolm A, Lee TH, Hoy MB, Scott SM, et al. Review of the indications, methods, and clinical utility of anorectal manometry and the rectal balloon expulsion test. Neurogastroenterology and Motility. 2022;**34**(9):e14335

[14] Van Koughnett JA, da Silva G. Anorectal physiology and testing. Gastroenterology Clinics of North America. 2013;**42**(4):713-728

[15] Dinning PG, Carrington EV, Scott SM. The use of colonic and anorectal high-resolution manometry and its place in clinical work and in research. Neurogastroenterology and Motility. 2015;**27**(12):1693-1708

[16] Rao SS, Azpiroz F, Diamant N, Enck P, Tougas G, Wald A. Minimum standards of anorectal manometry. Neurogastroenterology and Motility. 2002;**14**(5):553-559

[17] Schuster MM, Hookman P, Hendrix TR, Mendeloff AI. Simultaneous

manometric recording of internal and external anal sphincteric reflexes. Bulletin of the Johns Hopkins Hospital. 1965;**116**:79-88

[18] Sun WM, Rao SS. Manometric assessment of anorectal function. Gastroenterology Clinics of North America. 2001;**30**(1):15-32

[19] Lee TH, Bharucha AE. How to perform and interpret a high-resolution anorectal manometry test. Journal of Neurogastroenterology and Motility. 2016;**22**(1):46-59

[20] Robertson EV, Lee YY, Derakhshan MH, Wirz AA, Whiting JR, Seenan JP, et al. High-resolution esophageal manometry: Addressing thermal drift of the manoscan system. Neurogastroenterology and Motility. 2012;**24**(1):61-64, e11

[21] Jorge JM, Wexner SD. Anorectal manometry: Techniques and clinical applications. Southern Medical Journal. 1993;**86**(8):924-931

[22] Kiff ES, Swash M. Slowed conduction in the pudendal nerves in idiopathic (neurogenic) faecal incontinence. The British Journal of Surgery. 1984;**71**(8):614-616

[23] Rogers J, Henry MM, Misiewicz JJ. Disposable pudendal nerve stimulator: Evaluation of the standard instrument and new device. Gut. 1988;**29**(8):1131-1133

[24] Ricciardi R, Mellgren AF, Madoff RD, Baxter NN, Karulf RE, Parker SC. The utility of pudendal nerve terminal motor latencies in idiopathic incontinence. Diseases of the Colon and Rectum. 2006;**49**(6):852-857

[25] Lund JA, Sundstrom SH, Haaverstad R, Wibe A, Svinsaas M, Myrvold HE. Endoanal ultrasound is of little value in follow-up of anal carcinomas. Diseases of the Colon and Rectum. 2004;**47**(6):839-842

[26] Samdani T, Garcia-Aguilar J. Imaging in rectal cancer: Magnetic resonance imaging versus endorectal ultrasonography. Surgical Oncology Clinics of North America. 2014;**23**(1):59-77

[27] Cârţână ET, Pârvu D, Săftoiu A. Endoscopic ultrasound: Current role and future perspectives in managing rectal cancer patients. Journal of Gastrointestinal and Liver Diseases. 2011;**20**(4):407-413

[28] Krajewski KM, Kane RA. Ultrasound staging of rectal cancer. Seminars in Ultrasound, CT, and MR. 2008;**29**(6):427-432

[29] Wang Y, Zhou CW, Hao YZ, Li L, Liu SM, Feng XL, et al. Improvement in T-staging of rectal carcinoma: Using a novel endorectal ultrasonography technique with sterile coupling gel filling the rectum. Ultrasound in Medicine & Biology. 2012;**38**(4):574-579

[30] Ghoneem E, Shabana ASA, El Sherbini M, Zuhdy M, Eldamshety O, Gouda M, et al. Endoluminal ultrasound versus magnetic resonance imaging in assessment of rectal cancer after neoadjuvant therapy. BMC Gastroenterology. 2022;**22**(1):542

[31] MERCURY Study Group. Diagnostic accuracy of preoperative magnetic resonance imaging in predicting curative resection of rectal cancer: Prospective observational study. BMJ. 2006;**333**(7572):779

[32] Santoro GA, Pelizzo P, Grossi U, Cian R, Zanus G, Brusciano L. Role of ultrasonography for anal incontinence.

In: Docimo L, Brusciano L, editors. Anal Incontinence. Updates in Surgery. Cham: Springer; 2023

[33] Felt-Bersma RJ. Endoanal ultrasound in perianal fistulas and abscesses. Digestive and Liver Disease. 2006;**38**(8):537-543

[34] Huebner M, Margulies RU, Fenner DE, Ashton-Miller JA, Bitar KN, DeLancey JO. Age effects on internal anal sphincter thickness and diameter in nulliparous females. Diseases of the Colon and Rectum. 2007;**50**(9):1405-1411

[35] Thakar R, Sultan AH. Anal endosonography and its role in assessing the incontinent patient. Best Practice & Research. Clinical Obstetrics & Gynaecology. 2004;**18**(1):157-173

[36] Oberwalder M, Thaler K, Baig MK, Dinnewitzer A, Efron J, Weiss EG, et al. Anal ultrasound and endosonographic measurement of perineal body thickness: A new evaluation for fecal incontinence in females. Surgical Endoscopy. 2004;**18**(4):650-654

[37] Fuchsjäger MH, Maier AG. Imaging fecal incontinence. European Journal of Radiology. 2003;**47**(2):108-116

[38] Kirss J Jr, Huhtinen H, Niskanen E, Ruohonen J, Kallio-Packalen M, Victorzon S, et al. Comparison of 3D endoanal ultrasound and external phased array magnetic resonance imaging in the diagnosis of obstetric anal sphincter injuries. European Radiology. 2019;**29**(10):5717-5722

[39] Siddiqui MR, Ashrafian H, Tozer P, Daulatzai N, Burling D, Hart A, et al. A diagnostic accuracy meta-analysis of endoanal ultrasound and MRI for perianal fistula assessment. Diseases of the Colon and Rectum. 2012;**55**(5):576-585

[40] Kobi M, Flusberg M, Paroder V, Chernyak V. Practical guide to dynamic pelvic floor MRI. Journal of Magnetic Resonance Imaging. 2018;**47**(5):1155-1170

[41] Thapar RB, Patankar RV, Kamat RD, Thapar RR, Chemburkar V. MR defecography for obstructed defecation syndrome. Indian Journal Of Radiology And Imaging. 2015;**25**(1):25-30

[42] Welch EK, Ross W, Dengler KL, Gruber DD, Lamb S. The "ins and outs" of dynamic magnetic resonance imaging for female pelvic organ prolapse. International Urogynecology Journal. 2024;**35**(11):2223-2225

[43] El Sayed RF, Alt CD, Maccioni F, Meissnitzer M, Masselli G, Manganaro L, et al. Magnetic resonance imaging of pelvic floor dysfunction—Joint recommendations of the ESUR and ESGAR pelvic floor working group. European Radiology. 2017;**27**(5):2067-2085

[44] Kim AY. How to interpret a functional or motility test - defecography. Journal of Neurogastroenterology and Motility. 2011;**17**(4):416-420

[45] Jorge JM, Ger GC, Gonzalez L, Wexner SD. Patient position during cinedefecography. Influence on perineal descent and other measurements. Diseases of the Colon and Rectum. 1994;**37**(9):927-931

Section 5

Functional Disorders and Anorectal Infections

Chapter 13

Fecal Incontinence: How to Approach and Treat?

Damir Karlović, Lucia Klarica, Dorian Kršul, Nikola Simičić, Ante Jerković, Mario Milotić and Marko Zelić

Abstract

Main function of rectum and anal canal is to maintain fecal continence and allow defecation at an appropriate time and place. When patient has the unintentional loss of stool and inability to control bowel movements in socially acceptable situations, we talk about fecal incontinence (FI). This condition leads to distress and social difficulties for affected individuals. Different causes including neurological disorders, gastrointestinal diseases, and pelvic floor dysfunction can lead to FI. The condition is classified into different types: passive incontinence, where individuals are unaware of stool passage, and urge incontinence, characterized by a sudden, strong urge to defecate that cannot be controlled. Diagnosis typically involves a thorough medical history and physical examination and may include imaging studies (transrectal ultrasound and MRI defecography) or anorectal manometry to assess muscle function and rectal sensation. Management strategies range from dietary modifications and pelvic floor exercises to pharmacological treatment and surgical interventions.

Keywords: fecal incontinence, pelvic floor dysfunction, MRI defecography, anorectal manometry, sacral neuromodulation, LARS syndrome

1. Introduction

Fecal incontinence (FI), often referred to as bowel incontinence or encopresis, is the inability to control bowel movements, resulting in involuntary leakage of stool. In the newest diagnostic criteria (DSM-5), the definition of FI requires multiple criteria, which involves a 4-year period of complaints, at least one event occurring each month for at least a 3-month period, and the complaints not related to the physiological aspect of the disorder which occurs from pharmacological therapy [1].

In the Rome IV criteria, FI is now not part of the subclassification of anorectal disorders.

Preferred terms for FI are retentive FI and nonretentive FI [1].

It is a complex and multifactorial condition that affects individuals across all age groups, though it is more prevalent in older adults, particularly women [2].

The condition can range from occasional and minor leakage to complete loss of bowel control, severely impacting an individual's quality of life.

Despite its significant effects on the physical, psychological, and social well-being of those affected, fecal incontinence remains an underreported and often stigmatized issue, leading to delays in diagnosis and treatment [3].

The impact of fecal incontinence extends beyond its physical manifestations. It often leads to significant emotional distress, including embarrassment, social isolation, and reduced self-esteem. The inability to control bowel movements can cause individuals to withdraw from social activities, limit their mobility, and restrict their engagement in daily life, further contributing to the psychological burden. Consequently, the emotional and psychological toll of fecal incontinence can be as debilitating as the physical symptoms [2].

Fecal incontinence can be classified in various ways based on its severity, etiology, and pathophysiology. The most common classification method divides the condition into four types based on the degree of control:

1. *Minor incontinence*: This includes infrequent, small leaks of stool or mucus, often occurring in situations such as sneezing, coughing, or laughing. Minor incontinence is often a temporary condition and may be associated with transient factors like constipation, childbirth, or minor rectal trauma.

2. *Moderate incontinence*: In this category, individuals experience more frequent episodes of involuntary stool loss, though they may still retain some degree of control. This can include leakage of stool during certain activities or in response to a strong urge to defecate.

3. *Severe incontinence*: In individuals with severe fecal incontinence, there is a total loss of control, with the involuntary passage of stool occurring frequently and without warning. This often leads to social embarrassment, hygiene problems, and a significant decline in the individual's quality of life.

4. *Complete incontinence*: This is the most extreme form of fecal incontinence, where the individual experiences constant leakage or an inability to hold stool at all. Complete incontinence often requires significant medical intervention and management to maintain hygiene and comfort.

From a clinical perspective, the underlying cause of fecal incontinence can also inform treatment strategies. Common causes include *neurological disorders* (e.g., stroke and multiple sclerosis), *musculoskeletal damage* (e.g., anal sphincter injury following childbirth or surgery with developing of the LARS syndrome), *posttraumatic injuries of the pelvic floor* (OASIS), *pelvic floor dysfunction*, *chronic constipation*, *diarrhea*, and *rectal prolapse* [4–6].

In some cases, fecal incontinence may be idiopathic, with no clear underlying cause identified.

1.1 The etiology of fecal incontinence

The causes of fecal incontinence are diverse and can be broadly grouped into several categories: *neurological*, *musculoskeletal*, *structural*, and *functional*.

- *Neurological causes*: Nervous system plays a vital role in the regulation of bowel function. Conditions such as stroke, spinal cord injury, multiple sclerosis,

Parkinson's disease, and peripheral neuropathy can damage the nerves responsible for bowel control. Such conditions can impair both sensory and motor components of bowel function, leading to fecal incontinence.

- *Musculoskeletal causes*: Injury to the anal sphincters, particularly during childbirth, can weaken or damage muscles responsible for bowel control. Pelvic floor muscles, which support the rectum, may also be weakened or stretched, further contributing to fecal incontinence. Chronic constipation, anal surgery, and trauma can exacerbate these issues with developing of LARS syndrome.

- *Structural causes*: Structural abnormalities in gastrointestinal system, such as rectal prolapse, anal fissures, or hemorrhoids, may also contribute to fecal incontinence. These conditions can alter the anatomy of the anus or rectum, impairing the ability to retain stool.

- *Functional causes*: In some cases, fecal incontinence arises due to functional impairments in the bowel or rectum. Conditions like irritable bowel syndrome (IBS), chronic diarrhea, and inflammatory bowel disease (IBD) can disrupt normal bowel function, leading to leakage. Additionally, factors like pelvic floor dysfunction and aging can affect the ability to control defecation, even in the absence of structural damage.

Understanding the diverse etiology of fecal incontinence is crucial for developing effective treatment strategies, as the underlying cause will often guide management decisions [5, 6].

1.2 Impact on quality of life

The impact of fecal incontinence on an individual's quality of life is profound. Many individuals with this condition experience embarrassment, shame, and a fear of social stigma, which can lead to social withdrawal and depression. The psychological burden is often compounded by practical concerns such as managing incontinence episodes, maintaining hygiene, and avoiding triggering situations like travel or social events.

Studies have shown that individuals with fecal incontinence report lower scores on quality-of-life measures, particularly in areas related to physical function, emotional well-being, and social functioning. The condition may interfere with work, intimate relationships, and family life, further exacerbating the psychological distress.

The stigma surrounding fecal incontinence often leads to underreporting, as individuals may be reluctant to discuss their symptoms with healthcare providers. This delay in seeking medical attention can result in prolonged suffering and may prevent timely intervention [3].

2. Diagnostic evaluation of fecal incontinence

2.1 History

Like in most clinical situations, the evaluation of fecal incontinence starts with a thorough and detailed history and physical examination of the patient. Given the nature of the problem, it is to be expected that the patient will be reluctant to give information and speak about the condition in an open manner. It often occurs that patients do not realize that they are suffering from fecal incontinence and start describing problems with diarrhea. Therefore, it is of the utmost importance that the physician then leads the patient through specific questions to get to the diagnosis. To formulate the questions, the clinician must take into account the causes of fecal incontinence which can be subdivided into structural abnormalities like trauma, obstetric injuries, previous anorectal surgeries, rectal prolapse, hemorrhoidal disease, and similar. Another cause can be a functional disorder like diarrhea, IBD, radiation proctitis, rectal neoplasm, and psychiatric disorders. Neurologic disorders like pudendal neuropathy, multiple sclerosis, dementia, spina bifida, and diabetic neuropathy can also lead to FI.

To objectify the extent of incontinence, a large number of clinical scores have been developed. An example of a widely used scoring system is the Wexner or Cleveland Clinic Florida Incontinence Score, which evaluates the frequency of five parameters, namely incontinence for solid stool, liquid stool, gas, usage of protective pads and lifestyle alteration. To each of the categories listed a grade from 0 to 4 can be attributed. The results range from 0 (perfect continence) to 20 (total incontinence). The Vaizey, also known as St. Mark's Incontinence Score, also considers three types of leakage (solid stool, liquid stool, gas) and alteration of lifestyle [7, 8].

Each of these categories is graded based on frequency. The need to wear a pad or plug, the consummation of constipating medicines, and inability to defer evacuation for 15 minutes are answered in binary terms just by yes and no. A total score of 0 represents total continence, while a score of 24 means complete incontinence [9]. Additional scores like fecal incontinence severity index (FISI) [10], Rapid Assessment Fecal Incontinence Score [11], and others are described in **Table 1** [9].

2.1.1 Physical examination

A thorough and detailed physical examination is mandatory to get a complete insight into the patient's situation and decide the next diagnostic or therapeutic step. The examination starts with the inspection of the perianal and perineal areas. Episiotomy scars, keyhole deformities (a groove in the anal canal following fistula or fissure treatment), or skin changes due to constant soiling should be visible immediately. During a Valsalva maneuver, a rectal or vaginal prolapse may be visible. The anocutaneous reflex, which evaluates the perianal sensation and has the afferent and efferent pathways in the pudendal nerve, can be elicited by stroking the perianal skin and observing an anal sphincter contraction. The absence of this reflex indicates an anomaly at the S4 level. The next step is a digital rectal examination (DRE), during which the tone and function of the anal sphincter is assessed. The puborectalis function may also be examined by placing the finger at the top of the anal canal and feeling an elevation of the finger with the contraction of the muscle. During DRE, care must be taken to palpate for a tumor or impacted stool in the anal canal. In female patients, especially if there is a history of obstetric trauma, the integrity of the rectovaginal septum and perineal body must be examined. The clinician may feel a discontinuity resulting from a rectovaginal fistula. If the examiner is able to push the vaginal wall outside through the introitus while performing a DRE, a diagnosis of rectocele can be made. Finally, it is recommended to perform anoscopy for hemorrhoidal disease or the presence of fistulas and mucosal inflammation. Flexible sigmoidoscopy may reveal proctitis, secretory adenomas, or rectal cancer. If there is any suspicion of colon cancer during history, taking a complete colonoscopy is preferred [12].

Fecal incontinence scoring systems		
Name	**Parameters assessed**	**Result**
Pescatori incontinence score	Severity and frequency of incontinence for flatus, liquid, and solid stool	0 (complete continence)–6 (complete incontinence)
Wexner/Cleveland Clinic Florida Incontinence Score	Frequency of incontinence to gas, solid and liquid stool as well as lifestyle alteration, and pad-wearing	0 (complete continence)–20 (complete incontinence)
Fecal Incontinence Severity Index—FISI	Frequency of incontinence to gas, solid and liquid stool, and mucus	0 (complete continence)–61 (severe incontinence)
St. Mark's/Vaizey Incontinence Score	Frequency of incontinence to gas, solid and liquid stool, lifestyle alteration, necessity to wear a plug or pad, lack of ability to defer defecation for 15 minutes, constipating medicines consumption	0 (perfect continence)–24 (complete incontinence)
Rapid Assessment Fecal Incontinence Score	Frequency of incontinence to gas, solid and liquid stool, urgency, social and emotional impact	0 (complete continence and no impact)–18 (severe incontinence and significant impact)

Table 1.
Most used scoring systems.

2.1.2 Objective testing

A final diagnostic phase includes objective testing of the sphincter integrity and anorectal function, and it includes radiologic and anorectal physiology testing. This phase will be necessary in most patients that require surgical therapy and in cases in which the history and physical examination did not reveal the etiology of fecal incontinence.

2.1.2.1 Endoanal ultrasound

Considered the golden standard for sphincter evaluation, endoanal ultrasound has been gaining popularity since its first use in the 1990s by Law and Bartram. Many studies have described a 100% sensitivity in identifying defects of the anal sphincter [13].

The study is performed using a 360° rotating transducer with high resolution. Newer probes allow for a 3D representation of the scanned area. During the evaluation, an area from the upper part of the puborectalis muscle to the anal margin is taken into consideration. The layers seen on the screen depend on the level at which the probe is inserted, but generally, the internal anal sphincter is seen as a hypoechoic circular structure, while the external anal sphincter is seen as hyperechoic. Another distinct structure that can be identified is the muscle in the upper third of the anal canal, as well as the mucosa and subepithelial tissue [14]. A less invasive alternative to endoanal ultrasound may be transvaginal (TVUS) or transperineal ultrasound (TPUS). A review found that the incidence of occult anal sphincter damage in primiparous women is comparable between EAUS and TVUS (29%) but is significantly lower with TPUS (7.9%) [14].

TPUS, however, has a possibility of dynamic imaging, which can reveal the presence of a rectocele or enterocele during a Valsalva maneuver. The learning curve is greater in TPUS than in endoanal ultrasound since the scanned area is more complex (**Figure 1**) [15] .

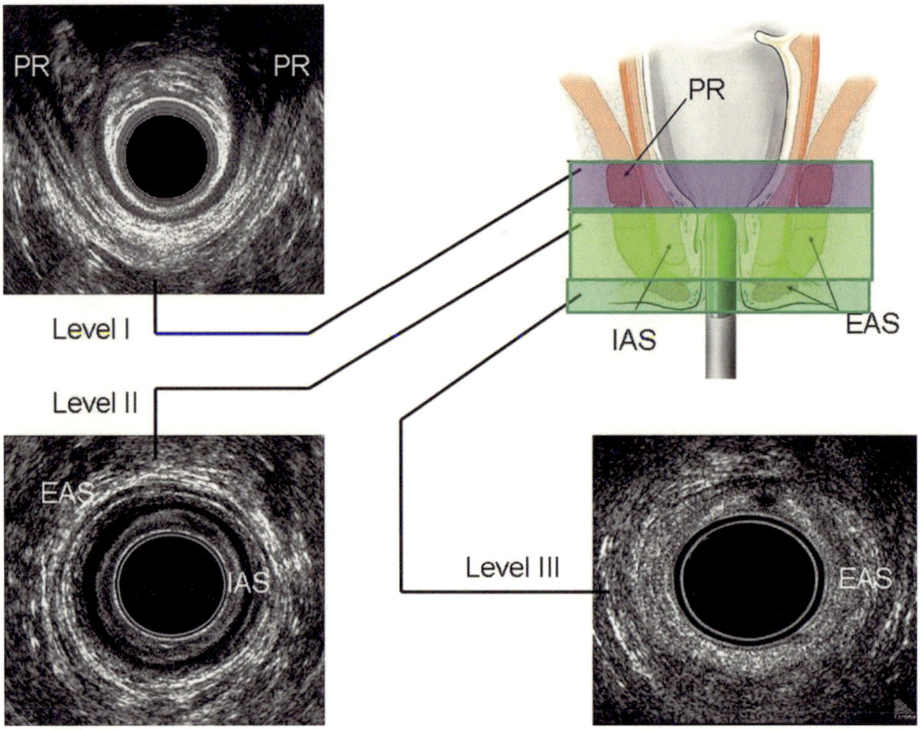

Figure 1.
Normal ultrasonographic anatomy of the anal canal. EAS, external anal sphincter; IAS, internal anal sphincter; PR, puborectalis muscle (with permission of Prof. Giulio A. Santoro).

2.1.2.2 Pudendal nerve terminal motor latency (PNTML)

To assess the integrity of the pudendal nerve, which brings motor innervation to the external anal sphincter as well as sensory innervation to the perineum, the pudendal nerve terminal motor latency is measured. The pudendal nerve may be injured by excessive traction, for example, during childbirth or if rectal prolapse is present. The test is conducted *via* an electrode mounted on the examiner's finger, which stimulates the pudendal nerve at the level of the ischial spine and then measures the activity of the external anal sphincter. Studies have shown that this method does not adequately address the pudendal nerve integrity since it depends on the fastest nerve fibers, which are less prone to injury; thus, it is not routinely administered [16, 17].

Back in 1993, Vernava et al. explained in their article the importance of electromyography (EMG) evaluation of fecal incontinence. They concluded that electromyographic examination specifically measuring PNTML is the best way to tell whether the patient has a neuropathy [18].

2.1.2.3 Defecography

Defecography is a radiologic study used to investigate pelvic floor anomalies such as a prolapse, rectocele or enterocele or postural instability. It can be performed by fluoroscopy or by means of MRI. The patient is administered a contrast enema (either barium paste or gadolinium), and real-time scans are recorded during defecation.

Additionally, an oral contrast solution or vaginal contrast may be used to opacify the small bowel or vagina. Although MRI defecography has the advantage of eliminating radiation, its use is limited by availability, non-physiological prone positioning (except in open MRI machines), and time consumption [19].

2.1.2.4 Manometry

Anorectal manometry is a noninvasive test of the anal sphincter function and the rectal sensitivity. The test can be done as an outpatient procedure and is conducted by placing a probe inside the patients' rectum. The equipment used varies according to the manufacturer but is usually comprised of a probe that contains sensors, a catheter that can be solid state, water perfused, or air charged, a balloon to test rectal sensitivity, and software to incorporate and analyze all the collected data.

Initially, there was no agreed protocol for anorectal manometry, but in 2019, the International Anorectal Physiology Working Group (IAPWG) released a standardized protocol for anorectal manometry [20].

The London classification describes several diagnoses based on the finding of high-resolution Anorectal Manometry Measures (HR-ARM). These diagnoses can be classified into four groups as follows:

1. Disorder of the rectoanal inhibitory reflex

2. Disorders of the anal tone and contractility

3. Disorders of rectoanal coordination

4. Disorders of rectal sensation

The results can then be subdivided into major, minor, and inconclusive findings based on their clinical relevance. Major findings are defined as manometry patterns that are not present in healthy individuals and can then be understood as causative of the patients' symptoms. They include rectoanal areflexia, anal hypotension with normal contractility, anal normotension with anal hypocontractility, combined anal hypotension and hypocontractility, rectal hyposensitivity, and rectal hypersensitivity. Minor findings like anal hypertension, abnormal expulsion with poor propulsion, abnormal expulsion with dyssynergia, and abnormal expulsion with poor propulsion and dyssynergia are patterns seen in symptomatic patients and occasionally in healthy individuals. Inconclusive findings are manometric patterns seen in symptomatic patients and in healthy people and their contribution to the symptomatology is yet to be defined. These findings include abnormal expulsion with normal manometric pattern of rectoanal coordination, normal expulsion with abnormal manometric pattern of rectoanal coordination, and borderline rectal hyposensitivity [21].

3. Treatment

Treatment of fecal incontinence should be individualized based on the types of symptoms and how much it affects patients' quality of life. The first step is usually a conservative treatment, which includes different dietary therapeutic strategies, pharmacological therapy, or biofeedback therapy.

3.1 Medical therapy

Medical treatment focuses on controlling diarrhea by slowing down or thickening the stool using agents like loperamide or diphenoxylate plus atropine. Loperamide decreases intestinal motility and secretion, while diphenoxylate with atropine slows down intestinal transit, similar to narcotics such as morphine. Together with dietary regimens and fiber intake, it can help with forming bulky stools.

3.2 Biofeedback

Biofeedback therapy has an impact on the voluntary phase of defecation by enhancing the sensation and tonus of the external anal sphincter muscle to keep the stool inside the rectum. This is accomplished by the instillation of progressively smaller quantities of air into a rectal balloon or anal plug, with the patient simultaneously monitoring the procedure. Patients then perceive rectal distension and coordinate contractions of pelvic floor muscles. In a retrospective study by Byrne et al. more than 70% of 513 patients treated with biofeedback therapy demonstrated improved short-term outcomes [22]. Biofeedback is painless, noninvasive, relatively inexpensive, and risk-free.

3.3 Injectable anal bulking agents

Injection of a bulking agent into the anal submucosal or intersphincteric space may theoretically help to increase resting pressures by augmenting the anal cushions or restoring anal symmetry (**Figure 2**). In 2011, the dextranomer-hyaluronic acid gel was approved by the United States Food and Drug Administration (FDA) in adult patients who have failed conservative therapy. Graf W et al., in their randomized controlled trial with 206 patients, compared injection with dextranomer-hyaluronic acid

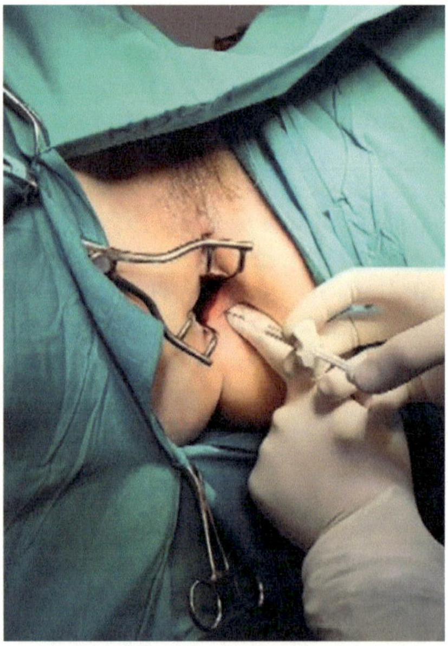

Figure 2.
Bulking agents procedure in CHC Rijeka.

with sham injections of no substance. After 6 months of follow-up, 52% of patients in the active treatment arm reported a 50% or greater reduction in incontinence episodes, compared with 32% in the sham arm [23].

There are debates about its efficiency. In a randomized, single-blinded, controlled trial by Dehli et al. in 2013, the efficacy of anal injections and biofeedback in treating anal incontinence did not differ [24].

This therapy is simpler and can be offered in outpatient settings. For better results, repeated injections may be necessary.

3.4 Sacral nerve stimulation (SNS)

Initially developed for urinary incontinence, sacral nerve stimulation has gained popularity and slowly became the first treatment option for selected candidates after its FDA approval in 2011.

The mechanism of action is explained in pertinent neuroanatomy and neurophysiology related to SNS. The mechanism of action, from a neurophysiological point of view, resides in the spinal cord and can be awakened by somatic and visceral afferent nerve stimulations [25–27].

Efferent outflow to the lower urinary tract is influenced by both spinal and brain input. Afferent pathways from the pelvic organs and somatic sensations from the perineum play a key role in regulating voiding [28–30].

Somatic afferents in the pudendal nerves transmit signals from the genital organs, urethra, prostate, and skin, modulating bladder function. Bladder afferents, which include A-delta fibers and C-fibers, send signals about bladder fullness and discomfort. A-delta fibers detect bladder wall tension, while C-fibers signal pain, especially during infections. C-fibers also contribute to reflex voiding, acting as a defense mechanism to eliminate irritants [28]. In conditions like spinal cord injury or multiple sclerosis, C-fiber dysfunction can trigger bladder hyperactivity and incontinence. This may be linked to the re-emergence of primitive reflexes or new reflex circuits and can potentially be treated by blocking C-fiber activity [31].

The procedure consists of placing an electrode using Selinger's technique under fluoroscopic guidance. The wire is placed in the foramina of the sacrum. Since sacral nerves have fibers that contribute to the innervation of the lower extremity as well as the pelvic floor, it is not uncommon during implantation to witness leg movements and pelvic floor muscle contractions. The surgeon must choose the foramina, which results in the lowest stimulation of the leg and the highest stimulation of the pelvic floor, and it is usually S3 (**Figure 3**).

During phase one of the procedure, the electrode wire is connected to a temporary generator, which can be regulated in an outpatient clinic. It is kept for 2–3 weeks, and the patient is asked to keep an incontinence journal. If the patient experiences a significant quality of life improvement and reduction of at least 50% of incontinence episodes, phase two of the procedure follows, during which a permanent stimulator is implanted subcutaneously. In today's market, there are different stimulators with either rechargeable or non-rechargeable batteries from which the patient can choose.

Recently, a one-phase procedure has been proposed in selected patients. In a study by Duelund-Jakobsen et al., 73 patients were offered an alternative technique consisting of a one-stage implant based on parameters measured intraoperatively. Ninety-two percent of patients experienced a reduction of at least 50% of incontinence episodes at a 23-week follow-up [32].

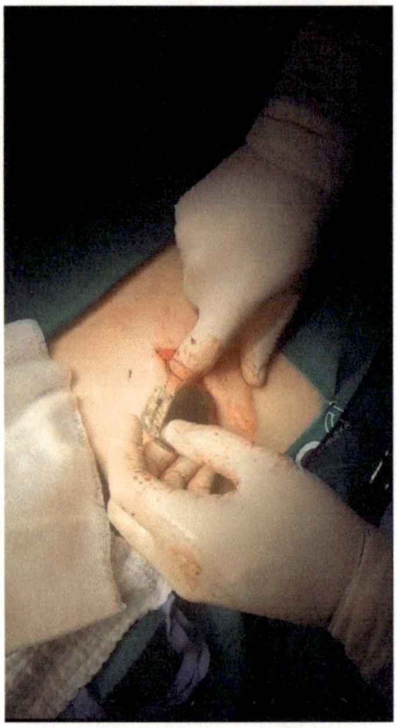

Figure 3.
Sacral nerve stimulator (SNS) placement in CHC Rijeka.

In a study by Wexner et al., from 2010, 120 patients received permanent implantation of the sacral nerve stimulator. After a period of 1 year, 83% of the patients had achieved therapeutic success, and 41% achieved complete continence [33].

SNS is a safe and potentially reversible treatment option with complications mainly consisting of pain at the implantation site and infection. These complications are treated by removal of the implant and infection control. After the infection has cleared, a new implantation can be attempted.

3.5 Sphincter reconstruction surgery

Sphincter defects most often occur during childbirth in the delivery room. The rupture of the sphincter is usually located at the thinnest anterior part. If such an injury is identified, a primary apposition with sutures can be attempted; however, if there is an infection, an associated severe pelvic injury, or if the patient is unstable, the sphincter repair is usually delayed. A diverting stoma to help clear the infection may be performed. The technique of overlapping anterior sphincteroplasty is performed with the patient in a jackknife or lithotomy position. Initially, a curvilinear transverse perineal incision is made. A skin and subcutaneous tissue flap is raised to allow visualization of the two sphincter edges. The scar tissue at the sphincter muscle is not excised as it holds sutures better than the muscle fibers. The sphincter muscles are then mobilized, usually en-block (internal and external sphincter together), and an overlap is created (**Figure 4**). The muscles are sutured together using PDS or Vycril sutures. Many surgeons perform a levatoroplasty as well to fortify the perineal body. Finally, the incision is closed in a T fashion, suturing the anterior part vertically and posterior transversely. Overlapping anterior sphincteroplasty demonstrates initially satisfactory results, but as the follow-up period extends the success rate diminishes. In a study by Karoui et al., 49% of patients

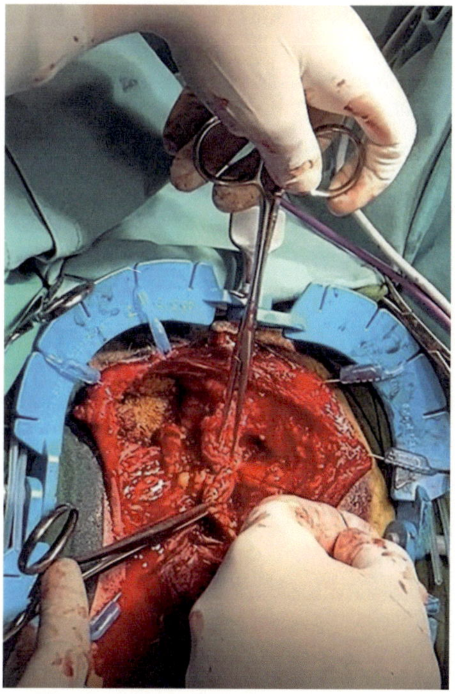

Figure 4.
Overlapping sphincteroplasty procedure in CHC Rijeka.

were completely continent at the 3-month follow-up, but only 28% at the 40-month follow-up [34]. Halverson and Hull showed that only 14% of patients were totally continent at a median of 69 months following sphincteroplasty [35]. Some surgeons opt to retry with sphincteroplasty after failure, but the results of a “redo sphincteroplasty” are also poor [36].

3.5.1 Dynamic (electrostimulated) graciloplasty

Graciloplasty, first described by Pickrell et al. over 50 years ago, has seen fluctuating popularity due to inconsistent results, mainly caused by reliance on the fatigable Type 2 muscle fibers for continence [37].

In the late 1980s, chronic muscle electrostimulation was introduced to convert these fibers into more fatigue-resistant Type 1 fibers suitable for sphincter function. Two methods of stimulation are used: intramuscular electrodes and direct stimulation of the neurovascular bundle, with intramuscular electrodes being more common due to their security [38, 39].

Dynamic graciloplasty has shown improvement in continence for over half of patients, with success rates ranging from 44% to 79% [40, 41].

The procedure has also been applied for anorectal reconstruction post-abdomiperineal resection (APER), but success rates are lower (40–80%), and complications, including infection and reoperations, are common [42–48].

Long-term outcomes of electrostimulation remain unclear, and studies in animal models suggest muscle degeneration may occur over time. Despite high costs, dynamic graciloplasty can be more cost-effective than stomas in some cases, though the cost of patient quality of life is difficult to quantify.

3.6 Malone anterograde continence enema (MACE) or appendicostomy

A right iliac fossa Gridiron incision is made, and if additional procedures are needed, a laparotomy is performed. The caecum and appendix are mobilized, preserving the blood supply to the appendix. The appendix is resected with a generous caecal cuff, and the caecal defect is closed. The distal end of the appendix is amputated. Patency is confirmed by catheter insertion into the appendix lumen [49].

A 5 cm submucosal tunnel is created in the caecum by sharp dissection of one taenia, and the mucosa is opened distally. The appendix is reversed and anastomosed to the caecal mucosa using absorbable sutures, ensuring a non-refluxing channel following the Mitrofanoff principle.

The stoma site is marked preoperatively. The appendix is brought through the abdominal wall, and the caecum is anchored to the anterior abdominal wall. A lateral skin flap is fashioned into a tube, anastomosed to the caecal cuff, to minimize discharge. This creates a continent stoma with a catheterizable channel for proximal colon access [50].

A catheter is left in place for 2–3 weeks to prevent kinking, and washouts can begin after 10 days without catheter removal. Saline irrigation is delivered *via* an intravenous set or with tap water containing salt (1 tsp. per pint) (**Figure 5**).

3.7 Diversion colostomy

When all other treatment options are depleted, the definitive therapy is diverting the fecal stream. The best solution for many patients is terminal sigmodostomy. While

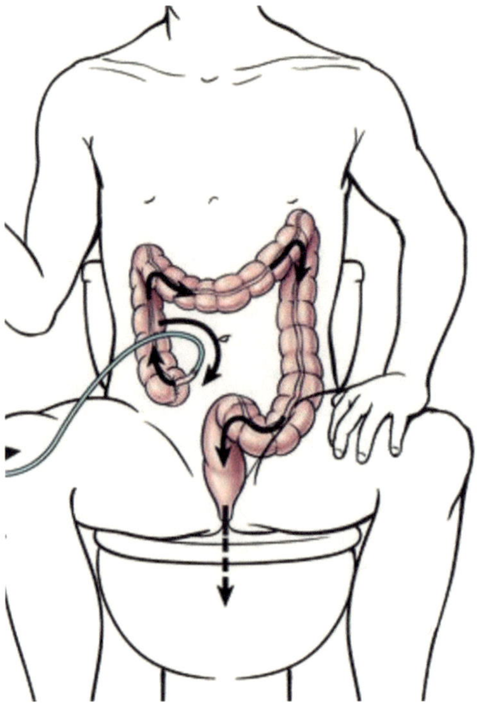

Figure 5.
MACE procedure.

many patients are reluctant to this treatment, they need to be educated by enterostomal therapist and explained the benefits of having a pouchable stoma on the abdomen than having unpouchable stoma between the buttocks.

3.8 Treatment approach in University Hospital Centre Rijeka

In our institution, we adopt a patient-centered approach to the management of fecal incontinence, recognizing that therapeutic strategies must be tailored to individual patient needs. Not all treatment modalities are universally applicable, and thus, a stepwise approach is employed to optimize patient outcomes.

Our initial therapeutic strategy focuses on conservative measures, which include dietary modifications, optimization of bowel habits using medications such as loperamide and micro-enema program, and targeted pelvic floor muscle training. These interventions aim to enhance sphincter function and improve continence, as well as control bowel movements. A key aspect of our conservative approach is patient education and destigmatization, as psychological barriers often hinder open discussions about symptoms. By normalizing the condition within the healthcare system and fostering a supportive environment, we encourage patients to articulate their concerns comprehensively, thereby facilitating more accurate diagnosis and treatment planning.

For patients who exhibit insufficient improvement with conservative measures, we proceed with minimally invasive therapeutic options. One such intervention involves the local injection of bulking agents, which have demonstrated promising efficacy in select patient populations especially those who suffer from inadequate function of internal anal sphincter muscle (responsible for resting anal pressure). These agents augment the volume and rigidity of the anal canal, thereby enhancing sphincter competence. While our experience suggests favorable outcomes in a subset of patients, further research is warranted to refine patient selection criteria and optimize long-term efficacy. Even though it is not first option in treatment for LARS syndrome, according to our experience some patients can have benefits after this treatment.

In cases where minimally invasive interventions yield suboptimal results, sacral neuromodulation (SNM) is considered for patients meeting the established very rigorous criteria. SNM modulates neural pathways governing anorectal function, offering significant symptomatic relief in appropriately selected individuals.

For patients who fail to achieve satisfactory continence with the aforementioned therapies, the formation of a permanent colostomy is presented as a definitive treatment option. This decision is made in close collaboration with the patient, taking into account their quality of life, comorbidities, and personal preferences. Our institution places a strong emphasis on perioperative counseling, ensuring that patients are well-informed and psychologically prepared for this transition. An important role in treating those patients is to have educated stoma therapists, which are specially educated nurses.

The successful management of fecal incontinence necessitates a multidisciplinary approach. We work in close collaboration with gastroenterologists, specialized stoma care nurses, psychologists, physical medicine and rehabilitation specialists, and radiologists to ensure comprehensive patient care. Our stoma care team plays a pivotal role in patient education and postoperative support, significantly improving patient adaptation and quality of life.

By integrating conservative, minimally invasive, and surgical approaches within a multidisciplinary framework, we strive to provide optimal, individualized care for patients with fecal incontinence. Future advancements in treatment modalities, patient selection algorithms, and long-term outcome assessments will further refine our approach, ultimately enhancing patient-centered care in this challenging clinical domain.

4. Discussion

Fecal incontinence (FI) is a complex condition that significantly affects individuals' physical, psychological, and social well-being. Its diverse etiology and impact on quality of life make it a challenging condition to address both from a diagnostic and therapeutic standpoint. As the prevalence of fecal incontinence increases, particularly among older adults and women, understanding the complexities of its classification, diagnosis, and treatment has become increasingly critical for improving patient outcomes.

The introduction to FI highlights the critical need for appropriate terminology and classification of the disorder. The distinction between retentive and nonretentive forms of FI, as outlined in the Rome IV criteria, offers a more nuanced approach to understanding the disorder, facilitating better treatment strategies. The condition's multifactorial nature, stemming from neurological, musculoskeletal, structural, and functional causes, underscores the importance of individualized treatment plans. However, while these classifications help guide clinical decision-making, they also emphasize the need for comprehensive evaluation, given that each patient's experience with FI may differ significantly in severity and underlying cause.

The impact of FI on quality of life is profound. As mentioned in the introduction, the emotional and psychological distress caused by FI can be as debilitating as its physical symptoms. The fear of social stigma and embarrassment leads many patients to avoid discussing their symptoms, resulting in delayed diagnoses and a prolonged course of suffering. Studies have consistently shown that individuals with FI report significantly lower quality-of-life scores, particularly in domains such as physical functioning, emotional well-being, and social interactions. The psychological burden can lead to social isolation, depression, and a diminished sense of self-worth. This highlights the importance of not only addressing the physical aspects of FI but also providing psychological and emotional support to affected individuals.

The diagnostic evaluation of FI, as detailed in the paper, emphasizes the necessity of a comprehensive approach. A thorough history and physical examination are crucial in uncovering potential causes, such as obstetric trauma, anorectal surgery, neurological disorders, and chronic gastrointestinal issues. Tools such as the Wexner and Vaizey scores aid in quantifying the severity of incontinence, but more objective tests like endoanal ultrasound, anorectal manometry, and defecography are often required to assess the structural and functional integrity of the anorectal region. The application of endoanal ultrasound, in particular, has been heralded as the gold standard for assessing sphincter integrity, with studies reporting high sensitivity in detecting anal sphincter defects. The ability to visualize defects, especially following obstetric trauma, offers invaluable information in tailoring interventions that may include surgical repair or biofeedback therapy.

However, despite the advances in diagnostic methods, challenges remain in identifying the precise etiology of fecal incontinence in some patients. A significant proportion of cases remain idiopathic, underscoring the complexity of the condition and the need for ongoing research into its pathophysiology. Furthermore, while diagnostic tools such as manometry and defecography provide essential insights into rectal function, the interpretation of results can be challenging due to variations in technique, patient compliance, and the complexity of anorectal function.

In terms of treatment, the paper highlights a range of options from conservative approaches to more invasive surgical interventions. Initial conservative treatments, including dietary modifications, pharmacological therapy, and biofeedback, can be effective for some individuals. Biofeedback, in particular, has shown promising results in improving sphincter function by enhancing the voluntary control of the external anal sphincter. Its noninvasive nature and positive short-term outcomes make it an attractive option for many patients.

For those who do not respond to conservative management, injectable anal bulking agents or sacral nerve stimulation (SNS) offer further options. Injectable agents such as dextranomer-hyaluronic acid gel have been FDA-approved and show efficacy in improving anal sphincter function and reducing incontinence episodes, though the debate over their long-term effectiveness persists. Sacral nerve stimulation, while a more invasive option, has gained widespread acceptance and FDA approval due to its ability to improve both the quality of life and the frequency of incontinence episodes. Although the exact mechanism remains unclear, the therapeutic success observed in patients who undergo SNS is promising, with significant improvements in clinical outcomes observed across multiple studies.

Sphincter reconstruction surgery, particularly in cases of obstetric trauma or anal sphincter defects, represents a more definitive approach. However, the success rates of sphincteroplasty diminish over time, with studies indicating a gradual decline in continence, even with well-conducted repairs. Given the limited long-term outcomes of surgical sphincter repair, further research is needed to refine surgical techniques and improve their efficacy.

When all other treatment options fail, diversion colostomy becomes the final therapeutic option. While a controversial solution, a colostomy provides an effective means of diverting the fecal stream, offering patients relief from the physical symptoms of FI. However, patient education is crucial, as many patients may initially be resistant to this approach due to the stigma associated with having a stoma. The role of enterostomal therapy and proper patient support is essential in ensuring that patients accept and adapt to the changes in their quality of life brought about by a stoma.

Ultimately, the treatment of fecal incontinence requires a multidisciplinary approach that considers not only the physical aspects of the disorder but also the psychological, social, and emotional impacts on the patient. The ongoing development of new diagnostic techniques and therapeutic options provides hope for improved management of this challenging condition. However, further research is needed to better understand the underlying causes, improve the long-term outcomes of treatments, and address the emotional burden that often accompanies this condition.

5. Conclusion

Fecal incontinence (FI) is a multifactorial condition with significant implications for an individual's physical, emotional, and social well-being. The classification of FI into various degrees of severity, such as minor, moderate, severe, and complete, underscores the diverse impact it has on affected individuals. Its etiology spans neurological, musculoskeletal, structural, and functional causes, each of which requires tailored diagnostic and therapeutic approaches.

The diagnostic process of FI relies heavily on thorough patient history, physical examination, and a range of objective tests, including endoanal ultrasound, manometry, and defecography. These diagnostic tools are essential for identifying the underlying cause and informing the treatment plan. Despite the availability of advanced diagnostic techniques, FI remains underreported due to the associated stigma, contributing to delays in diagnosis and treatment.

Treatment strategies for FI are primarily focused on symptom management and improving quality of life. Conservative options such as medical therapy, biofeedback, and injectable bulking agents are often effective for patients with less severe symptoms. For more severe cases, interventions like sacral nerve stimulation and sphincter reconstruction surgery have shown promising results, although their long-term success can be variable. In cases where conservative and surgical treatments fail, a diversion colostomy may offer a definitive solution.

In conclusion, the management of fecal incontinence is complex and should be personalized based on the severity of symptoms, the underlying cause, and the patient's preferences. Timely diagnosis and appropriate intervention are critical for improving the quality of life of those affected by this debilitating condition. Further research into the long-term efficacy of available treatments and the development of less invasive interventions is necessary to optimize care for individuals suffering from fecal incontinence.

Author details

Damir Karlović, Lucia Klarica*, Dorian Kršul, Nikola Simičić, Ante Jerković, Mario Milotić and Marko Zelić
Department of Digestive Surgery, Centre for Digestive and Metabolic Medicine, University Hospital Rijeka, Croatia

*Address all correspondence to: lklarica@gmail.com

References

[1] Andrews Christine B, Kasper V. Fecal Incontinence (Encopresis). Ferri's Clinical Advisor. 2025;**447**:e1-447.e2

[2] Bharucha AE, Fletcher JG, Harper CM, et al. Relationship between symptoms and disordered continence mechanisms in women with idiopathic fecal incontinence. Gut. 2005;**54**:546-555

[3] Heymen S, Palsson O, Simren M, et al. Patient preferences for endpoints in fecal incontinence treatment studies. Neurogastroenterology and Motility. 2017;**29**:e13032

[4] Bordeianou L, Amy T, Keller D, et al. The American Society of colon and rectal surgeons' clinical practice guidelines for the management of fecal incontinence. Diseases of the Colon and Rectum. 2023;**66**:647-661

[5] Bharucha AE, Dunivan G, Goode PS, et al. Epidemiology, pathophysiology, and classification of fecal incontinence: State of the science summary for the national institute of diabetes and digestive and kidney diseases (NIDDK) workshop. The American Journal of Gastroenterology. 2015;**110**:127-136

[6] Thekkinkattil DK, Lim M, Stojkovic SG, et al. A classification system for faecal incontinence based on anorectal investigations. The British Journal of Surgery. 2008;**95**:222-228

[7] Jorge JM, Wexner SD. Etiology and management of fecal incontinence. Diseases of the Colon and Rectum. 1993;**36**:77-97

[8] Vaizey CJ, Carapeti E, Cahill JA, Kamm MA. Prospective comparison of faecal incontinence grading systems. Gut. 1999;**44**:77-80

[9] Liptak P, Duricek M, Banovcin P. Diagnostic tools for fecal incontinence: Scoring systems are the crucial first step. World Journal of Gastroenterology. 2024;**30**(6):516-522

[10] Rockwood TH, Church JM, Fleshman JW, Kane RL, Mavrantonis C, Thorson AG, et al. Patient and surgeon ranking of the severity of symptoms associated with fecal incontinence: The fecal incontinence severity index. Diseases of the Colon and Rectum. 1999;**42**(12):1525-1532

[11] de la Portilla F, Calero-Lillo A, Jiménez-Rodríguez RM, Reyes ML, Segovia-González M, Maestre MV, et al. Validation of a new scoring system: Rapid assessment faecal incontinence score. World Journal of Gastrointestinal Surgery. 2015;7(9):203-207

[12] Bliss D, Mimura T, Berghmans B, et al. Clinical assessment, conservative management, specialized diagnostic testing, and quality of life for fecal incontinence: Update on research and practice recommendations. Continence. 2024;**9**:101063. ISSN:2772-9737. Available from: https://www.sciencedirect.com/science/article/pii/S2772973723009219

[13] Albuquerque A. Endoanal ultrasonography in fecal incontinence: Current and future perspectives. World Journal of Gastrointestinal Endoscopy. 2015;7(6):575-581

[14] Santoro GA, Pelizzo P, Grossi U, Cian R, Zanus G, Brusciano L. Role of ultrasonography for anal incontinence. In: Docimo L, Brusciano L, editors. Anal Incontinence. Updates in Surgery. Springer; 10 October 2023

[15] Abdool Z, Sultan AH, Thakar R. Ultrasound imaging of the anal sphincter

complex: A review. The British Journal of Radiology. 2012;**85**(1015):865-875

[16] Sultan AH, Monga A, Lee J, Emmanuel A, Norton C, Santoro G, et al. An International Urogynecological Association (IUGA)/International Continence Society (ICS) joint report on the terminology for anorectal dysfunction in women. International Urogynecology Journal. 2017;**28**(1):5-31

[17] Hibner M, Desai N, Robertson LJ, et al. Pudendal neuralgia. Journal of Minimally Invasive Gynecology. 2010;**17**:148-153

[18] Vernava AM III, Longo WE, Daniel GL. Pudendal neuropathy and the importance of EMG evaluation of fecal incontinence. Diseases of the Colon & Rectum;**36**(1):23-27

[19] Kim AY. How to interpret a functional or motility test—Defecography. Journal of Neurogastroenterology and Motility. 2011;**17**(4):416-420

[20] Carrington EV, Heinrich H, Knowles CH, Fox M, Rao S, Altomare DF, et al. The international anorectal physiology working group (IAPWG) recommendations: Standardized testing protocol and the London classification for disorders of anorectal function. Neurogastroenterology and Motility. 2020;**32**(1):e13679

[21] Scott SM, Carrington EV. The London classification: Improving characterization and classification of anorectal function with anorectal manometry. Current Gastroenterology Reports. 2020;**22**(11):55

[22] Byrne CM, Solomon MJ, Young JM, Rex J, Merlino CL. Biofeedback for fecal incontinence: Short-term outcomes of 513 consecutive patients and predictors of successful treatment. Diseases of the Colon and Rectum. 2007;**50**(4): 417-427

[23] Graf W, Mellgren A, Matzel KE, Hull T, Johansson C, Bernstein M, et al. Efficacy of dextranomer in stabilised hyaluronic acid for treatment of faecal incontinence: A randomised, sham-controlled trial. Lancet. 2011;**377**(9770):997-1003

[24] Dehli T, Stordahl A, Vatten LJ, Romundstad PR, Mevik K, Sahlin Y, et al. Sphincter training or anal injections of dextranomer for treatment of anal incontinence: A randomized trial. Scandinavian Journal of Gastroenterology. 2013;**48**(3):302-310

[25] de Groat WC, Ryall RW. The identification and antidromic responses of sacral preganglionic parasympathetic neurons. Journal of Physiology (London). 1968;**196**:533

[26] de Groat WC, Ryall RW. Recurrent inhibition in sacral parasympathetic pathways to the bladder. Journal of Physiology (London). 1968;**196**:579

[27] de Groat WC. Nervous control of the urinary bladder of the cat. Brain Research. 1975;**87**:201

[28] Yoshimura N, de Groat WC. Neural control of the lower urinary tract. International Journal of Urology. 1997;**4**:111

[29] de Groat WC. Central nervous system control of micturition. In: O'Donnell PD, editor. Urinary in-Continence. St. Louis (MO): Mosby; 1997. pp. 33-47

[30] de Groat WC, Araki I, Vizzard MA, et al. Developmental and injury induced plasticity in the micturition reflex

pathway. Behavioural Brain Research. 1997;**92**:127

[31] de Groat WC. Changes in the organization of the micturition reflex pathway of the cat after transection of the spinal cord. In: Veraa RP, Grafstein B, editors. Cellular Mechanisms for Recovery from Nervous Systems Injury: A Conference Report. Experimental Neurology. Vol. 71. 1981. p. 22

[32] Duelund-Jakobsen J, Buntzen S, Lundby L, Laurberg S, Sørensen M, Rydningen M. One-stage implant in sacral neuromodulation for faecal incontinence—Short-term outcome from a prospective study. Colorectal Disease. 2024;**26**:968-973

[33] Wexner SD, Coller JA, Devroede G, Hull T, McCallum R, Chan M, et al. Sacral nerve stimulation for fecal incontinence: Results of a 120-patient prospective multicenter study. Annals of Surgery. 2010;**251**(3):441-449

[34] Karoui S, Leroi AM, Koning E, Menard JF, Michot F, Denis P. Results of sphincteroplasty in 86 patients with anal incontinence. Diseases of the Colon and Rectum. 2000;**43**(6):813-820

[35] Halverson AL, Hull TL. Long-term outcome of overlapping anal sphincter repair. Diseases of the Colon and Rectum. 2002;**45**(3):345-348

[36] Hong K, Dasilva G, Dollerschell JT, Maron D, Wexner SD. Redo sphincteroplasty: Are the results sustainable? Gastroenterology Report. 2016;**4**(1):39-42

[37] Pickrell KL, Broadbent TR, Masters FW, Metzger JT. Construction of a rectal sphincter and restoration of anal continence by transplanting the gracilis muscle: A report of four cases in children. Annals of Surgery. 1952;**135**:853-862

[38] Salmons S, Vrbová G. The influence of activity on some contractile characteristics of mammalian fast and slow muscles. The Journal of Physiology. 1969;**201**(3):535-549

[39] Hallan RI, Williams NS, Hutton MR, Scott M, Pilot MA, Swash M, et al. Electrically stimulated sartorius neo-sphincter: Canine model of activation and skeletal muscle transformation. The British Journal of Surgery. 1990;**77**(2):208-213

[40] Madoff RD, Rosen HR, Baeten CG, LaFontaine LJ. Safety and efficacy of dynamic muscle plasty for anal incontinence: Lessons from a prospective, multicenter trial. Gastroenterology. 1999;**116**(3):549-556

[41] Altomare DF, Rinaldi M, Pannarale OC, Memeo V. Electrostimulated gracilis neosphincter for faecal incontinence and in total anorectal reconstruction: Still an experimental procedure? International Journal of Colorectal Disease. 1997;**12**(5):308-312

[42] Seccia M, Menconi C, Balestri R, Cavina E. Study protocols and functional results in 86 electrostimulated graciloplasties. Diseases of the Colon and Rectum. 1994;**37**(9):897-904

[43] Mander BJ, Abercrombie J, George B, Williams NS. The electrically stimulated gracilis neosphincter incorporated as part of total anorectal reconstruction after abdominoperineal excision of the rectum. Annals of Surgery. 1996;**224**(6):702-711

[44] Geerdes BP, Zoetmulder FA, Heineman E, Vos EJ, Rongen MJ, Baeten CG. Total anorectal

reconstruction with a double dynamic graciloplasty after abdominoperineal reconstruction for low rectal cancer. Diseases of the Colon and Rectum. 1997;**40**(6):698-705

[45] Rosen HR, Novi G, Zoech G, Feil W, Urbarz C, Schiessel R. Restoration of anal sphincter function by single-stage dynamic graciloplasty with a modified (split sling) technique. American Journal of Surgery. 1998;**175**(3):187-193

[46] Rullier E, Laurent C, Zerbib F, Garrelon JL, Caudry M, Saric J. Anorectal reconstruction by coloperineal anastomosis and dynamic double graciloplasty after abdominoperineal resection [English abstract]. Annales de Chirurgie. 1998;**52**(9):905-912

[47] Cavina E, Seccia M, Banti P, Zocco G. Anorectal reconstruction after abdominoperineal resection: Experience with double-wrap graciloplasty supported by low-frequency electrostimulation. Diseases of the Colon and Rectum. 1998;**41**(8):1010-1016

[48] Rouanet P, Senesse P, Bouamrirene D, Toureille E, Veyrac M, Astre C, et al. Anal sphincter reconstruction by dynamic graciloplasty after abdominoperineal resection for cancer. Diseases of the Colon and Rectum. 1999;**42**(4):451-456

[49] Malone PS, Ransley PG, Kiely EM. Preliminary report: The antegrade continence enema. The Lancet. 1990;**336**(8725):1217-1218

[50] Mitrofanoff P. Cystostomie continente trans-appendiculare dans le traitement des vessies neurologiques. Chirurgie Pédiatrique. 1980;**21**:297-305

Chapter 14

Internal Anal Sphincter Achalasia: A Rare Cause of Chronic Constipation

Farah Slaczka and Mateusz Slaczka

Abstract

Internal anal sphincter achalasia (IASA) is a rare anorectal disorder that presents as chronic refractory constipation in pediatrics. With poor response to conventional constipation-based therapy, it is often misdiagnosed as other conditions such as ultra-short segment Hirschsprung disease. A case report discussed in this chapter describes a rare case of IASA in an adolescent female, emphasizing the importance of ruling out other differentials including Hirschsprung disease via rectal biopsy, and thus allowing for early targeted therapy to improve lifestyle conditions. IASA's physiological basis involves altered innervation, absence of nitrergic nerves, and defective neuromuscular junctions in the internal anal sphincter. Diagnosis requires anorectal manometry and rectal suction biopsy. Treatment options include botulism toxin injections and posterior internal anal sphincter myectomy. Botulism injections offer temporary relief, while myectomy provides long-term improvement. Also discussed in this chapter are other disorders that must be ruled out before arriving at a diagnosis of IASA. These conditions include Hirschsprung's disease, congenital hypothyroidism, and functional constipation. These diseases can present with similar symptoms of chronic constipation in children, and therefore should be ruled out. Early recognition and diagnosis of IASA is crucial, given its potential misdiagnosis as any of these other conditions. Treatment decisions of IASA should consider the patient's age, symptoms, and response to conservative therapies. Diet changes that may help relieve symptoms of constipation are also discussed.

Keywords: chronic constipation, pediatrics, internal anal sphincter achalasia, gastroenterology, botulism toxin

1. Introduction

Anorectal disorders are relatively common in children, with constipation being the most prevalent. Initial presentations of constipation in children are typically handled conservatively with dietary changes, stool softeners, and laxatives. However, when constipation does not respond to conventional treatment methods, the underlying condition should be explored further. In a small subset of children with persistent constipation, the diagnosis of internal anal sphincter achalasia (IASA) has been made. This relatively rare condition is similar to Hirschsprung disease, with the major difference of having the presence of ganglionic cells in the rectum. Due to the similarity in patient presentation, some cases of IASA had been misdiagnosed as ultra-short segment Hirschsprung and treated surgically [1].

IASA is a relatively understudied topic and therefore the prevalence and incidence of this condition is not widely known. One report cites the incidence as 4.5% among children investigated for chronic constipation [2]. A retrospective study done in 2020 reviewed 1072 anorectal manometry studies (ARMs) done on children <18 years of age at the Nationwide Children's Hospital between August 2010 and April 2019. Of these reviewed ARMs, 109 patients had absent rectoanal inhibitory reflex (RAIR), which is the reflex that normally causes relaxation of the internal anal sphincter in response to distention of the rectum by gas or feces. Of these 109 patients with absent RAIR, 28 of them were diagnosed with IASA due to presence of ganglion cells on rectal biopsy, giving a less than 3% diagnosis rate of IASA among this study [3]. This case report focuses on an adolescent female patient who has suffered from chronic constipation since childhood and received the diagnosis of IASA in her teenage years, with limited relief of symptoms from semiannual botulism injections.

2. Case presentation

A 20-year-old female with a history of internal anal sphincter achalasia (IASA) presented to the pre-operative area of the hospital in June 2023 for her semiannual botulism toxin injections procedure. She last underwent Botox treatment in December 2022, after which she had significant relief of her constipation. However, over the last month she noticed increasing return of her constipation symptoms, with her last bowel movement being 6 days ago. Laxative therapy with Dulcolax and MiraLax provided her with no relief in the past few weeks. She has no other medical history and complained of no other symptoms.

The patient was initially referred for her symptoms of severe, refractory constipation to the Children's National Colorectal Center for further workup and diagnosis in December 2020. At that time, she was on Bisacodyl 20 mg and MiraLax 34 g daily, which enabled her to have a bowel movement approximately twice a week. In January of 2021, she underwent colonic and anorectal manometry with exam under anesthesia and Botox injection therapy. Post-Botox treatment, she was able to have a bowel movement every other day. She was also advised to take two tablets of 10 mg Dulcolax, which may be increased to three tablets the next day if constipation persists. In March 2021, she underwent contrast enema of the colon, which revealed a large colon and sigmoid colon with no transition zone identified, which ruled out a diagnosis of Hirschsprung disease (**Figure 1**). In a follow-up visit with the Colorectal Center in April of 2021, she described gradual return of her constipation symptoms, with her last bowel movement being 10 days ago. The colorectal surgeon and gastrointestinal motility specialist reviewed her medical history and manometry results and concluded that she has overall normal colonic manometry, but rectoanal inhibitory reflex was inconsistently seen. They recommended that a biopsy should be performed to make a diagnosis of internal anal sphincter achalasia.

A full-thickness rectal biopsy was performed in June 2021 by her local pediatric surgeon. The biopsy was approximately 1–1.5 cm proximal to the dentate line extending proximal towards the rectum. The specimen was secured to a tongue depressor and labeled proximal and distal. The specimen was sent to pathology for gross and

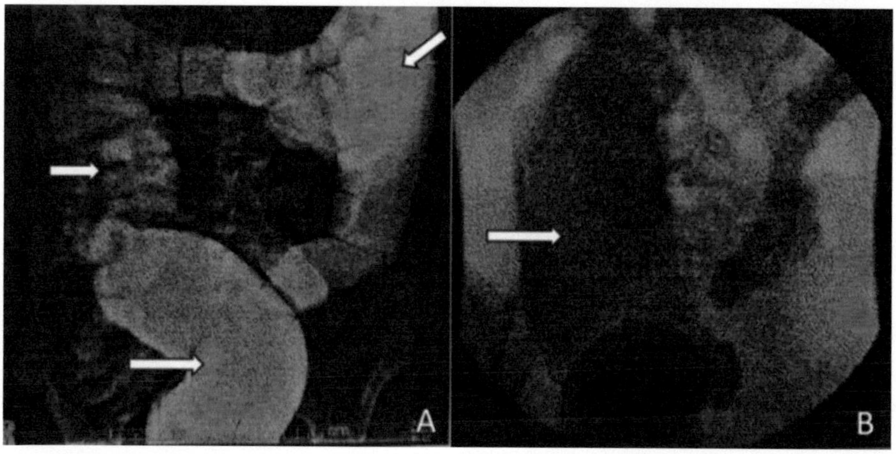

Figure 1.
(A/B) Contrast enema showed a large colon and sigmoid colon (A). No transition zone was identified to suggest Hirschsprung's disease. No clear obstructive lesions or strictures seen. Post evacuation film shows good evacuation of contrast from the colon (B). These findings are suggestive of IASA by eliminating other potential causes of chronic constipation. Source is Ref. [4].

microscopic analysis. Results of the biopsy showed presence of ganglionic cells, ruling out Hirschsprung and leading to a diagnosis of internal anal sphincter achalasia.

She has continued therapy with four quadrant injections of 100 units total of Botox (25 units in each quadrant) to treat her symptoms of intractable constipation at her local hospital. Each round of injections has provided her with relief of symptoms for approximately 6 months, with gradual return of constipation. Between injections, she takes two tablets of Dulcolax orally every evening, but will still go several days to a week without a bowel movement. She has had episodes of severe abdominal distention with associated pain as a result.

3. Pathophysiology of IASA

Internal anal sphincter achalasia was first described in 1958 by Davidson and Bauer, who reported three cases of constipation since birth with no zone of narrowing seen on barium enema. They also examined histological specimen samples of the colon and identified the presence of ganglia in all regions of the colon. They therefore described this phenomenon as "achalasia of the rectal distal segment." Over time, this terminology eventually changed to "ultra-short segment Hirschsprung disease" and finally to "internal anal sphincter achalasia" [5].

It is essential to understand the physiology and innervation of the internal anal sphincter to fully appreciate what occurs in IASA. The internal anal sphincter is crucial for fecal continence and responds to rectal distention via the rectosphincteric inhibitory reflex. Nitric oxide is a significant mediator to cause relaxation of the internal anal sphincter in response to adequate rectal distention. IASA may be the result of several pathological issues, including altered innervation, absence of nitrergic nerves, defective neuromuscular junctions, and abnormal distribution of interstitial cells of Cajal which are important for electrical pacemaker activity and neurotransmission. Absence of interstitial cells of Cajal (ICC) may result in impaired nitric-oxide mediated signaling resulting in a lack of relaxation to the internal anal sphincter. In one study done by Piotrowska et al. in 2003, they found that normal internal anal sphincter samples contained abundant and uniformly distributed peripherin-immunoreactive nerve fibers as well as a large number of ICC cells. In contrast, samples of the internal anal sphincter in patients with IASA has markedly reduced peripherin-immunoreactive nerve fibers and ICCs, while these nerve fibers and ICCs were absent or sparse in Hirschsprung disease patient samples [6]. Therefore, to make a definitive diagnosis of IASA, anorectal manometry and rectal suction biopsy are required to rule out other potential causes of chronic constipation in children [1].

4. Comparison of IASA with other causes of constipation

As internal anal sphincter achalasia is a diagnosis of exclusion, it is important to understand the key differences between IASA and other causes of constipation, particularly pediatric constipation. Two causes of pediatric constipation will be discussed here: Hirschsprung disease, congenital hypothyroidism, and functional constipation.

4.1 Hirschsprung disease

Hirschsprung disease is a congenital abnormality of the distal colon due to a lack of ganglion neural cells. There has been association of this disease with the male sex, Down syndrome, and MEN type 2 [7]. This disease is caused by a failure of enteric neural crest-derived cell proliferation, migration, or differentiation [8]. These enteric neural crest-derived cells must migrate rostrocaudally along the embryonic gut mesenchyme during development in order for the enteric nervous system to adequately innervate the gastrointestinal system. Hirschsprung disease is due to incomplete rostrocaudal migration of these cells, resulting in aganglionosis of the distal colon. The lack of neural cells disrupts the normal signaling that is required to ensure appropriate intestinal motility. Without adequate motility in the distal colon region, the result is fecal retention leading to constipation.

Patients typically present with symptoms such as delayed passing of meconium (not passed in the first 24 hours after birth) with explosive expulsion of feces upon rectal exam in neonates, while young children may present with chronic constipation and abdominal distention. The age on onset of symptoms depends on the severity of the colonic aganglionosis; more severe colonic involvement results in earlier onset of symptoms [9]. It can be more difficult to diagnose Hirschsprung disease in children ages 1–5 years who present with chronic constipation, due to the vast number of pathologies that may lead to pediatric constipation. Diagnostic workup includes abdominal x-ray, barium enema, and anorectal manometry, but the most accurate test is a rectal suction biopsy to confirm the absence of the Auerbach and Meissner plexuses [7]. The rectal biopsy is the main distinguishing feature between Hirschsprung disease and IASA, since in IASA there is presence of neural cells.

4.2 Congenital hypothyroidism

Congenital hypothyroidism is a disorder of the thyroid in neonates in which it does not produce sufficient amounts of T3 and T4. It is critical to diagnose this disorder early to avoid major complications such as cretinism, intellectual disability, and constipation. About 12% of babies born with congenital hypothyroidism suffer from constipation, and this condition can sometimes mimic the symptoms of Hirschsprung disease [10]. Some of other distinguishing symptoms of congenital hypothyroidism are the 6 Ps: pot-bellied, protruding umbilicus, pale, puffy-faced, protuberant tongue, and poor brain development [7].

This condition needs to be diagnosed in neonates as quickly as possible to avoid severe symptoms. Diagnostic workup includes measurement of TSH and T4 levels. A repeat workup is recommended in certain situations, such as infants with low-birth weight, preterm, and infants admitted into the neonatal intensive care unit. A confirmed diagnosis of congenital hypothyroidism is when labs show low free T4 and elevated TSH levels [11]. Treatment for this condition includes prompt administration of levothyroxine (T4), which may start to improve symptoms of constipation within a month. It is important to note that a large majority of patients born with congenital hypothyroidism show no or minimum symptoms, which emphasizes the importance of neonatal screenings for this disorder [10].

4.3 Functional constipation

Functional constipation is defined as infrequent or difficult bowel movements without any identifiable organic cause. Patients may also experience painful defecation, passing hard stools, and a sensation of incomplete bowel evacuation. This is a relatively common issue in the pediatric population, with peak incidence of constipation occurring between the ages of 2–4 years old [12]. There are a variety of causal events or triggers that can cause functional constipation in children. Some of these include toilet training, anxiety, starting preschool, dietary changes, fear of defecating in public places, and voluntary withholding while playing. Once the child holds onto the stool, the colon draws in more and more water from it, causing it to become drier and harder [13]. This leads to a cycle of constipation, due to the pain caused by passing hard stools. If this continues as a chronic cycle, the child's rectum will become full of hardened stool, which then leads to a decreased sensation of needing to defecate [13]. Oftentimes softer liquid stools can pass around the hard plug resulting in encopresis, and may cause embarrassment for the child.

To make a diagnosis of functional constipation, a thorough history and physical exam must be done. History should include duration of symptoms, consistency and frequency of stools, any associated life changes, and if there are any other associated symptoms such as abdominal pain, vomiting, or urinary symptoms [13]. Physical exam should include vitals, growth parameters, and assessment of possible causes of

For Infants up to 4 Years
Must include 1 month of at least 2 of the following or 2 or fewer defecations per week
1. History of excessive stool retention
2. History of painful or hard bowel movements
3. History of large-diameter stools
4. Presence of a large fecal mass in the rectum
In toilet-trained children, the following additional criteria may be used:
1. At least 1 episode/week of incontinence after the acquisition of toileting skills
2. History of large-diameter stools that may obstruct the toilet

Table 1.
Rome IV criteria for a diagnosis of functional constipation in infants-4 years old.

constipation such as hypothyroidism (exophthalmos and lid lag), appendicitis (pain on palpation of abdomen), or a neural tube defect such as myelomeningocele (hair tuft or dimples in the lumbar region). Once these other potential causes are ruled out, the Rome IV definition can be used to diagnose a child with functional constipation. These definitions can be seen in **Tables 1** and **2** [14]:

Some pediatricians recommend parents keep a stool diary of their child to track consistency and frequency of bowel movements to assist with the diagnosis of functional constipation. Another tool that can be used to assess fecal consistency is the Bristol stool scale (**Figure 2**), which categorizes 7 types of stool consistencies [15]:

For Children Older than 4 Years
Must include 2 or more of the following occurring at least once per week for a minimum of 1 month with insufficient criteria for a diagnosis of irritable bowel syndrome:
1. Two or fewer defecations in the toilet per week in a child of a developmental age of at least 4 years
2. At least 1 episode of fecal incontinence per week
3. History of retentive posturing or excessive volitional stool retention
4. History of painful or hard bowel movements
5. Presence of a large fecal mass in the rectum
6. History of large-diameter stools that can obstruct the toilet

Table 2.
Rome IV criteria for a diagnosis of functional constipation for children ages >4 years old.

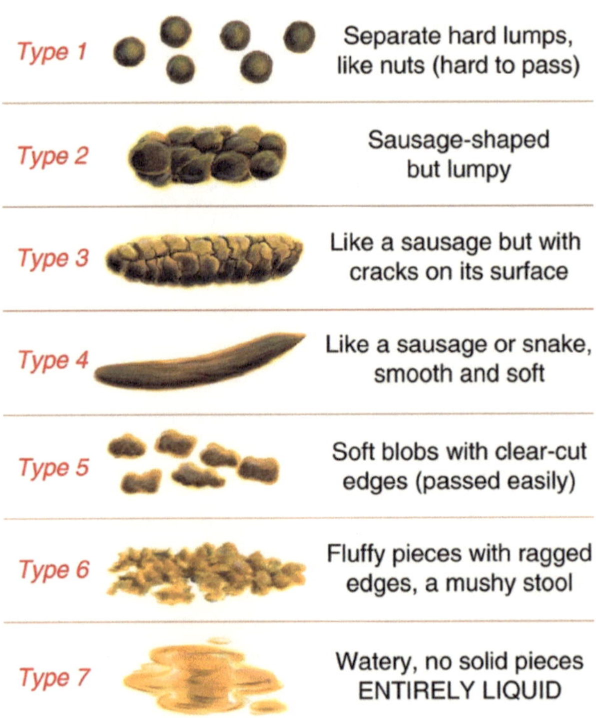

Figure 2.
Bristol stool scale.

Management of functional constipation starts with disimpaction, or the removal of the hardened stool from the child's bowel. First-line treatment for clearing of the fecal impaction is a solution of polyethylene glycol (PEG 3350), which may be taken in the outpatient setting over several hours. If there is no response to the solution after the second day of treatment, the child may require alternative method such as enema [13]. The second part of management is maintenance of soft stools, to avoid reaccumulation and rehardening of stools in the rectum. Oral administration of laxatives and stool softeners should be used; however, it is critical to advise parents to ensure the child has adequate fiber and fluid intake in their daily diet, along with regular physical activity [13].

5. Treatment options for IASA

Treatment options are currently limited to 4-quadrant botulism toxin injections and posterior internal anal sphincter myectomy. As was described previously in this case report, the patient only found relief of her constipation and abdominal bloating symptoms after receiving botulism toxin injections. While she schedules these injections biannually, she only finds significant relief of symptoms for approximately 4 months after the injections, after which she has gradual return of constipation and bloating despite use of various laxatives. There are several risk factors associated with botulism toxin injections, including urinary incontinence, pelvic muscle paresis, perianal abscess formation, pruritis ani, and rectal prolapse [16]. While the occurrence of these adverse effects is relatively rare, they are still important aspects to consider when deciding upon an appropriate treatment plan for patients with IASA.

The definitive treatment for IASA is posterior internal anal sphincter (IAS) myectomy. In a study done in 2000 by Caluwe et al., 15 patients between the ages of 2–12 with IASA underwent myectomy of the internal anal sphincter. Of these patients, seven had regular bowel movements without the use of laxatives, six stay regular on low dose laxatives, one requires regular enemas to stay regular, and one required resection of dilated redundant sigmoid colon but has regular bowel habits since then [16]. In 2012, Friedmacher and Puri conducted a meta-analysis of 16 prospective and retrospective studies published between 1973 and 2009 to compare the effectiveness of botulism toxin injections versus myectomy. They concluded that the rate of transient fecal incontinence was significantly higher after Botox injections, as were subsequent surgical treatments. Short and long-term improvement were significantly more frequent after IAS myectomy [17]. However, as some of the detrimental effects of IAS myectomy, such as fecal incontinence, rectal bleeding, rectal urgency, and wound healing issues, may not become apparent for several years after the procedure, many pediatric surgeons avoid performing this procedure for as long as possible [3], as is the case with this patient. Due to her young age and active lifestyle, she did not want to risk having side effects such as fecal incontinence, and has so far deferred treatment with a myectomy in preference to continuing botox injection treatment.

In the study done in 2020, they noticed that IASA typically had a later onset of symptoms, likely had normal meconium passing at birth, and are diagnosed later in childhood compared to Hirschsprung disease patients [3]. It is therefore essential to perform a thorough work-up of children presenting with a history of chronic constipation refractory to traditional treatments of lifestyle and diet modifications. This would help to avoid cases of rarer conditions such as IASA going undiagnosed, or being misdiagnosed and treated incorrectly. Once a diagnosis of IASA is made, the pros and cons of all treatment options should be discussed with the patient and family to decide the best course of action for that particular patient. With more education about this topic, we can hope to identify more cases of IASA and the effectiveness of the various treatment methods in providing these patients with a more comfortable lifestyle.

6. Diet to help with constipation symptoms

Patients with IASA typically have abdominal pain because of the back-up stool that cannot be expelled. Aside from laxative use to try and release some of this discomfort, patients may also be encouraged to adjust their diet to try and relieve their constipation as well.

6.1 Increased water intake

One of the first aspects of dietary management of constipation includes adequate water intake. Mineral water rich in magnesium and sulfates are the most ideal due the laxative effects of these compounds. Magnesium hydroxide has long been used to help with constipation due to its osmotic laxative effects. Once consumed, it is converted into magnesium carbonate by the gut which draws water into the intestinal lumen, thus hydrating and softening the stool to allow for easier passing [18].

6.2 Increased dietary fiber intake

Dietary fiber is commonly suggested to patients to help with constipation symptoms, and therefore may give some benefit to IASA patients as well. Dietary fiber is a class of carbohydrates and polysaccharides that are unable to be broken down by gastrointestinal enzymes. This class has a variety of colonic benefits. Firstly, some fiber gets fermented in the gut to produce short chain fatty acids such as butyrate, which in turn helps increase gut motility. Secondly, fiber can also act as stool-bulking agent by retaining water and therefore hydrating the stool to allow easier bowel movements. An amount as small as 2% change in the water content of stool can affect the consistency dramatically [18].

There are several subclassifications of fiber based on solubility, viscosity, and fermentability, all of which will not be discussed here. A few of the more common fiber types include: psyllium husk, rice, potatoes, wheat bran, and cellulose. In addition to this, whole grains, vegetables, and fruits high in fiber are also rich in prebiotic benefits. Prebiotics have a multitude of benefits in the gut, including promoting the growth and maintenance of healthy gut bacteria [19]. Some high fiber vegetables include broccoli, green leafy vegetables, carrots, and sweet potatoes. Some of the higher fiber fruits are bananas, apples, any berries and many other fruits.

These recommendations are appropriate for most patients suffering from constipation or other gastrointestinal distress, including patients with IASA, although excessive intake may have undesirable side effects. The most common side effect is bloating, flatulence, or diarrhea, and patients with certain malabsorption conditions must be cautious. Additionally, patient should also be reminded that the higher the fiber intake, the higher the water intake must also be to reduce the risk of dehydration or intestinal obstruction [19].

6.3 Foods/beverages to avoid

It is important for patients who suffer from constipation to avoid foods and drinks that cause dehydration. These include alcohol and coffee, which pull water from the body and increase urination. Additionally, foods high in salt and/or sugar may have the same effect of pulling water from the body leading to dehydration [20].

7. Conclusion

This chapter highlights the critical diagnostic challenges in distinguishing internal anal sphincter achalasia from phenotypically similar conditions, such as Hirschsprung disease and other causes of chronic constipation. The case study presented in this chapter comprehensively explores the patient's history, diagnostic trajectory, and treatment response to emphasize all the steps involved in diagnosing and managing this rare anorectal disorder. The pivotal role of rectal biopsy to make a definitive diagnosis of internal anal sphincter achalasia is absolutely crucial to distinguish this disease from other causes of chronic constipation. Conditions like Hirschsprung disease, congenital hypothyroidism, and functional constipation all present with symptoms of chronic constipation in young patients, just as internal anal sphincter achalasia does. The differentiating features of each disease as described in this chapter are essential to obtain in patient work-up in order to rule these out, as internal anal sphincter achalasia is a diagnosis of exclusion.

The definitive diagnosis of internal anal sphincter achalasia is essential in order to provide patients with the appropriate treatment options. Some management techniques may apply to all causes of chronic constipation, such as the diet strategies elucidated in this chapter. While these may provide temporary relief of constipation symptoms in patients with internal anal sphincter achalasia, this is not a definitive treatment, and further management is necessary to provide longer relief of symptoms. The patient case displays the temporality of relief associated with botulism toxin injections for internal anal sphincter achalasia patients, providing a nuanced understanding of the treatment's efficacy and its limitations. The subsequent consideration of posterior internal anal sphincter myectomy as the definitive treatment underlines the gravity of decision-making in managing IASA, with careful weighing of risks and benefits. It is essential to discuss all of this with patients, and provide them with a full understanding of their condition and options for treatment.

It is in our opinion, due to the rarity of this condition, there is a strong need for ongoing research on this topic. More case reports of patients with internal anal sphincter achalasia would greatly increase our understanding of the nuances of this anorectal disorder. There are many challenges with regards to diagnosing and treating this disease, due to the numerous differential diagnoses that are possible, and the limited treatment options once diagnosed. Some strategies that should be implemented to improve patient outcomes include ongoing research and education. This is definitely needed so that more pediatric patients will benefit from early diagnosis and management of such disorders to improve patient quality of life as soon as possible. It is our hope that bringing more awareness to this disease may help prevent it from being overlooked, and give physicians the ability to identify more of these patient cases and provide the appropriate management plan.

Acknowledgements

This article was previously presented as a poster at the 2024 Georgia Association of Physicians of Indian Heritage (GAPI) on March 9, 2024.

We would like to acknowledge the contributions of Dr. Roshan Uruthirakumar and Dr. Andrew Bozeman towards their work on the original article entitled "Refractory Chronic Constipation in an Adolescent Female Later Diagnosed with Internal Anal Sphincter Achalasia" [4].

We would like to give special acknowledgement to our sponsoring institution Trinity School of Medicine for providing us with the opportunity to work with such unique patient cases and thus expand our medical knowledge.

Author details

Farah Slaczka* and Mateusz Slaczka
Trinity School of Medicine, Warner Robins, USA

*Address all correspondence to: farah.azam.20@tmsu.edu.vc

References

[1] Ciamarra P, Nurko S, Barksdale E, Fishman S, Di Lorenzo C. Internal anal sphincter achalasia in children: Clinical characteristics and treatment with clostridium botulinum toxin. Journal of Pediatric Gastroenterology and Nutrition. 2003;**37**(3):315-319. Available from: https://journals.lww.com/jpgn/_layouts/15/oaks.journals/downloadpdf.aspx?an=00005176-200309000-00020&casa_token=y7T9ngQOa7MAAAAA:0ILLST7eVVS3XlmMcMor75F8gd6_yfb9pwWnvH8rp5uAYGxCj0Am_0vcWaqTRyFcW2vEgoFs9V53VcXFpwSWsQ

[2] Doodnath R, Puri P. Internal anal sphincter achalasia. Seminars in Pediatric Surgery (WB Saunders). Science Direct. 2009;**18**(4):246-248. Available from: https://www.sciencedirect.com/science/article/pii/S1055858609000444?casa_token=7vuSzU2SSAUAAAAA:VXMZQHQIid8f1yUEQXeH1eGQHKIH4Yu9hc7_PY6gid2_3cDJUKQpMSLPAt6eK4uERBa5TW9m

[3] Baaleman DF et al. The not-so-rare absent RAIR: Internal anal sphincter achalasia in a review of 1072 children with constipation undergoing high-resolution anorectal manometry. Neurogastroenterology and Motility. 2020;**33**(4):2021. DOI: 10.1111/nmo.14028

[4] Slaczka F, Uruthirakumar R, Slaczka M, et al. Refractory chronic constipation in an adolescent female later diagnosed with internal anal sphincter achalasia. Cureus. 2024;**16**(3):e57135. DOI: 10.7759/cureus.57135

[5] Ueno S. Internal anal sphincter achalasia. In: Hirschsprung's Disease and the Allied Disorders. 2019. pp. 261-268. Available from: https://link.springer.com/chapter/10.1007/978-981-13-3606-5_41

[6] Piotrowska AP, Solari V, Puri P. Distribution of interstitial cells of Cajal in the internal anal sphincter of patients with internal anal sphincter achalasia and Hirschsprung disease. Archives of Pathology and Laboratory Medicine. 2003;**127**(9):1192-1195. Available from: https://meridian.allenpress.com/aplm/article/127/9/1192/454652/Distribution-of-Interstitial-Cells-of-Cajal-in-the

[7] Le TT, Bhushan V, Griffin D, et al. First Aid for the USMLE Step 2 CK. 11th ed. United States: McGraw Hill; 2023

[8] Mueller JL, Goldstein AM. The science of Hirschsprung disease: What we know and where we are headed. Seminars in Pediatric Surgery. 2022;**31**(2). Available from: https://www.sciencedirect.com/science/article/abs/pii/S105585862200018X

[9] Palissei AS, Faruk AM. Hirschsprung's disease: Epidemiology, diagnosis, and treatment in a retrospective hospital-based study. Journal of the Medical Sciences. 2021;**53**(2):127-134. DOI: 10.19106/JMedSci005302202103

[10] Tahan S, Siviero-Miachon AA, de Faria Soares MF, et al. Untreated congenital hypothyroidism mimicking Hirschsprung disease: A puzzling case in a one-year-old child. Case Reports in Pediatrics (Wiley Online Library). 2018. Available from: https://pmc.ncbi.nlm.nih.gov/articles/PMC6046164/

[11] Sasigarn AB, Marina G. Congenital hypothyroidism. In: StatPearls. 2023. Available from: https://www.ncbi.nlm.nih.gov/books/NBK558913/

[12] Bashir SK, Khan MB. Pediatric functional constipation: A new challenge. In: Advanced Gut and

Microbiome Research. 2024. Available from: https://onlinelibrary.wiley.com/doi/full/10.1155/2024/5569563

[13] Allen P, Setya A, Lawrence VN. Pediatric functional constipation. In: StatPearls. 2024. Available from: https://www.ncbi.nlm.nih.gov/books/NBK537037/

[14] Zeevenhooven J, Koppen IJ, Benninga MA. The new Rome IV criteria for functional gastrointestinal disorders in infants and toddlers. Pediatric Gastroenterology, Hepatology and Nutrition. 2017;**20**(1):1-13

[15] Nicolais S, Weaver C, Saarie D, et al. Pediatrics Associates. Image Accessed 2025. Available from: https://www.pediatricassociatesny.com/bristol-stool-chart

[16] De Caluwe D, Yoneda A, Akl U, Puri P. Internal anal sphincter achalasia: Outcome after internal sphincter myectomy. Journal of Pediatric Surgery. 2001;**36**(5):736-738. Available from: https://www.sciencedirect.com/science/article/pii/S0022346801298388?casa_token=SlYYKaMzAqUAAAAA:8RzHDtpgWcnf2aFbcfMCxz_vPOYUlB-_aJQSocg47ETaaTKd6gziEbWK1eOYruUf_hbScY8y

[17] Friedmacher F, Puri P. Comparison of posterior internal anal sphincter myectomy and intrasphincteric botulism toxin injection for treatment of internal anal sphincter achalasia: A meta-analysis. Pediatric Surgery International. 2012;**28**:765-771. Available from: https://link.springer.com/article/10.1007/s00383-012-3123-5

[18] Bellini M, Tonarelli S, Barracca F, et al. Chronic constipation: Is a nutritional approach reasonable? Nutrients. 2021;**13**(10):3386. DOI: 10.3390/nu13103386

[19] Ioniță-Mîndrican CB, Ziani K, Mititelu M, et al. Therapeutic benefits and dietary restrictions of fiber intake: A state of the art review. Nutrients. 2022;**14**(13):2641. DOI: 10.3390/nu14132641

[20] Unknown. Dehydration. Cleveland Clinic; Health Library; 2023. Available from: https://my.clevelandclinic.org/health/diseases/9013-dehydration#living-with

Chapter 15

Perianal Abscesses

Eleni Polyzou, Maria Gavatha, Despoina Papageorgiou, Francesk Mulita and Karolina Akinosoglou

Abstract

Perianal abscesses constitute a common perianal infection frequently encountered in emergency medical settings. Their development is influenced by several predisposing factors, including inflammatory bowel disease, smoking, and HIV infection, with peak incidence typically observed in individuals around the age of 40. The pathogenesis of perianal abscesses is attributed to obstruction of the ducts of the anal glands, which facilitates bacterial proliferation and subsequent inflammation. Anatomically, perianal abscesses are classified into ischiorectal, intersphincteric, supralevator, and perianal; the latter being the most frequently encountered. The predominant clinical manifestation is localized perianal pain, although systemic symptoms may also be present. While medical history and physical examination are generally sufficient for diagnosing uncomplicated perianal abscesses, imaging modalities should be employed in cases with atypical presentations, suspected occult supralevator abscesses, complex anal fistulas, or perianal Crohn's disease. The primary treatment for perianal abscesses is surgical incision and drainage. Perioperative antibiotic prophylaxis is indicated for patients with specific comorbidities, in accordance with current clinical guidelines. Antibiotic therapy is generally reserved for cases complicated by cellulitis, systemic infection, or immunosuppression, with empiric antimicrobial regimens determined based on patient risk stratification and local antimicrobial resistance patterns. Although perianal abscesses are considered benign, their clinical course is complicated by variable rates of recurrence and fistula formation. Therefore, patients undergoing drainage procedures require meticulous follow-up and close clinical monitoring to identify and manage potential complications effectively.

Keywords: perianal infections, ischiorectal abscess, intersphincteric abscess, supralevator abscess, perianal abscesses, surgical management, antibiotic therapy, fistula formation

1. Introduction

Perianal abscesses are localized infections occurring in the perianal region. This condition is prevalent and represents a frequent presentation in emergency general surgery. It is estimated that perianal abscess and anal fistula affect 8–23 individuals per 100,000 [1]. The true prevalence remains unclear, as many patients treated with antibiotics, leading to spontaneous regression of the abscess, are not included in the statistics, resulting in an underestimated overall incidence. It is important to note that certain individuals exhibit a higher susceptibility to developing perianal abscesses. Specifically, male sex is a significant factor, as perianal abscesses occur twice as often in males as in females [2]. Conditions such as inflammatory bowel disease (IBD), for instance, Crohn's disease, smoking, and HIV infection, as well as other conditions that cause immunosuppression, also seem to be risk factors for developing these abscesses [3]. The mean age for the development of perianal abscesses for both genders is approximately 40 years [3]. Through direct medical costs and indirect expenses such as lost workdays and diminished quality of life, perianal abscess remains a major economic burden and challenge for healthcare systems. It is important for physicians in acute care settings to remain vigilant; hence advancing knowledge in the field to improve diagnosis, treatment, and outcomes for this common condition is crucial.

2. Etiology and pathogenesis

2.1 Anatomy

The anal canal is the terminal part of the gastrointestinal tract and typically measures approximately 2.5–4 cm in length [4]. It is connected to the rectum, which plays a critical role as storage for feces, while the anal canal serves as a critical muscular structure, primarily essential for fecal continence [5]. The main contributor to fecal continence, along with the puborectalis sling, is the anal sphincter. The anal sphincter consists of two muscle groups, the internal and the external anal sphincter, which together form a circular ring around the anus [6]. The internal anal sphincter is composed of smooth muscle, while the external anal sphincter is a striated muscle. Of note, the internal anal sphincter contributes approximately 60–70% of the resting anal tone, and the external anal sphincter, working in conjunction with the puborectalis sling, contributes around 20% of the resting anal tone, offering additional support in terms of fecal continence and voluntary control [5, 6]. The anal canal is divided into superior and inferior parts by the dentate line, which is a significant anatomical landmark, as it marks the transitional zone from the columnar epithelium of the superior anal canal to the squamous epithelium of the inferior anal canal [7]. Furthermore, the upper part of the anal canal is characterized by vertical mucosal folds, referred to as the anal columns of Morgagni [5].

At the base of the columns of Morgagni, the anal crypts are located, playing a crucial role in infection development in the region. Those crypts communicate with adjacent anal glands via ducts, where they secrete their substance. The continuous secretion of those substances facilitates the integrity and function of the anal canal. The interruption of constant secretion by the obstruction of the anal gland ducts creates an ideal environment for bacterial proliferation. It can lead to inflammation development and the formation of perianal abscesses. This mechanism is called the cryptoglandular theory of perianal abscess formation [8].

The blood supply of the anal canal is provided mainly by three arteries: the superior rectal artery, the middle rectal (hemorrhoidal) arteries, and the inferior rectal (hemorrhoidal) arteries. More specifically, the superior rectal artery, i.e., the final branch of the inferior mesenteric artery, provides blood supply to the upper third of the anal canal and the rectum. The distal rectum and the proximal anal canal are supplied by the middle rectal (hemorrhoidal) arteries, branches of the internal iliac arteries. However, the middle rectal arteries are not present in every individual due to anatomical variations. The lower part of the anal canal and the sphincter muscles are supplied by the inferior (hemorrhoidal) arteries, which originate from the internal pudendal artery [9]. The lymphatic drainage of the anal canal follows its arterial supply, with distinct pathways above and below the dentate line. Above the dentate line, lymph drains to the inferior mesenteric lymph nodes via the superior rectal lymphatics. Below the pectinate line, lymphatic fluid primarily drains to the superficial inguinal lymph nodes. Additionally, lymph from the lower part of the anal canal can drain laterally to the internal iliac nodes through the ischio-anal fossa [4, 9]. The venous drainage of the anal canal is divided into two parts. The superior part of the anal canal, located above the dentate line, is drained by the superior rectal veins, which ultimately empty into the inferior mesenteric vein. These veins are part of the hepatic portal venous system. In contrast, the venous drainage of the inferior part of the anal canal is provided by the internal pudendal veins, which drain into the internal iliac vein. These veins are part of the systemic venous system [4, 9]. It is also important to note that innervation differs between the inferior and superior parts of the anal canal. Especially, the superior part receives autonomic innervation from the inferior hypogastric plexus. The parasympathetic innervation aims to inhibit the tone of the internal anal sphincter and to stimulate a peristaltic contraction to allow defecation. In contrast, the sympathetic innervation seeks to maintain the tone of the internal anal sphincter and preserve continence [4, 7].

2.2 Types of abscesses

Anorectal abscesses are classified anatomically into perianal, ischiorectal, intersphincteric, and supralevator abscesses, among which perianal remains the most common subtype [10] (**Figure 1**). Perianal abscesses develop adjacent to the anal verge and manifest as localized pain, with systemic symptoms such as fever and malaise potentially occurring. Ischiorectal abscesses extend through the external anal sphincter into the ischiorectal space, presenting as vague pelvic or perianal pain along with a region of diffuse tenderness and induration within the gluteal region.

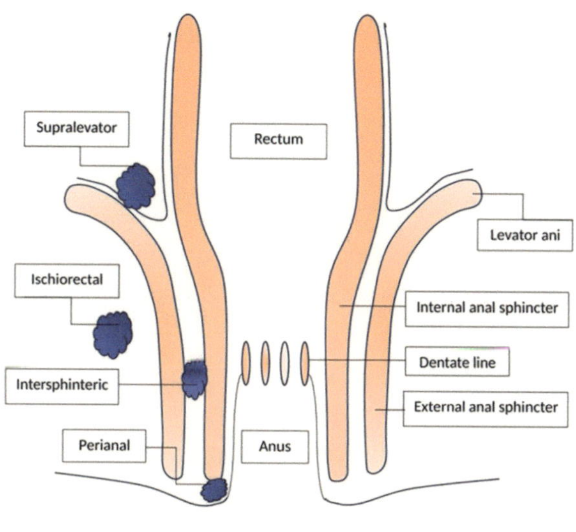

Figure 1.
Types of abscesses.

Ischiorectal abscesses can take a longer time to manifest externally. Intersphincteric abscesses are localized between the internal and external anal sphincters within the intersphincteric groove and are mainly associated with pain. Supralevator abscesses are situated superior to the levator ani muscle and are characterized by severe perianal pain accompanied by systemic symptoms [11].

2.3 Microbiology

A perianal abscess may result from a single pathogen or, more commonly, a polymicrobial infection involving multiple microorganisms. The most prevalent pathogen responsible for perianal abscess formation is *Escherichia coli (E. coli)*, a pathogen that is part of the normal intestinal flora and can be found in up to 69.9% of positive cultures. Anaerobic bacteria, which have the ability to survive in low-oxygen environments, such as *Streptococcus* species, can be present in 36.7%, and *Bacteroides*, particularly *Bacteroides fragilis*, in 13.2% of cases [12]. Other pathogens include *Klebsiella pneumoniae* and *Peptostreptococcus* species, which can be found in smaller proportions [3]. *Staphylococcus* species, particularly *Staphylococcus aureus*, are also identified [13].

3. Clinical manifestation

The characteristic symptom of a perianal abscess is pain, which is typically constant. The pain is usually localized to the anus and may depend on the site of its development. It may be dull, sharp, or throbbing, depending on how extensive the abscess is and the surrounding tissue involvement. Noteworthy is that some individuals experience significant discomfort during defecation, whereas others report persistent pain independent of bowel movement. Pain is the main symptom that raises the patient's concern to seek medical attention for further evaluation. Physical examination in the perianal area often reveals erythema and swelling, as well as purulent discharge, which typically drains from the abscess cavity. This discharge may be accompanied by blood loss from the rectum. Patients may also experience systematic symptoms, such as fever and malaise. Systematic symptoms indicate a more extensive and severe condition with potential spread of the infection [13].

4. Differential diagnosis

In the differential diagnosis, several other medical conditions that affect the anal region present with similar symptoms (**Table 1**).

- *Anal fissure*: A longitudinal tear or crack in the lining of the anal canal, extending from the dentate line to the anal verge. These fissures are typically located in the posterior midline (90% of cases), and the mean age of diagnosis is 30 years, with no significant sex difference.

- *Anal fistula:* Often coexists with or results from abscesses; careful assessment is required.

- *Rectal prolapse:* Typically involves a complete displacement of the rectal wall, and in some cases, the sigmoid colon, through the anal opening. In true or type III

Condition	Clinical features
Perianal abscess	Gradual pain, discomfort, +/− systematic symptoms (fever, malaise), perianal erythema and swelling, purulent discharge.
Thrombosed external hemorrhoid	Acute pain, discomfort, constipation, absence of systematic symptoms, rectal bleeding, blue-purple mass, tenderness.
Anal malignancy	Rare, painless, slowly growing, ulcerating mass, rectal bleeding, advanced stages: anal obstruction, weight loss.
Anal fistula	Skin opening around the anus, perianal erythema, discharge of pus/blood/feces from the tunnel opening, fever.
Anal fissure	Acute or chronic, perianal pain (worsening during defecation, persistent after defecation), +/− rectal bleeding.
Perianal Crohn's disease	Edematous, skin-colored, or cyanotic "elephant ear" tags, fissures, and usually an absence of pain and drainage are more common in children.
Rectal prolapse	Rectal wall/sigmoid colon complete displacement through the anal opening.
Proctitis	Rectal pain and discomfort, need for frequent bowel movement, rectal bleeding, and mucous discharge.
HIV/AIDS	Common anal condylomata acuminata caused by HPV due to immunological status: Itchy perianal gray-tan cauliflower-like lesion, pain may be present. Other common conditions due to immunosuppression: perianal herpes, fungal infections, anal malignancy, etc.
Hidradenitis suppurativa	Commonly affecting areas with sweat glands and hair follicles, pain, recurrent abscesses, cysts, and scarring.
Fournier's gangrene	Pain in the genital/perianal region, erythema and swelling in the genital/perianal region, and discoloration of the skin.

HPV: Human Papilloma Virus; HIV: Human Immunodeficiency Virus; AIDS: Acquired Immunodeficiency Syndrome.

Table 1.
Differential diagnosis.

prolapses, the entire rectal wall, including all layers, externally protrudes. This may result from weakened pelvic floor muscles, chronic straining, or neurological disorders affecting anorectal function [13].

- *Fournier's gangrene*: A rare, life-threatening necrotizing infection involving the fascia and subcutaneous tissues of the perineal, genital, or perianal region.

- *Thrombosed external hemorrhoid:* Hemorrhoids are swollen blood vessels in the anorectal region, often categorized as internal or external. Complicated hemorrhoids typically present with acute anal pain (hemorrhoidal crisis) or anorectal bleeding.

- *Crohn's disease*

- Malignancy

- *Proctitis*

- *HIV/AIDS*

- *Mpox virus infection*

- *Other sexually transmitted diseases*
- *Hidradenitis suppurativa:* A chronic and painful inflammatory skin condition characterized by recurrent abscesses, cysts, and scarring, often affecting areas with sweat glands and hair follicles, such as the armpits, groin, buttocks, and breasts.

5. Diagnosis and workup

As with any medical condition, obtaining a detailed medical history and performing a thorough physical examination are the two most important key factors for establishing the diagnosis. A thorough history should include details about prior anorectal issues, recurrent infections, pain patterns, discharge, systemic symptoms such as fever or urinary retention, and any history or risk factors for any state of immunocompromization or other pertinent risk factors, including smoking or pre-existing conditions like Crohn's disease, as these elements significantly contribute to the likelihood of developing a perianal abscess [11, 14]. A complete medical history can reveal important information about risk factors or other causes for fistula formation, which could alter treatment decisions [15].

In addition, the physical examination for an anorectal abscess should include a careful inspection of the perianal area to identify external signs such as a tender, fluctuant mass, swelling, or fluctuance, as well as any external openings suggestive of a fistula or other anorectal pathology indicative of Crohn's disease. Palpation of the perianal region is essential to assess tenderness, fluctuance, or signs of deeper abscesses. A digital rectal examination should be performed to evaluate pelvic or rectal tenderness and fluctuance, particularly in cases of intersphincteric or supralevator abscesses where external findings may not be apparent. Careful probing of any tracts can help define the presence and anatomy of a fistula [16].

Medical history and physical examination should suffice for the diagnosis of a superficial uncomplicated perianal abscess. In patients presenting with signs of systemic infection or sepsis, white blood cell count, creatinine serum levels, and inflammatory markers (procalcitonin, c-reactive protein, lactates) must also be assessed [14]. Further investigations in order to detect previously undiagnosed diabetes mellitus, including, serum glucose, hemoglobin A1c, and urine ketones, should also be ordered. Additionally, serological testing for HIV infections or other causes of immunocompromise should be performed. Blood cultures should be obtained only in immunocompromised patients or in the presence of hypotension, tachypnea, delirium, or risk factors for antibiotic-resistant microorganisms [17].

Imaging investigations are not mandatory for the diagnosis of an uncomplicated perianal abscess and are usually performed in cases of atypical presentation, suspected occult supralevator abscesses, complex anal fistulas, or perianal Crohn's disease. The techniques that are used in clinical practice include CT scans, Magnetic resonance imaging (MRI), and ultrasonography.

Endoanal ultrasound can identify fistulas and anorectal abscesses, especially horseshoe abscess extensions, achieving rates of 80–89%. On the other hand, it requires specialized skills and is impractical for awake patients in the emergency room due to severe anal pain. Endoanal ultrasound seemed to be, in some studies, more accurate than MRI in evaluating an anal fistula, mostly in cases associated with underlying Crohn's disease. Similarly, point-of-care transperineal ultrasound is becoming an increasingly useful method for identifying perineal and perirectal abscesses in emergency care. Its benefits include immediate imaging, minimal invasiveness, and bedside accessibility. However, its accuracy heavily depends on the operator's expertise, given the intricate regional anatomy and variations in abscess location. While recent findings show encouraging diagnostic potential, the current evidence is insufficient to support formal guidelines for routine use [14].

Computed tomography can offer several advantages, especially in the emergency department, including rapid image acquisition and widespread availability. It remains a rapid and readily available option to differentiate abscesses from severe cellulitis or identify supralevator extension. However, its accuracy in pelvic imaging is limited due to poor spatial resolution. Additionally, distinguishing between fistula tracts and inflamed tissue can be challenging, as these structures often share similar characteristics [18].

Magnetic resonance imaging (MRI) avoids radiation exposure and provides excellent tissue resolution in complex cases or patients with IBD. Conversely, its long acquisition time and limited availability make it incompetent for the emergency department [18].

Anoscopy and *sigmoidoscopy* are indicated for identifying any mucosal abnormalities associated with Crohn's disease [14].

Fistulography due to a low accuracy rate (of 16%) is not used as a radiological method [14].

6. Surgical management

Trainees often perform perianal abscess drainage procedures, which may be complex due to the intricate anatomy involved. Nonetheless, this practice is considered safe, with recurrence rates consistent with those reported in current literature [13]. As anticipated, recurrence or fistula formation is more common in patients with comorbidities like IBD or conditions associated with immunosuppression, such as malignancy or diabetes. The prompt identification of high-risk patients is of utmost importance, as those patients may benefit from early consultation with an experienced surgeon, as evidence indicates this can improve the identification and definitive treatment of underlying fistula tracts [19].

From a practical point of view, making skin incisions close to the anal verge ensures that any potential fistula that may occur will be shorter. The careful use of anal retractors and Lockhart-Mummery probes is essential to avoid creating false tracts during the search for fistula tracts [20]. Wound packing is usually at the proceduralist's discretion and depends on the cavity size; however, randomized trials have not demonstrated significant benefits from packing apart from increased postoperative pain [21].

Performing a fistulotomy or inserting a seton during abscess drainage remains a controversial approach. Several studies report conflicting outcomes, and traditional teachings suggest delaying fistula management until acute inflammation and edematous tissue have subsided [22]. Although benefits such as faster wound healing and reduced recurrence or fistula formation are proposed, these must be weighed against the threefold increased risk of incontinence. Hence, these procedures are typically considered on a case-by-case basis after consultation with an experienced surgeon [23].

Cultures from the site of the wound should not be routinely obtained when draining a perianal abscess. Nevertheless, they can be useful in identifying whether the bacterial infection originates from the colon or from the skin. Cryptoglandular-origin abscesses were historically believed to pose a greater risk of recurrence or fistula formation, though this has not been consistently demonstrated [24].

Surgical examination under anesthesia is widely regarded as the gold standard for identifying abscesses or fistula tracts. Imaging, in selected patients with suspected complex pathology, can provide a detailed anatomical roadmap to avoid sphincter damage or the creation of false tracts [24].

6.1 Perioperative prophylaxis

Based on current data, perioperative antibiotic prophylaxis is not routinely indicated. However, the American Heart Association recommends preoperative antibiotic administration for individuals with prosthetic valves, a history of bacterial endocarditis, congenital heart disease, or heart transplant recipients with valve pathology [25]. Overall, according to the World Society of Emergency Surgery and American Association for the Surgery of Trauma (WSES-AAST) guidelines, there is insufficient evidence to support preoperative antibiotic treatment even in patients with bicuspid aortic valves or mitral valve prolapse [14]. This aligns with the European Society of Coloproctology (ESCP) guidelines, which do not recommend antibiotic administration prior to the surgical management of anal fistula.

In case perioperative prophylaxis is recommended, options include both parenteral and oral regimens. For parenteral administration, cefazolin combined with metronidazole is the preferred regimen. Alternative parenteral options include cefoxitin, cefotetan, or ampicillin-sulbactam. For oral prophylaxis, the recommended regimen includes neomycin combined with either erythromycin base or metronidazole. For patients with allergies to penicillins or cephalosporins, we prefer clindamycin or vancomycin in combination with either gentamicin, ciprofloxacin, levofloxacin, or aztreonam. Alternatively, metronidazole can be combined with an aminoglycoside or fluoroquinolone, although metronidazole combined with aztreonam is not recommended due to a lack of aerobic gram-positive activity. Local resistance patterns should always be reviewed due to increased resistance of pathogens such as *E. coli* for regimens like ampicillin-sulbactam and fluoroquinolones. The use of carbapenems should be avoided to prevent antimicrobial resistance. Prophylactic antibiotics should be initiated as a single IV dose within 60 minutes before surgery to ensure adequate tissue levels at the time of incision. If vancomycin or fluoroquinolone is used, administration should begin 60–120 minutes prior to surgery to minimize infusion-related reactions and ensure adequate drug levels [15].

7. Antibiotic therapy

The primary treatment for perianal abscess is prompt surgical drainage to achieve source control, but medical management with antibiotics is also indicated in certain situations. Antibiotic treatment following abscess drainage has been shown in a few meta-analyses to reduce the risk of fistula formation and abscess recurrence, particularly in cases of sepsis or surrounding soft tissue infections [26]. However, according to the ESCP guidelines, routine use of antibiotics after abscess drainage is not recommended to prevent fistula or abscess recurrence, due to the high risk of promoting antibiotic resistance [15]. Similarly, the American Society of Colon and Rectal Surgeons (ASCRS) guidelines advise against the routine use of antibiotics

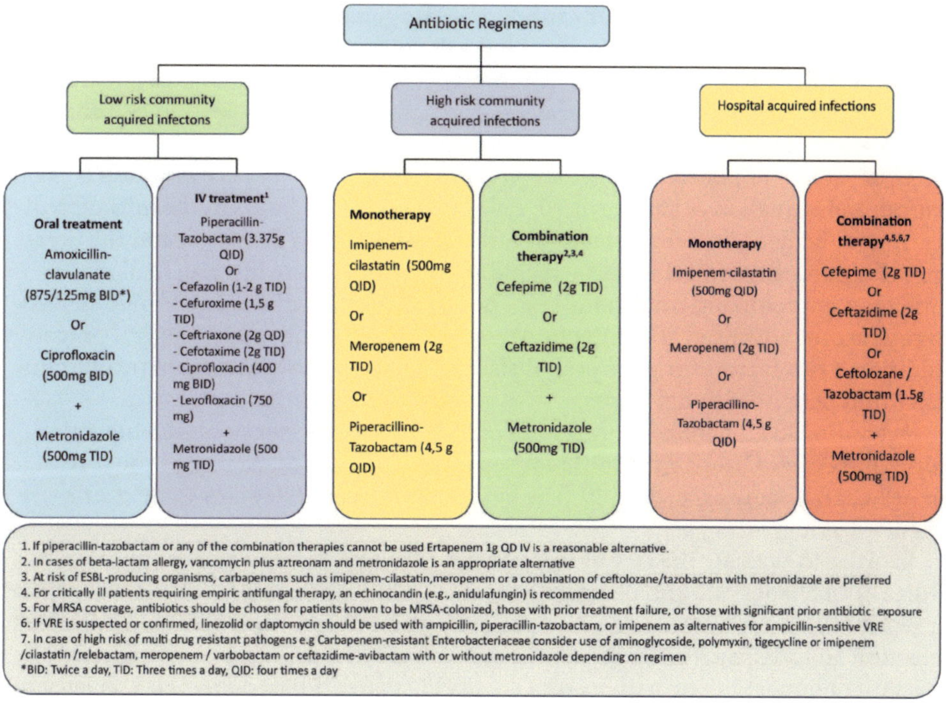

Figure 2.
Antibiotic regimens.

in healthy patients with uncomplicated anorectal abscesses, as it does not improve healing outcomes or reduce recurrence rates [2]. The antibiotic regimens that are preferred are derived from guidelines on intra-abdominal infections, with their approach extrapolated to anorectal abscess treatment (**Figure 2**).

In line with all guidelines, antibiotic administration is indicated in cases of anorectal abscess complicated by cellulitis, systemic signs of infection such as fever, chills, or leukocytosis, or in patients with underlying immunosuppression, including low neutrophil counts, atypical infections like tuberculosis or HIV infection where drainage alone would not suffice [2, 14, 15]. Empiric therapy should target the most common pathogens while guided by local resistance patterns, unless or until culture results, are available [2]. Following culture results targeted treatment and immediate de-escalation are imperative.

7.1 General principles

When selecting the optimal antibiotic regimen, decision-making should follow several key principles.

Risk stratification is essential in determining the necessity for broader empiric antimicrobial coverage. The risk assessment should distinguish between community-acquired and healthcare-associated infections while identifying specific risk factors for antimicrobial resistance [14, 17]. Such risk factors include hospitalization for more than 48 hours within the past 90 days, residence in a skilled nursing or long-term care facility within the preceding 30 days, and recent receipt of intravenous infusion therapy, wound care, or renal replacement therapy. Additional considerations include prior exposure to broad-spectrum antimicrobial agents for several days within the past 90 days, postoperative infections, and a documented history of colonization or infection with resistant pathogens [27]. Moreover, local epidemiological data regarding antibiotic-resistant *Enterobacteriaceae* and surveillance colonization culture data should always be integrated into the assessment.

Identification of patients at high risk for adverse outcomes and poor prognosis is equally critical. Individuals over the age of 70, delays exceeding 24 hours in the initiation of treatment, inadequate debridement or infection control via drainage, and the presence of significant comorbidities—including renal or hepatic disease, malignancy, or immunocompromizing conditions (e.g., poorly controlled diabetes, chronic corticosteroid use, or advanced HIV infection)—are associated with worse clinical outcomes. Additional risk factors for poor prognosis include organ dysfunction, hypoalbuminemia, and poor nutritional status.

According to guidelines for intra-abdominal infections, patients who meet the Surviving Sepsis Campaign criteria for sepsis or septic shock, as well as those with an APACHE II score exceeding 10 (the preferred scoring system for evaluation), are classified as high-risk [27].

In order to evaluate the risk of treatment failure and mortality, it is important to utilize both phenotypic and physiologic factors. Those factors include signs of sepsis or septic shock, extremes of age, and patient comorbidities; the extent of abdominal infection and adequacy of initial source control; and the presence or persistence of resistant or opportunistic pathogens. Classifying patients based on their risk level for treatment failure or mortality and determining whether their infection is community-acquired or healthcare-associated, (including postoperative ones) is pivotal so as to design a proper source control and empiric antibiotic therapy strategy.

In any case, the selected regimen should provide effective coverage against the most commonly encountered pathogens at the site, including enteric streptococci, coliforms, and anaerobes. However, consider drug toxicities, drug-drug interactions, patient-associated tolerance, and allergies, and avoid antibiotics administered <3 months prior to diagnosis. Last, strict adherence to antimicrobial stewardship principles remains imperative to mitigate the spread of resistance and preserve the efficacy of available antimicrobial agents [14].

Pus cultures are generally not required in patients with uncomplicated perianal abscesses. However, they are indicated in high-risk individuals, such as when there are risk factors for multidrug-resistant (MDR) bacteria, recurrent or non-healing infections, or in immunocompromised patients, including those with HIV infection [14]. This is important, as studies have reported methicillin-resistant *Staphylococcus aureus* (MRSA) prevalence as high as 35% in anorectal abscesses [28].

7.2 Treatment of low-risk community-acquired infections

Treatment options include both single-agent and combination regimens. Single-agent choices are ertapenem or piperacillin-tazobactam. For combination regimens, a b-lactam (cefazolin, cefuroxime, ceftriaxone, cefotaxime) or a quinolone (ciprofloxacin, or levofloxacin) can be used in combination with metronidazole. In certain cases, an oral regimen, such as fluoroquinolone combined with metronidazole or amoxicillin-clavulanate, may also be a suitable treatment option.

Cefotetan and clindamycin are not recommended for use because of *Bacteroides fragilis* increasing resistance rates to these agents. Aminoglycosides are not recommended for routine use in adults with community-acquired intra-abdominal infections due to their toxicity [27, 29]. For low-risk community-acquired infections, an empiric antimicrobial regimen does not have to include specific activity against enterococci or fungi.

7.3 Treatment of high-risk community-acquired infections

Treatment should target Gram-negative bacteria, including *Pseudomonas aeruginosa* and *Enterobacteriaceae* resistant to non-pseudomonal cephalosporins, coverage against enteric streptococci, and (in most cases) anaerobes. Empiric antifungal therapy is generally not warranted but may be reasonable for critically ill patients. Coverage for MRSA is typically unnecessary, even if the patient is known to be MRSA-colonized.

If local resistance is under 10%, single-agent options include imipenem-cilastatin, meropenem, or piperacillin-tazobactam. Combination regimens include cefepime or ceftazidime, each administered with metronidazole. For patients at risk of ESBL-producing organisms, carbapenems such as imipenem-cilastatin, meropenem, or a combination of ceftolozane/tazobactam with metronidazole are preferred. Vancomycin or ampicillin may be added for enterococcal coverage when using regimens other than imipenem-cilastatin or piperacillin-tazobactam, though this is not routinely recommended for community-acquired infections.

In cases of beta-lactam or carbapenem allergy, vancomycin plus aztreonam and metronidazole is an appropriate alternative. For critically ill patients requiring empiric antifungal therapy, an echinocandin (e.g., anidulafungin) is recommended. Amphotericin B is generally avoided as initial therapy due to its toxicity.

When beta-lactams or carbapenems are selected, a prolonged infusion dosing strategy should be used for optimal efficacy [27, 29, 30].

7.4 Treatment of hospital-acquired infections

In healthcare-associated infections, the likelihood of drug resistance is high. Therefore, coverage should further include *Pseudomonas aeruginosa* and *Enterobacteriaceae* resistant to non-pseudomonal third-generation cephalosporins and fluoroquinolones. Anti-enterococcal coverage should be considered, especially for immunocompromised patients or patients with postoperative infections, previous administration of cephalosporins, or other antibiotic regimens active against *Enterococcus* species, patients with valvular heart disease, or prosthetic intravascular materials. Empiric coverage for vancomycin-resistant *Enterococcus* (VRE) is not typically needed unless the patient is a liver transplant recipient or known to be colonized. For MRSA coverage, antibiotics should be chosen for patients known to be MRSA-colonized, those with prior treatment failure, or those with significant prior antibiotic exposure. Antifungal treatment is recommended for patients with severe infections or heavy colonization with *Candida* or yeast identified in gram stains of infected tissue. The preferred antifungal is an echinocandin (e.g., anidulafungin), though fluconazole may be used if *Candida* isolates are sensitive.

For highly resistant Gram-negative bacteria, adding an aminoglycoside, polymyxin, tigecycline, colistin, or a novel beta-lactam combination (e.g., imipenem/cilastatin/relebactam, meropenem/varbobactam or ceftazidime-avibactam) with or without metronidazole (depending on the selected regimen) to an empiric regimen is recommended. If VRE is suspected or confirmed, linezolid or daptomycin should be used with ampicillin, piperacillin-tazobactam, or imipenem as alternatives for ampicillin-sensitive VRE [27, 29, 30].

7.5 Treatment duration

Treatment should begin as soon as possible, ideally within an hour. If adequate source control is achieved, antibiotics should be continued for 4–5 and 7–8 days if there is secondary bacteremia or if the patient is critically ill. If the duration is uncertain, a longer course of 7–10 days may be considered. The duration of antibiotic therapy could be longer, based on clinical judgment, inflammatory markers, and imaging. There is inadequate evidence to recommend a specific duration for immunosuppressed patients [27, 30].

7.6 Adjunctive management

Adjunctive therapies for treating perianal abscesses primarily include pain management and the use of laxatives. Alternative non-surgical therapies include herbal sitz baths, which have shown promise in improving postoperative outcomes for patients with perianal abscesses [31]. According to recent studies, sitz baths contribute to relief of postoperative pain and increase wound healing by modulating the wound's microbial environment and specifically by reducing harmful bacteria like *Enterococcus* and increasing beneficial genera such as *Bifidobacterium*, *Faecalibacterium*, and *Ruminococcus* [31].

8. Follow-up

Currently, there are no universally accepted guidelines or protocols specifying the timing and frequency of follow-up visits after the initial management. After initial surgical intervention, a scheduled follow-up visit is not required in individuals diagnosed with a first episode of perianal abscess according to the Association of Coloproctology of Great Britain and Ireland (ACPGBI) [32]. In the absence of underlying medical conditions, surgical draining in these patients should be followed by discharge and advice to seek medical reevaluation in cases of healing failure or sustained exudation from the abscess. Contrarily, a review appointment can be offered to patients with recurrent abscesses for further investigation or treatment of an underlying fistula [11]. According to the American Society of Colon and Rectal Surgeons, approximately 30–50% of patients who undergo abscess drainage will ultimately be diagnosed with a fistula-in-ano within months to years following the procedure [16]. Hence, due to the high recurrence rate, it is suggested that all patients need to receive a thorough follow-up and close monitoring for any potential complications until there is a complete recovery, which may take up to 8 weeks [13]. Routine imaging after surgical management of the perianal abscess is usually not recommended, although on special occasions an imaging follow-up may be of importance. Such cases include symptoms or signs of recurrence or fistula and/or persistent non-resolving wound and suspected inflammatory bowel disease [14].

9. Prognosis

Perianal abscess is a benign condition with a favorable therapeutic outcome when identified and treated promptly and adequately. For this purpose, the patient should not dismiss characteristic symptoms, since following appropriate surgical and medical management, mortality from perianal abscess remains low. However, in special populations, including immunocompromised patients and those with Crohn's disease, as well as in cases where the abscess was not detected early enough and progressed to a potentially fatal infection such as necrotizing fasciitis, morbidity, and mortality increase significantly [16, 33]. Complications associated with perianal abscesses and their treatment may include systemic infection and sepsis, recurrence of the abscess, fistula formation, fecal incontinence, and also urinary retention [13]. In fact, patients with Crohn's disease have an increased complication incidence rate of 24% compared to 4.8% of healthy individuals presenting with perianal abscess [11].

Laboratory markers may be of use in stratifying patients with poor prognoses. More specifically, mean platelet volume has been recognized as a potential additional marker for assessing disease severity, providing further insights into the disease prognosis [34], whereas in patients presenting with Fournier's gangrene, risk assessment and prognosis can be evaluated by using the Laboratory Risk Indicator for Necrotising Fasciitis (LRINEC) score or similarly the Fournier's Gangrene Severity Index (FGSI) [14].

The published incidence of perianal abscess recurrence varies from 1.6% to 88% with a recent study stating that half of the patients with perianal abscess will relapse and 40% will develop a fistula during the first year of follow-up [35]. In another recent study, the location and the extent of perianal abscess were identified as associated factors with the prognosis of the disease, with larger and deeper abscesses tending to have a poorer outcome in terms of recurrence, healing, and fistula formation. Additionally, an elevated preoperative white blood cell count was associated with postoperative recurrence [34]. Recurrence episodes seem to occur after the first year. A recent study including 205 patients found that the recurrence rate of anorectal abscesses was 36%, with 74 out of 205 patients experiencing recurrence, while the cumulative cure rates were 68.7% at 1 year, 64.2% at 2 years, and 63.5% at 3 years, indicating a gradual decline in recurrence-free patients over time [36].

10. Preventive measures and patient education

Although current literature lacks evidence-based data on potential preventive measures for perianal abscesses, several strategies may still be beneficial. Maintaining good personal hygiene and keeping the perianal area clean and dry to avoid skin breakdown can be helpful [13]. Following a diet high in fiber may theoretically reduce the chance of anal gland blockage and subsequently perianal abscess formation. However, one can argue that a high-fiber diet can increase stool bulk and frequency, leading to more stools that need to be passed; hence, not making a strong case for its protective effect against perianal conditions like abscesses [37]. Also, treatment of underlying etiology, including Crohn's disease or HIV infection, as well as making lifestyle changes such as quitting smoking and engaging in physical activity, can help reduce the risk of developing a perianal abscess [13].

11. Conclusion

Perianal abscesses represent a critical medical condition and need to be recognized and treated in the proper time and way. Patients often seek medical attention after experiencing significant and constant pain in the perianal region. The suspicion of a perianal abscess formation should rise when specific risk factors such as inflammatory bowel disease, HIV infection, etc., are present. The cornerstone of perianal abscess treatment is surgical management, primarily involving incision and drainage. Antibiotic treatment is required in complicated cases, whereas patients with hospital-acquired infections need even more extensive coverage. Antimicrobial stewardship is essential to avoid further antimicrobial resistance. Complementary interventions such as pain management and sitz baths accelerate the recovery. Further research should focus on preventing the formation of abscesses and thus reduce rates of resistant and recurrent infections.

Author details

Eleni Polyzou[1,2], Maria Gavatha[1], Despoina Papageorgiou[1,2], Francesk Mulita[3] and Karolina Akinosoglou[1,2,4]*

1 Department of Medicine, University of Patras, Rio, Greece

2 Department of Internal Medicine, University General Hospital of Patras, Rio, Greece

3 Department of Surgery, General Hospital of Eastern Achaia—Unit of Aigio, Egio, Greece

4 Division of Infectious Diseases, University General Hospital of Patras, Rio Greece

*Address all correspondence to: akin@upatras.gr

References

[1] Hokkanen SR, Boxall N, Khalid JM, Bennett D, Patel H. Prevalence of anal fistula in the United Kingdom. World Journal of Clinical Cases. 2019;7(14):1795-1804

[2] Steele SR, Kumar R, Feingold DL, Rafferty JL, Buie WD. Practice parameters for the management of perianal abscess and fistula-in-ano. Diseases of the Colon and Rectum. 2011;**54**(12):1465-1474

[3] Alabbad J, Abdul Raheem F, Alkhalifa F, Hassan Y, Al-Banoun A, Alfouzan W. Retrospective clinical and microbiologic analysis of patients with anorectal abscess. Surgical Infections. 2019;**20**(1):31-34

[4] Ahmed A, Arbor TC, Qureshi WA. Anatomy, Abdomen and Pelvis: Anal Canal. Treasure Island (FL): StatPearls Publishing LLC; 2025

[5] Bazira PJ. Anatomy of the rectum and anal canal. Surgery (Oxford). 2023;**41**(1):7-14

[6] Kumar L, Emmanuel A. Internal anal sphincter: Clinical perspective. The Surgeon. 2017;**15**(4):211-226

[7] Lee JM, Kim NK. Essential anatomy of the anorectum for colorectal surgeons focused on the gross anatomy and histologic findings. Annals of Coloproctology. 2018;**34**(2):59-71

[8] Gosselink MP, van Onkelen RS, Schouten WR. The cryptoglandular theory revisited. Colorectal Disease. 2015;**17**(12):1041-1043

[9] Barleben A, Mills S. Anorectal anatomy and physiology. The Surgical Clinics of North America. 2010;**90**(1):1-15. Table of Contents

[10] Ma X, Li Y, Xu S, Wang B, Wang C. The analysis of different types of anorectal abscesses was conducted using the MRI 3D reconstruction technique. Scientific Reports. 2024;**14**(1):18473

[11] Sahnan K, Adegbola SO, Tozer PJ, Watfah J, Phillips RK. Perianal abscess. BMJ. 2017;**356**:j475

[12] Paran M, Dagan J, Hameiri G, Dudkiewicz M, Kessel B. Does microbiology of perianal abscesses affect the length of hospital stay? The American Journal of the Medical Sciences. 2024;**368**(4):320-324

[13] Sigmon DF, Emmanuel B, Tuma F. Perianal Abscess. Treasure Island (FL): StatPearls Publishing LLC; 2025

[14] Tarasconi A, Perrone G, Davies J, Coimbra R, Moore E, Azzaroli F, et al. Anorectal emergencies: WSES-AAST guidelines. World Journal of Emergency Surgery : WJES. 2021;**16**(1):48

[15] Reza L, Gottgens K, Kleijnen J, Breukink S, Ambe PC, Aigner F, et al. European Society of Coloproctology: Guidelines for diagnosis and treatment of cryptoglandular anal fistula. Colorectal Disease. 2024;**26**(1):145-196

[16] Gaertner WB, Burgess PL, Davids JS, Lightner AL, Shogan BD, Sun MY, et al. The American Society of colon and rectal surgeons clinical practice guidelines for the management of anorectal abscess, fistula-in-ano, and rectovaginal fistula. Diseases of the Colon and Rectum. 2022;**65**(8):964-985

[17] Bonomo RA, Chow AW, Edwards MS, Humphries R, Tamma PD, Abrahamian FM, et al. Clinical practice

guideline update by the Infectious Diseases Society of America on complicated intra-abdominal infections: Risk assessment, diagnostic imaging, and microbiological evaluation in adults, children, and pregnant people. Clinical Infectious Diseases. 2024, 2024;**79** (Suppl. 3):S81-S87

[18] Choe J, Wortman JR, Sodickson AD, Khurana B, Uyeda JW. Imaging of acute conditions of the perineum. Radiographics. 2018;**38**(4):1111-1130

[19] Malik A, Hall D, Devaney R, Sylvester H, Yalamarthi S. The impact of specialist experience in the surgical management of perianal abscesses. International Journal of Surgery. 2011;**9**(6):475-477

[20] Perera AP, Howell AM, Sodergren MH, Farne H, Darzi A, Purkayastha S, et al. A pilot randomised controlled trial evaluating postoperative packing of the perianal abscess. Langenbeck's Archives of Surgery. 2015;**400**(2):267-271

[21] Tonkin DM, Murphy E, Brooke-Smith M, Hollington P, Rieger N, Hockley S, et al. Perianal abscess: A pilot study comparing packing with nonpacking of the abscess cavity. Diseases of the Colon and Rectum. 2004;**47**(9):1510-1514

[22] Shi Y, Zhi C, Cheng Y, Zheng L. A systematic review and meta-analysis of incision and seton drainage in the treatment of high perianal abscess. Annals of Palliative Medicine. 2021;**10**(9):9830-9840

[23] Malik AI, Nelson RL, Tou S. Incision and drainage of perianal abscess with or without treatment of anal fistula. Cochrane Database of Systematic Reviews. 2010;(7):CD006827

[24] Xu RW, Tan KK, Chong CS. Bacteriological study in perianal abscess is not useful and not cost-effective. ANZ Journal of Surgery. 2016;**86**(10):782-784

[25] Wilson W, Taubert KA, Gewitz M, Lockhart PB, Baddour LM, Levison M, et al. Prevention of infective endocarditis: Guidelines from the American Heart Association: A guideline from the American Heart Association Rheumatic Fever, Endocarditis, and Kawasaki Disease Committee, Council on Cardiovascular Disease in the Young, and the Council on Clinical Cardiology, Council on Cardiovascular Surgery and Anesthesia, and the Quality of Care and Outcomes Research Interdisciplinary Working Group. Circulation. 2007;**116**(15):1736-1754

[26] Mocanu V, Dang JT, Ladak F, Tian C, Wang H, Birch DW, et al. Antibiotic use in prevention of anal fistulas following incision and drainage of anorectal abscesses: A systematic review and meta-analysis. American Journal of Surgery. 2019;**217**(5):910-917

[27] Sartelli M, Chichom-Mefire A, Labricciosa FM, Hardcastle T, Abu-Zidan FM, Adesunkanmi AK, et al. The management of intra-abdominal infections from a global perspective: 2017 WSES guidelines for management of intra-abdominal infections. World Journal of Emergency Surgery : WJES. 2017;**12**:29

[28] Brown SR, Horton JD, Davis KG. Perirectal abscess infections related to MRSA: A prevalent and underrecognized pathogen. Journal of Surgical Education. 2009;**66**(5):264-266

[29] Solomkin JS, Mazuski JE, Bradley JS, Rodvold KA, Goldstein EJ, Baron EJ, et al. Diagnosis and management of complicated intra-abdominal infection in adults and children: Guidelines by

the Surgical Infection Society and the Infectious Diseases Society of America. Clinical Infectious Diseases. 2010;**50**(2):133-164

[30] Mazuski JE, Tessier JM, May AK, Sawyer RG, Nadler EP, Rosengart MR, et al. The surgical infection society revised guidelines on the management of intra-abdominal infection. Surgical Infections. 2017;**18**(1):1-76

[31] Chen X, Guo X. Microbiome analysis reveals the potential mechanism of herbal sitz bath complementary therapy in accelerating postoperative recovery from perianal abscesses. IET Systems Biology. 2024;**19**(1):e12114

[32] Arokianathar D, Lingam G, Sivarajah V. FP3.7—Do we need to follow up perianal abscesses in clinic? The British Journal of Surgery. 2024;**111**(Suppl 8)

[33] Solis E, Liang Y, Ctercteko G, Toh JWT. Dangers of delayed diagnosis of perianal abscess and undrained perianal sepsis in Fournier's gangrene: A case series. BML Case Reports. 4 Oct 2020;**13**(10):e236503

[34] Dong S, Chen B, Zhang J. Study on the factors influencing the prognosis after perianal abscess surgery. BMC Gastroenterology. 2023;**23**(1):334

[35] Chaveli Díaz C, Esquiroz Lizaur I, Eguaras Córdoba I, González Álvarez G, Calvo Benito A, Oteiza Martínez F, et al. Recurrence and incidence of fistula after urgent drainage of an anal abscess. Long-term results. Cirugía Española (English Edition). 2022;**100**(1):25-32

[36] Yano T, Asano M, Matsuda Y, Kawakami K, Nakai K, Nonaka M. Prognostic factors for recurrence following the initial drainage of an anorectal abscess. International Journal of Colorectal Disease. 2010;**25**(12):1495-1498

[37] Tan KY, Seow-Choen F. Fiber and colorectal diseases: Separating fact from fiction. World Journal of Gastroenterology. 2007;**13**(31):4161-4167